Clinical Consequences of COVID-19

Clinical Consequences of COVID-19

Editors

**Francesco Pugliese
Francesco Alessandri
Giovanni Giordano**

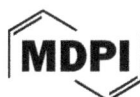

Basel • Beijing • Wuhan • Barcelona • Belgrade • Novi Sad • Cluj • Manchester

Editors
Francesco Pugliese
Sapienza University of Rome
Rome, Italy

Francesco Alessandri
Sapienza University of Rome
Rome, Italy

Giovanni Giordano
Sapienza University of Rome
Rome, Italy

Editorial Office
MDPI
St. Alban-Anlage 66
4052 Basel, Switzerland

This is a reprint of articles from the Special Issue published online in the open access journal *Journal of Clinical Medicine* (ISSN 2077-0383) (available at: https://www.mdpi.com/journal/jcm/special_issues/Clinical_Consequences_COVID).

For citation purposes, cite each article independently as indicated on the article page online and as indicated below:

Lastname, A.A.; Lastname, B.B. Article Title. *Journal Name* **Year**, *Volume Number*, Page Range.

ISBN 978-3-0365-9855-0 (Hbk)
ISBN 978-3-0365-9856-7 (PDF)
doi.org/10.3390/books978-3-0365-9856-7

© 2024 by the authors. Articles in this book are Open Access and distributed under the Creative Commons Attribution (CC BY) license. The book as a whole is distributed by MDPI under the terms and conditions of the Creative Commons Attribution-NonCommercial-NoDerivs (CC BY-NC-ND) license.

Contents

Giovanni Giordano, Francesco Alessandri and Francesco Pugliese
Special Issue "Clinical Consequences of COVID-19": Taking a Look at Complexity
Reprinted from: *J. Clin. Med.* **2023**, *12*, 7756, doi:10.3390/jcm12247756 1

Magdalena Chlabicz, Aleksandra Szum-Jakubowska, Paweł Sowa, Małgorzata Chlabicz, Sebastian Sołomacha, Łukasz Kiszkiel, et al.
The Effect of the COVID-19 Pandemic on Self-Reported Health Status and Smoking and Drinking Habits in the General Urban Population
Reprinted from: *J. Clin. Med.* **2023**, *12*, 6241, doi:10.3390/jcm12196241 3

Giancarlo Ceccarelli, Francesco Alessandri, Giuseppe Migliara, Valentina Baccolini, Giovanni Giordano, Gioacchino Galardo, et al.
Reduced Reliability of Procalcitonin (PCT) as a Biomarker of Bacterial Superinfection: Concerns about PCT-Driven Antibiotic Stewardship in Critically Ill COVID-19 Patients—Results from a Retrospective Observational Study in Intensive Care Units
Reprinted from: *J. Clin. Med.* **2023**, *12*, 6171, doi:10.3390/jcm12196171 15

Justine Benoit-Piau, Karine Tremblay, Alain Piché, Frédéric Dallaire, Mathieu Bélanger, Marc-André d'Entremont, et al.
Long-Term Consequences of COVID-19 in Predominantly Immunonaive Patients: A Canadian Prospective Population-Based Study
Reprinted from: *J. Clin. Med.* **2023**, *12*, 5939, doi:10.3390/jcm12185939 25

Maciej Koźlik, Maciej Kaźmierski, Wojciech Kaźmierski, Paulina Lis, Anna Lis, Weronika Łowicka, et al.
Quality of Life 6 Months after COVID-19 Hospitalisation: A Single-Centre Polish Registry
Reprinted from: *J. Clin. Med.* **2023**, *12*, 5327, doi:10.3390/jcm12165327 39

Maurizio Di Marco, Nicoletta Miano, Simona Marchisello, Giuseppe Coppolino, Giuseppe L'Episcopo, Sabrina Scilletta, et al.
Indirect Effects of the COVID-19 Pandemic on In-Hospital Outcomes among Internal Medicine Departments: A Double-Center Retrospective Study
Reprinted from: *J. Clin. Med.* **2023**, *12*, 5304, doi:10.3390/jcm12165304 51

Samy Talha, Sid Lamrous, Loic Kassegne, Nicolas Lefebvre, Abrar-Ahmad Zulfiqar, Pierre Tran Ba Loc, et al.
Early Hospital Discharge Using Remote Monitoring for Patients Hospitalized for COVID-19, Regardless of Need for Home Oxygen Therapy: A Descriptive Study
Reprinted from: *J. Clin. Med.* **2023**, *12*, 5100, doi:10.3390/jcm12155100 61

Grzegorz Kobelski, Katarzyna Naylor, Robert Ślusarz and Mariusz Wysokiński
Post-Traumatic Stress Disorder among Polish Healthcare Staff in the Era of the COVID-19 Pandemic
Reprinted from: *J. Clin. Med.* **2023**, *12*, 4072, doi:10.3390/jcm12124072 73

Edyta Sutkowska, Agata Stanek, Katarzyna Madziarska, Grzegorz K. Jakubiak, Janusz Sokołowski, Marcin Madziarski, et al.
Physical Activity Modifies the Severity of COVID-19 in Hospitalized Patients—Observational Study
Reprinted from: *J. Clin. Med.* **2023**, *12*, 4046, doi:10.3390/jcm12124046 87

Aleksandra Kwaśniewska, Krzysztof Kwaśniewski, Andrzej Skorek, Dmitry Tretiakow,
Anna Jaźwińska-Curyłło and Paweł Burduk
Correlation of ENT Symptoms with Age, Sex, and Anti-SARS-CoV-2 Antibody Titer in Plasma
Reprinted from: *J. Clin. Med.* **2023**, *12*, 610, doi:10.3390/jcm12020610 97

Tamara Nikolic Turnic, Ivana Vasiljevic, Magdalena Stanic, Biljana Jakovljevic,
Maria Mikerova, Natalia Ekkert, et al.
Post-COVID-19 Status and Its Physical, Nutritional, Psychological, and Social Effects in Working-Age Adults—A Prospective Questionnaire Study
Reprinted from: *J. Clin. Med.* **2022**, *11*, 6668, doi:10.3390/jcm11226668 107

Vincent Tarazona, David Kirouchena, Pascal Clerc, Florence Pinsard-Laventure and
Bastien Bourrion
Quality of Life in COVID-19 Outpatients: A Long-Term Follow-Up Study
Reprinted from: *J. Clin. Med.* **2022**, *11*, 6478, doi:10.3390/jcm11216478 123

Shahrzad Ahangarzadeh, Alireza Yousefi, Mohammad Mehdi Ranjbar, Arezou Dabiri,
Atefeh Zarepour, Mahmoud Sadeghi, et al.
Association of Clinical Features with Spike Glycoprotein Mutations in Iranian COVID-19 Patients
Reprinted from: *J. Clin. Med.* **2022**, *11*, 6315, doi:10.3390/jcm11216315 133

Maximilian Kutschera, Valentin Ritschl, Berthold Reichardt, Tanja Stamm, Hans Kiener,
Harald Maier, et al.
Impact of COVID-19 Pandemic on Initiation of Immunosuppressive Treatment in Immune-Mediated Inflammatory Diseases in Austria: A Nationwide Retrospective Study
Reprinted from: *J. Clin. Med.* **2022**, *11*, 5308, doi:10.3390/jcm11185308 141

Valeria Calcaterra, Veronica Maria Tagi, Raffaella De Santis, Andrea Biuso, Silvia Taranto,
Enza D'Auria and Gianvincenzo Zuccotti
Endocrinological Involvement in Children and Adolescents Affected by COVID-19: A Narrative Review
Reprinted from: *J. Clin. Med.* **2023**, *12*, 5248, doi:10.3390/jcm12165248 153

Rosaria De Luca, Mirjam Bonanno and Rocco Salvatore Calabrò
Psychological and Cognitive Effects of Long COVID: A Narrative Review Focusing on the Assessment and Rehabilitative Approach
Reprinted from: *J. Clin. Med.* **2022**, *11*, 6554, doi:10.3390/jcm11216554 173

Iwona Jannasz, Michal Pruc, Mansur Rahnama-Hezavah, Tomasz Targowski,
Robert Olszewski, Stepan Feduniw, et al.
The Impact of COVID-19 on Carotid–Femoral Pulse Wave Velocity: A Systematic Review and Meta-Analysis
Reprinted from: *J. Clin. Med.* **2023**, *12*, 5747, doi:10.3390/jcm12175747 197

Nicoleta Anton, Camelia Margareta Bogdănici, Daniel Constantin Brănișteanu,
Ovidiu-Dumitru Ilie, Irina Andreea Pavel and Bogdan Doroftei
The Implications of SARS-CoV-2 Infection in a Series of Neuro-Ophthalmological Manifestations—Case Series and Literature Review
Reprinted from: *J. Clin. Med.* **2023**, *12*, 3795, doi:10.3390/jcm12113795 209

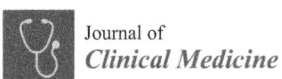

Editorial

Special Issue "Clinical Consequences of COVID-19": Taking a Look at Complexity

Giovanni Giordano *, Francesco Alessandri and Francesco Pugliese

Department of General and Specialistic Surgery, Sapienza University of Rome, Policlinico Umberto I, 00161 Rome, Italy; francesco.alessandri@uniroma1.it (F.A.); f.pugliese@uniroma1.it (F.P.)
* Correspondence: giordano.gj@gmail.com

Citation: Giordano, G.; Alessandri, F.; Pugliese, F. Special Issue "Clinical Consequences of COVID-19": Taking a Look at Complexity. *J. Clin. Med.* 2023, *12*, 7756. https://doi.org/10.3390/jcm12247756

Received: 7 December 2023
Accepted: 14 December 2023
Published: 18 December 2023

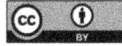

Copyright: © 2023 by the authors. Licensee MDPI, Basel, Switzerland. This article is an open access article distributed under the terms and conditions of the Creative Commons Attribution (CC BY) license (https://creativecommons.org/licenses/by/4.0/).

The consequences of SARS-CoV-2 infection are far from being fully understood or accounted for. The most common and dangerous acute clinical features of the disease affect the respiratory system, and can be involved in the wide spectrum of severity at presentation; the evolution of the disease can vary enormously, ranging from asymptomatic or mild disease to critical illness with multi-organ failure and high mortality rates [1,2]. In addition to this, and soon after the outbreak of the pandemic, it became clear that several other organs were involved in the multiform clinical presentation of COVID-19, including neurological, ear, nose, and throat, gastrointestinal, ophthalmic, dermatological, cardiac, and rheumatologic manifestations. The persistence of mild symptoms and disorders for up to several months after testing negative has been designated a new nosological identity called "long covid" or "post-acute COVID-19 syndrome" [3].

In this Special Issue we collected 17 high-quality and innovative papers investigating several factors that have contributed to the clinical complexity of COVID-19: from host–pathogen interactions to different clinical manifestations, including the impact on healthcare systems and post-COVID-19 consequences.

Differences in the clinical manifestation of the disease might be influenced by intricate interactions between the virus and the patient. For example, mutations in specific SARS-CoV-2 proteins are reported to potentially influence the clinical course of the disease [4]. Additionally, demographic characteristics and lifestyle might have an impact on the severity of COVID-19 [5].

The peculiarity of patient–virus interaction may further influence the clinical management of COVID-19. In the pre-pandemic era, PCT represented a useful laboratory tool for the diagnosis and management of bacterial infections [6]. However, the study by Ceccarelli and colleagues showed that, in critically ill COVID-19 patients, abnormal procalcitonin levels do not necessarily indicate the presence of a bacterial superinfection [7]. This is particularly relevant when dealing with highly complicated patients, who are potentially susceptible to deterioration and in which a rapid differential diagnosis is crucial.

The pandemic had a significant impact on healthcare systems worldwide, and alongside COVID-19 patients, non-COVID patients also suffered different kinds of consequences [8]. For instance, the rapid spread and the severity of infection raised concerns over the safety of using immunosuppressive drugs to treat immune-mediated inflammatory diseases [9]. In addition, medical departments that were not directly managing COVID-19 patients have also experienced the consequences of the COVID-19 pandemic [10]. In fact, the need to expand bed capacity in order to accept the (un)expected, and outstanding, number of patients, led to unprecedented intra-hospital organizational efforts at the expense of reducing resources in departments that had not been converted to COVID-19 wards. Other solutions have been proposed: in order to reduce the number of beds being used at any given time, some authors explored whether early hospital discharge would have been safe or useful [11]. Last but not least, the impact of the pandemic on healthcare personnel was overwhelming [12].

Moreover, several articles published in this Special Issue focus on the post disease and long-term effects of COVID-19, including the Quality of Life of hospitalized or non-hospitalized patients, and also the physical, psychological, and social effects of the pandemic.

As Guest Editors we want to thank all of the authors, the reviewers, and the Journal of Clinical Medicine team for their precious work and support.

Conflicts of Interest: The authors declare no conflict of interest.

Abbreviations

SAR-CoV-2	severe acute respiratory syndrome coronavirus-2
COVID-19	coronavirus disease 2019
PCT	procalcitonin

References

1. Berlin, D.A.; Gulick, R.M.; Martinez, F.J. Severe COVID-19. *N. Engl. J. Med.* **2020**, *383*, 2451. [CrossRef] [PubMed]
2. Huang, C.; Wang, Y.; Li, X.; Ren, L.; Zhao, J.; Hu, Y.; Zhang, L.; Fan, G.; Xu, J.; Gu, X.; et al. Clinical features of patients infected with 2019 novel coronavirus in Wuhan, China. *Lancet* **2020**, *395*, 497. [CrossRef] [PubMed]
3. Luchian, M.L.; Higny, J.; Benoit, M.; Robaye, B.; Berners, Y.; Henry, J.P.; Colle, B.; Xhaët, O.; Blommaert, D.; Droogmans, S.; et al. Unmasking Pandemic Echoes: An In-Depth Review of Long COVID's Unabated Cardiovascular Consequences beyond 2020. *Diagnostics* **2023**, *13*, 3368. [CrossRef] [PubMed]
4. Mendiola-Pastrana, I.R.; López-Ortiz, E.; Río de la Loza-Zamora, J.G.; González, J.; Gómez-García, A.; López-Ortiz, G. SARS-CoV-2 variants and clinical outcomes: A systematic review. *Life* **2022**, *12*, 170. [CrossRef] [PubMed]
5. Pijls, B.G.; Jolani, S.; Atherley, A.; Derckx, R.T.; Dijkstra, J.I.R.; Franssen, G.H.L.; Hendriks, S.; Richters, A.; Venemans-Jellema, A.; Zalpuri, S.; et al. Demographic risk factors for COVID-19 infection, severity, ICU admission and death: A meta-analysis of 59 studies. *BMJ Open* **2021**, *11*, e044640. [CrossRef] [PubMed]
6. Schuetz, P.; Beishuizen, A.; Broyles, M.; Ferrer, R.; Gavazzi, G.; Gluck, E.H.; González Del Castillo, J.; Jensen, J.U.; Kanizsai, P.L.; Kwa, A.L.H.; et al. Procalcitonin (PCT)-guided antibiotic stewardship: An international experts consensus on optimized clinical use. *Clin. Chem. Lab. Med.* **2019**, *57*, 1308–1318. [CrossRef] [PubMed]
7. Ceccarelli, G.; Alessandri, F.; Migliara, G.; Baccolini, V.; Giordano, G.; Galardo, G.; Marzuillo, C.; De Vito, C.; Russo, A.; Ciccozzi, M.; et al. Reduced Reliability of Procalcitonin (PCT) as a Biomarker of Bacterial Superinfection: Concerns about PCT-Driven Antibiotic Stewardship in Critically Ill COVID-19 Patients—Results from a Retrospective Observational Study in Intensive Care Units. *J. Clin. Med.* **2023**, *12*, 6171. [CrossRef] [PubMed]
8. Clerk, A.M. Beware of Neglect of Non-COVID Patients in COVID Era. *Indian J. Crit. Care Med.* **2021**, *25*, 837–838. [CrossRef] [PubMed]
9. Giuliani, F.; Gualdi, G.; Amerio, P. Effect of immunosuppressive drugs in immune-mediated inflammatory disease during the coronavirus pandemic. *Dermatol. Ther.* **2020**, *33*, e14204. [CrossRef] [PubMed]
10. Santi, L.; Golinelli, D.; Tampieri, A.; Farina, G.; Greco, M.; Rosa, S.; Beleffi, M.; Biavati, B.; Campinoti, F.; Guerrini, S.; et al. Non-COVID-19 patients in times of pandemic: Emergency department visits, hospitalizations and cause-specific mortality in Northern Italy. *PLoS ONE* **2021**, *16*, e0248995. [CrossRef] [PubMed]
11. Grutters, L.A.; Majoor, K.I.; Mattern, E.S.K.; Hardeman, J.A.; van Swol, C.F.P.; Vorselaars, A.D.M. Home telemonitoring makes early hospital discharge of COVID-19 patients possible. *J. Am. Med. Inform. Assoc.* **2020**, *27*, 1825–1827. [CrossRef] [PubMed]
12. Gupta, N.; Dhamija, S.; Patil, J.; Chaudhari, B. Impact of COVID-19 pandemic on healthcare workers. *Ind. Psychiatry J.* **2021**, *30*, S282–S284. [CrossRef] [PubMed]

Disclaimer/Publisher's Note: The statements, opinions and data contained in all publications are solely those of the individual author(s) and contributor(s) and not of MDPI and/or the editor(s). MDPI and/or the editor(s) disclaim responsibility for any injury to people or property resulting from any ideas, methods, instructions or products referred to in the content.

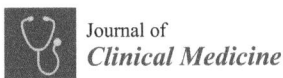

Article

The Effect of the COVID-19 Pandemic on Self-Reported Health Status and Smoking and Drinking Habits in the General Urban Population

Magdalena Chlabicz [1], Aleksandra Szum-Jakubowska [1], Paweł Sowa [1], Małgorzata Chlabicz [1,2], Sebastian Sołomacha [1], Łukasz Kiszkiel [3], Łukasz Minarowski [4], Katarzyna Guziejko [4], Piotr P. Laskowski [3], Anna M. Moniuszko-Malinowska [5] and Karol A. Kamiński [1,6,*]

[1] Department of Population Medicine and Lifestyle Diseases Prevention, Medical University of Bialystok, 15-269 Bialystok, Poland; chlabicz.m@gmail.com (M.C.); aleksandra.szum-jakubowska@umb.edu.pl (A.S.-J.); mailtosowa@gmail.com (P.S.); mchlabicz@op.pl (M.C.); sebastian.solomacha@sd.umb.edu.pl (S.S.)
[2] Department of Invasive Cardiology, Medical University of Bialystok, 15-276 Bialystok, Poland
[3] Society and Cognition Unit, Institute of Sociology, University of Bialystok, 15-420 Bialystok, Poland; lukaszkiszkiel@gmail.com (Ł.K.); p.laskowski@uwb.edu (P.P.L.)
[4] 2nd Department of Lung Diseases and Tuberculosis, Medical University of Bialystok, Zurawia 14, 15-540 Bialystok, Poland; lukasz.minarowski@umb.edu.pl (Ł.M.); kguziejko@wp.pl (K.G.)
[5] Department of Infectious Diseases and Neuroinfection, Medical University of Bialystok, 15-540 Bialystok, Poland; annamoniuszko@op.pl
[6] Department of Cardiology, Medical University of Bialystok, 15-276 Bialystok, Poland
* Correspondence: fizklin@wp.pl

Citation: Chlabicz, M.; Szum-Jakubowska, A.; Sowa, P.; Chlabicz, M.; Sołomacha, S.; Kiszkiel, Ł.; Minarowski, Ł.; Guziejko, K.; Laskowski, P.P.; Moniuszko-Malinowska, A.M.; et al. The Effect of the COVID-19 Pandemic on Self-Reported Health Status and Smoking and Drinking Habits in the General Urban Population. *J. Clin. Med.* **2023**, *12*, 6241. https://doi.org/10.3390/jcm12196241

Academic Editors: Francesco Pugliese, Francesco Alessandri, Giovanni Giordano, Sukhwinder Singh Sohal and Francisco Guillen-Grima

Received: 12 August 2023
Revised: 20 September 2023
Accepted: 26 September 2023
Published: 27 September 2023

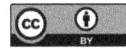

Copyright: © 2023 by the authors. Licensee MDPI, Basel, Switzerland. This article is an open access article distributed under the terms and conditions of the Creative Commons Attribution (CC BY) license (https:// creativecommons.org/licenses/by/ 4.0/).

Abstract: The coronavirus disease 2019 pandemic created a significant crisis in global health. The aim of the study was to compare the impact of the COVID-19 pandemic on self-rated health status and smoking and alcohol habits. The Bialystok PLUS cohort study was conducted in 2018–2022. A total of 1222 randomly selected city residents were examined and divided into two groups: before and during the COVID-19 pandemic. The participants' lifestyle habits and medical history were collected from self-reported questionnaires. The Alcohol Use Disorders Identification Test (AUDIT) and the Fagerström Test for Nicotine Dependence (FTND) were used to assess the degree of alcohol and nicotine dependence. The survey revealed a reduced frequency of reported allergies vs. an increased frequency of reported sinusitis and asthma; increased incidence of declared hypercholesterolemia and visual impairment; a reduced number of cigarettes smoked per day, lower FTND score, and a greater desire to quit smoking in the next six months; and an increase in hs-CRP and FeNO levels in the population during the pandemic compared to the pre-pandemic population. The COVID-19 pandemic had a measurable impact on the general population's prevalence of certain medical conditions and lifestyle habits. Further research should continue to examine the long-term health implications of the pandemic.

Keywords: COVID-19; smoking habits; alcohol habits; health status

1. Introduction

Coronavirus disease 2019 (COVID-19) is a respiratory infection induced by severe acute respiratory syndrome coronavirus 2 (SARS-CoV-2), also known as coronavirus [1]. The outbreak began in China, but has spread to all countries around the world, and the number of cases outside of East Asia exceeded those in China by 15 March 2020, and rose exponentially. The number of fatalities in several countries now exceeds the total in the epidemic focus [2]. The COVID-19 pandemic remains a primary concern for global health and society. Clinicians must keep up with the data generated from across the globe, since SARS-CoV-2 emerged in December 2019 [3]. In Poland, from January 2020 to December 2022, 6,364,708 confirmed cases of COVID-19, including 118,467 deaths, were reported to the WHO [4]. The introduction of lockdown in Poland has significantly affected the nature of citizens' work and human relations by limiting social interactions and mobility.

Health complications and lifestyle habits associated with the COVID-19 pandemic are currently being investigated. The percentage of daily tobacco smokers in 2019 in Poland was 24% among men and 18% among women [5]. Smoking is a significant risk factor for major causes of premature mortality, such as cancer and cardiovascular disease. Using cigarettes also increases the risk of heart attack, stroke, lung cancer, and cancers of the larynx and mouth. In addition, smoking is an essential contributor to respiratory diseases. Alcohol abuse also causes significant mortality and morbidity. Alcohol use disorders are usually linked to depressive episodes, severe anxiety, and insomnia. They can increase the incidence of heart disease, stroke, cancer, and cirrhosis by affecting the cardiovascular, digestive, and immune systems [6]. According to a 2019 analysis, the average level of alcohol consumption in Poland was 11 L of pure alcohol per capita (a person aged 15 years or older) [7].

The aim of the study was to compare the impact of pandemic COVID-19 on self-rated health status and smoking and alcohol habits. We used the Bialystok PLUS cohort, that started enrollment in 2018 and continued during pandemic, which allows for reliable data analysis before and during the pandemic. Therefore, we compared both populations—before and during the pandemic—studied using the same methodology.

2. Materials and Methods

The Bialystok PLUS cohort study was conducted in 2018–2022 on a sample of Bialystok (Poland) citizens. Based on a representative sample of the residents of Bialystok city, the Bialystok PLUS study describes the health status of the adult population in northeastern Poland. The survey not only addresses the present health status of the people, thus providing valuable data on risk factors and the development of diseases, but also examines the sociological and psychological determinants that may influence them [8]. Researchers received a pseudonymized list of residents aged 20–79 from the Bialystok City Hall each year. They were then assigned categories by gender and 5-year ranges. Subsequently, samples of citizens from each subcategory were randomly selected separately, in such numbers as to obtain a distribution of proportions similar to that of the city's population. The exact drawing procedure is described elsewhere [9]. The analyzed population, a total of 1222 respondents (570 men and 652 women), was divided into two groups: before the COVID-19 pandemic and during the COVID-19 pandemic. The beginning of the pandemic in Poland was considered to be 20 March 2020, when an epidemic state was imposed in Poland. A total of 713 probands tested between 5 November 2018 and 17 March 2020 were classified as a pre-pandemic group, and 509 probands tested between 14 July 2020 (the study had to be interrupted during lockdown between March and July) and 13 May 2022 were analyzed during the pandemic.

The participants' lifestyle habits and medical history were collected from self-reported questionnaires. All study participants underwent laboratory assessment, spirometry, and nitric oxide (NO) measurement in the exhaled air–fractional nitric oxide (FeNO) using nitric oxide analyzer FeNO+ from Medisoft. Anthropometric measurements included measurement of height and weight. Body mass index (BMI) was calculated as weight in kilograms divided by height in meters squared. The waist-to-hip ratio (WHR) was calculated as the circumference ratio between the waist and hips. From all patients, peripheral intravenous fasting blood samples were collected for laboratory tests, at the time of visit in the morning after eight hours of fasting. High-sensitivity C-reactive protein (hs-CRP) and a complete blood count with differential were established to assess the inflammatory state.

The Alcohol Use Disorders Identification Test (AUDIT) was used to assess the degree of alcohol dependence. AUDIT is a practical and simple screening test for unhealthy alcohol use, defined as risky or hazardous drinking or any alcohol use disorder. Following its publication in 1989 by the World Health Organization, AUDIT has become the most widely used alcohol use screening tool in the world [10]. In addition to questions about alcohol use scored on a scale of 0 to 4, the AUDIT asks about common alcohol-related problems that patients might face, including general symptoms of alcohol dependence [11].

The Fagerström Test for Nicotine Dependence (FTND) was used to assess ordinal measures of nicotine dependence related to cigarette smoking. FTND was developed by Karl-Olov Fagerström in 1978. The instrument was modified in 1991 by Todd Heatherton et al. to form the Fagerström Test for Nicotine Dependence [12]. When assessing nicotine dependence in the Fagerström Test, yes/no questions were scored on a scale of 0 to 1, and multiple-choice questions were scored on a scale of 0 to 3. The higher the summed Fagerström score, the more intense the patient's physical dependence on nicotine.

The Satisfaction with Life Scale (SWLS) has been used to measure a life satisfaction component of subjective well-being. SWLS was developed in 1959 by Diener [13] and has been shown to correlate with mental health measures and predict future behavior.

The questionnaire interview included an assessment of health status at the time of the study, including questions from AUDIT, FTND, and SWLS, lifestyle habits, education level, earnings, and medical history.

3. Statistical Analysis

The statistical analysis was performed using Stata 13.0 statistical software. Descriptive statistics for quantitative variables were presented as means and standard deviations (SD). The normality of distributions was assessed using the Shapiro–Wilk test. Values of normally distributed data were compared by unpaired t-test, whereas not-normally distributed continuous data were compared by Mann–Whitney U test. Categorical variables are displayed as frequency distributions (n) and simple percentages (%). The Chi^2 test was used for the univariate comparison between the groups for categorical variables. Spearman correlation was used to analyze the dependence between the variables. The statistical significance was considered when $p \leq 0.05$.

4. Results

The analyzed populations did not differ in terms of age (p = 0.487), sex (p = 0.219), height (p = 0.179), weight (p = 0.072), or body mass index (p = 0.388). In contrast, WHR was statistically significantly lower in the population during the pandemic (p = 0.006). In the population during the COVID-19 pandemic, examination of exhaled air from the respiratory tract showed higher concentrations of FeNO (21.3 ± 18.8 ppb vs. 18.7 ± 15.4 ppb, p < 0.001) and higher levels of high-sensitivity C-reactive protein (1.7 ± 3.1 mg/L vs. 1.5 ± 3.6 mg/L, p = 0.001) compared to the pre-pandemic group. Detailed data can be found in Table 1.

Table 1. Characteristics of the population before and during the COVID-19 pandemic; comparisons variables between subgroups.

Variable	Population before the COVID-19 Pandemic N = 713	Population during the COVID-19 Pandemic N = 509	p
Age, years	48.7 ± 15.4	49.3 ± 14.5	0.487
Male sex, n (%)	322 (45.2)	248 (48.7)	0.219
Height, cm	170.1 ± 10.1	170.8 ± 9.5	0.179
Weight, kg	77.9 ± 16.7	79.3 ± 16.2	0.072
BMI, kg/m^2	26.8 ± 4.9	27.2 ± 5.2	0.388
WHR	0.88 ± 0.1	0.86 ± 0.1	0.006

Table 1. Cont.

Variable	Population before the COVID-19 Pandemic N = 713	Population during the COVID-19 Pandemic N = 509	p
Laboratory parameters			
hs-CRP, mg/L	1.5 ± 3.6	1.7 ± 3.1	0.001
FeNO, ppb	18.7 ± 15.4	21.3 ± 18.8	<0.001
WBC, 10^3/uL	6.25 ± 1.6	5.8 ± 1.5	<0.001
Hgb, g/dL	14.1 ± 1.4	13.9 ± 1.3	0.057
Hct, %	41.1 ± 3.8	40.9 ± 3.7	0.396
PLT × 10^9/L	236 ± 62.8	235.9 ± 60.3	0.821
Spirometry			
FVC, L	4.3 ± 1.2	4.3 ± 1.1	0.678
FEV1/FVC, %	79.1 ± 6.9	78.9 ± 6.6	0.302

The data are shown as n (%), mean ± SD. BMI: body mass index; hs-CRP: high-sensitivity C-reactive protein; WBC: white blood cells; Hct: hematocrit; Hgb: hemoglobin; PLT: platelet count; kg: kilogram; cm: centimeter; mg: milligram; L: liter; dL: deciliter; ft: femtoliter; mmHg: millimeters of mercury; SD: standard deviation; ppb: parts per billion; mg/L: milligrams per liter; mg/dL: milligrams per deciliter; FVC: forced vital capacity; FEV1: forced expiratory volume in 1 s.

A significantly lower number of reported allergies was observed in the population during the pandemic (22.8%) compared to the pre-pandemic period (23.6%; p = 0.042). In contrast, the incidence of reported asthma and sinusitis was significantly higher during the pandemic (6.3% and 24.6%) than before the pandemic (2.9%; p < 0.001 and 24.0%; p = 0.006). In addition, visual impairment and hypercholesterolemia were declared more frequently in the population during the COVID-19 pandemic. Detailed data can be found in Figure 1 and Table 2.

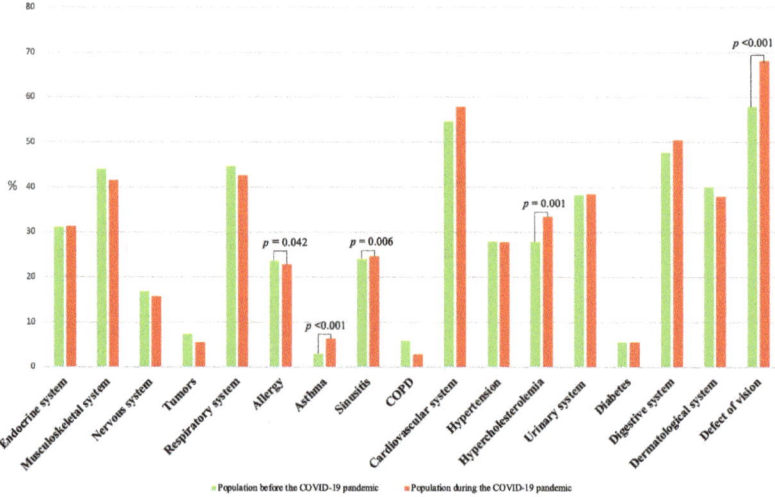

Figure 1. Percentage of reported diseases in the general population before and during the COVID-19 pandemic.

Table 2. The incidence of reported diseases in the general population before the pandemic COVID-19 and during the pandemic COVID-19.

Disease	Population before the COVID-19 Pandemic N = 713	Population during the COVID-19 Pandemic N = 509	p
Endocrine system	222 (31.1)	159 (31.2)	0.901
Musculoskeletal system	314 (44.0)	211 (41.5)	0.369
Nervous system	120 (16.8)	80 (15.7)	0.636
Tumors	53 (7.4)	28 (5.5)	0.184
Respiratory system	318 (44.6)	217 (42.6)	0.678
Allergy	168 (23.6)	116 (22.8)	0.042
Asthma	21 (2.9)	32 (6.3)	<0.001
Sinusitis	171 (24.0)	125 (24.6)	0.006
COPD	41 (5.8)	14 (2.8)	0.076
Cardiovascular system	389 (54.6)	294 (57.8)	0.262
Hypertension	199 (27.9)	141 (27.7)	0.469
Hypercholesterolemia	198 (27.8)	170 (33.4)	0.001
Urinary system	273 (38.3)	196 (38.5)	0.941
Diabetes	39 (5.5)	28 (5.5)	0.168
Digestive system	340 (47.7)	257 (50.5)	0.270
Dermatological system	285 (40.0)	193 (37.9)	0.506
Defect of vision	413 (57.9)	346 (68.0)	<0.001

The data are shown as n (%); COPD: chronic obstructive pulmonary disease.

The prevalence of smoking history remained similar between the two groups. At the same time, numerically fewer individuals reported current smoking in the COVID-19 population compared to the pre-pandemic population, although without statistical significance. The average number of cigarettes smoked per day decreased during the pandemic compared with the pre-pandemic period (10.7 ± 7.1 vs. 14.0 ± 9.1; $p = 0.005$). In addition, more individuals declared planning to quit smoking in the next six months during the pandemic (39.4%) than before it (33.8%; $p = 0.049$), which was also reflected in the FTND results. In the population during the pandemic, the FTND score was statistically significantly lower than before the pandemic (2.4 ± 2.2 vs. 3.2 ± 2.3; $p = 0.007$).

Alcohol consumption patterns were generally not different between the study groups. Only the frequency of drinking liquors, fruit liqueurs, and drinks in the past 30 days was lower during the pandemic than before the pandemic (2.3 ± 2.3 vs. 2.9 ± 2.7; $p = 0.018$), while other drinking frequencies remained unchanged. The results of the Alcohol Use Disorder Identification Test also remained consistent ($p = 0.329$) between both cohorts.

These results suggest a moderate change in smoking habits during the COVID-19 pandemic, while no differences were shown regarding alcohol drinking.

Subjective well-being, as measured by the SWLS scale, did not statistically differ between the study groups. Detailed data can be found in Table 3.

The analysis aimed to determine the relationship between the declared intention to quit smoking and various variables, such as age, sex, BMI, education, income, and FeNO levels. Results revealed no significant associations between the intention to quit smoking and any of these variables, which may suggest that the intention to quit smoking may be independent of these factors. Detailed data can be found in Table 4.

Table 3. Population behavior of the population before and during the COVID-19 pandemic.

Lifestyle Habits	Population before the COVID-19 Pandemic N = 713	Population during the COVID-19 Pandemic N = 509	p
Smoking habits			
Ever smoked cigarettes	402 (56.4)	289 (56.8)	0.998
Currently smoking	136 (19.1)	94 (18.5)	0.795
Number of cigarettes smoked during the day	14.0 ± 9.1	10.7 ± 7.1	0.005
The highest number of cigarettes smoked during the day	20.7 ± 10.6	16.7 ± 7.4	0.117
Individuals planning to quit smoking within 6 months	46 (33.8)	37 (39.4)	0.049
Fagerström Test for Nicotine Dependence score	3.2 ± 2.3	2.4 ± 2.2	0.007
Drinking habits			
Drinking alcoholic beverages in the last 30 days	512 (71.8)	361 (70.9)	0.564
Drinking beer in the last 30 days	326 (45.7)	195 (38.3)	0.404
Drinking alcohol in the last 30 days	232 (32.5)	147 (28.9)	0.930
Drinking liqueurs, fruit liqueurs, drink in the last 30 days	115 (16.1)	70 (13.8)	0.808
Drinking wine in the last 30 days	222 (31.1)	152 (29.9)	0.300
How many times have a beer been drunk in the last 30 days	5.9 ± 6.7	9.6 ± 5.4	0.908
Beer quantity in milliliters drunk in the last 30 days	2243.5 ± 3221.5	1327.8 ± 1337.2	0.991
How many times has alcohol been drunk in the last 30 days	2.7 ± 2.5	3.0 ± 3.7	0.720
Alcohol quantity in milliliters drunk in the last 30 days	331.9 ± 417.9	324.2 ± 364.4	0.4366
How many times has liqueurs, fruit liqueurs, drinks drunk in the last 30 days	2.9 ± 2.7	2.3 ± 2.3	0.018
Liqueurs, fruit liqueurs, drink quantity in milliliters drunk in the last 30 days	195.8 ± 282.2	339.9 ± 449.5	0.052
How many times have wine been drunk in the last 30 days	4.9 ± 4.1	2.6 ± 2.2	0.153
Wine quantity in milliliters drunk in the last 30 days	343.7 ± 427	389.4 ± 403.7	0.144
Alcohol Use Disorders Identification Test score	4 ± 3.7	3.6 ± 3.0	0.329
The Satisfaction with Life Scale (SWLS)			
SWLS	22.7 ± 5.2	22.4 ± 5.2	0.407

The data are shown as n (%), mean ± SD.

Table 4. Dependence between declared intention to quit smoking and the variables.

Variable	p
Age	0.724
Sex	0.327
BMI	0.184
Education	0.493
Income	0.482
FeNO, ppb	0.722

5. Discussion

The current study provides data on the incidence of major diseases, as well as smoking and drinking habits in the population during the COVID-19 pandemic compared to the pre-pandemic population. The survey revealed: (1) a reduced frequency of reported allergies vs. an increased frequency of reported sinusitis, asthma; (2) an increased incidence of declared hypercholesterolemia and visual impairment; (3) a reduced number of cigarettes smoked per day, lower FTND score, and a greater desire to quit smoking in the next six months; and (4) an increase in hs-CRP and FeNO levels in the population during the pandemic compared to the pre-pandemic COVID-19 population. No differences were found in alcohol consumption habits. The current study found that the COVID-19 pandemic had a measurable impact on the general population's prevalence of certain diseases and lifestyle habits.

Smoking is a leading factor in preventable morbidity and mortality worldwide. More than a billion people smoke, and without a significant increase in smoking cessation, at least half of them will die prematurely from tobacco-related complications [14]. Tetik B. K. et al. [15] studied patients who attended smoking cessation clinics in 2018 and were asked about their smoking cessation status after one year and after the COVID-19 pandemic. They investigated whether the pandemic had an impact on smoking cessation. When the success of those who quit smoking before the pandemic and those who quit smoking after the pandemic was compared, a statistically significant relationship was found ($p < 0.001$): the cessation rate after one year was 23.7%. In contrast, the cessation rate during the pandemic period was 31.1%. Nyman, A.L. et al. [16] conducted a study in which a sample of 1223 US adult cigarette smokers participated in an online survey in October–November 2020 to assess their perceptions of COVID-19 risk and changes in smoking, willingness to quit, and quit attempts during the COVID-19 pandemic. More smokers believed that smoking could increase COVID-19 severity than believed that smoking made them more susceptible to COVID-19. Greater perceptions of overall COVID-19 severity were associated with an increased likelihood of reduced smoking, greater readiness to quit smoking, and a greater chance of attempting to quit smoking. Gül Nur Çelik F. et al. [17] included a total of 749 respondents between the ages of 19 and 35 in the study. The degree of nicotine dependence was examined using the FTND. The mean nicotine dependence scores before the pandemic and COVID-19 were 3.03 and 2.97, respectively. A difference was observed before the pandemic ($p = 0.002$) and during the pandemic ($p = 0.005$) for health sciences students and others. Compared to before and during the pandemic, the mean addiction score was significantly lower for students whose parents were non-smokers during the pandemic. Our findings also showed a decrease in the FTND score, which can be reflected in the reduction in the average number of cigarettes smoked per day during the pandemic and the increased desire to quit smoking. This may result from increased awareness of the harmful effects of smoking on respiratory health. Smokers may also perceive increased susceptibility to and severity of COVID-19 infection, potentially increasing motivation to quit [1].

A systematic review by Roberts A. et al. [18] showed a mixed picture of alcohol use during the COVID-19 pandemic. Overall, there was a trend toward increased alcohol consumption. The percentage of people consuming alcohol during the pandemic ranged from 21.7% to 72.9% in the general population samples. Mental health-related factors were the most common correlates or triggers of increased alcohol use. Killgore W.D.S. et al. [19] evaluated whether COVID-19-related lockdown, in the form of stay-at-home orders and social isolation, was associated with changes in high-risk alcohol use. A total of 5931 people completed the AUDIT at one of six-time points between April and September 2020. Over the six-month period, hazardous alcohol use and probable dependence increased month after month for those on lockdown compared to those not on restriction. The current study found no differences in alcohol consumption between the study populations, reflected in the lack of differences in AUDIT test scores.

Based on recent literature, there is scientific and clinical evidence on the subacute and long-term implications of COVID-19, which may affect numerous organ systems [20]. The prevalence of allergic diseases was increasing globally before COVID-19. Choi, H.G. et al. [21] analyzed the frequency rate of self-reported and physician-diagnosed allergic diseases of asthma, atopic dermatitis, and allergic rhinitis in the Korean population. A total of 15,469 individuals were analyzed in the National Health and Nutrition Examination Survey dataset. There were no statistically relevant differences found between the prevalence of physician-diagnosed and present allergic diseases in 2019 and 2020 (asthma, $p = 0.667$ and $p = 0.268$; atopic dermatitis, $p = 0.268$ and $p = 0.973$; allergic rhinitis, $p = 0.691$ and $p = 0.942$, respectively). Among the Korean population, the prevalence of allergic diseases: asthma, atopic dermatitis, and allergic rhinitis did not decrease in 2019–2020. In comparison, the current study showed a decrease in the incidence of declared allergy, but increased reports of asthma and sinusitis. A particularly interesting finding is the increased awareness of hypercholesterolemia. More common contact with healthcare due to COVID-19 probably increased the number of blood labs. However, this may also be an effect of a preventive "40+" program, which has been introduced in Polish healthcare system and includes a packet of lab measurements, including cholesterol concentrations, available free of charge to all adults above the age of 40.

Additionally, the current survey also analyzed nitric oxide (NO) and C-reactive protein (CRP). NO is exhaled in human breath and is a marker of airway inflammation [22]. Increased exhaled nitric oxide (NO) is associated with the effects of cytokines and inflammatory mediators in various lung diseases [23]. In asthma, increased FeNO reflects moderately well the inflammatory pathways induced by eosinophils in the central and/or peripheral airways. In COPD, airway/alveolar NO concentrations may be normal, and the role of FeNO monitoring is less clear and therefore less established than in asthma. In addition, concurrent cigarette smoking decreases FeNO [23]. CRP belongs to the pentraxin protein and is often used in clinical practice as a marker of infection and inflammation because its synthesis rapidly and dramatically increases after infection or tissue injury [24]. There is evidence that CRP is not only a marker of inflammation, but also that destabilized isoforms of CRP have pro-inflammatory properties [25]. Data from a cross-sectional study by Meryam Maamar et al. [26] of 121 patients three months after COVID-19 infection showed an association between post-COVID-19 syndrome (PCS) and the upper ranges of neutrophil count, neutrophil/lymphocyte ratio (NLR), fibrinogen, and CRP, suggesting an association between low-grade inflammation (LGI) and PCS [26]. Gul M. et al. [27] compared cardiac and inflammatory markers and echocardiographic parameters between COVID-19 patients (n = 126) and controls (n = 98). The mean follow-up period in the COVID-19 group was 58.39 ± 39.1 days. The value of CRP was significantly higher in the COVID-19 group than the control group. The researchers suggest that although the clinical and prognostic significance of cardiac and other inflammatory markers in the acute phase of COVID-19 is well known, the biomarkers can also be used to observe cardiac damage in the medium term after infection [27]. Results from the current study on CRP are in line with other studies from the COVID-19 pandemic period and indicate an association between the COVID-19 pandemic on elevated CRP in the general population.

Wang W. et al. [28] surveyed a total of 1733 and 1728 students in 2020 and 2019, respectively. The Vision Behavior Questionnaire, including exposure to a digital screen, was used to investigate the association between the eye parameter and eye health behavior. The percentage of respondents with myopia was 55.02% in 2020, which was higher than in 2019 (44.62%). The authors showed that increased exposure to a digital screen contributes to the myopia progression in children and adolescents during the COVID-19 pandemic. The current study also shows similar results. In the population surveyed during the COVID-19 pandemic, a higher percentage of people reported vision deterioration compared to the pre-COVID population.

The current study showed a reduced incidence of reported allergies compared to an increased incidence of reported sinusitis and asthma. In addition, the study showed a significant difference in FeNO concentrations and CRP levels in the studied populations. Increased concentrations were shown in the population during the COVID-19 pandemic which might be associated with a higher prevalence of declared asthma and sinusitis. Further research should be conducted to analyze this phenomenon more deeply.

6. Conclusions

The COVID-19 pandemic had a measurable impact on the general population's prevalence of certain medical conditions and lifestyle habits. Future studies must be pursued to examine the long-term health impact of the pandemic, as well as the effectiveness of targeted interventions to mitigate these effects.

7. Study Limitation

This study has limitations. It is a single-center, cross-sectional study with a limited sample size of residents of a medium-sized city in the eastern part of the country. Nevertheless, the study has the advantage of analyzing the general population before and during the pandemic, carried out according to the same procedures, in the same research center, and by the same trained staff.

Author Contributions: Conceptualization, M.C. (Magdalena Chlabicz), M.C. (Małgorzata Chlabicz) and K.A.K.; Methodology, M.C. (Magdalena Chlabicz) and K.A.K.; Formal Analysis, M.C. (Magdalena Chlabicz) and A.S.-J.; Investigation, M.C. (Magdalena Chlabicz), S.S. and P.S.; Resources, K.A.K.; Data Curation, K.A.K.; Writing—Original Draft Preparation, M.C. (Magdalena Chlabicz), M.C. (Małgorzata Chlabicz) and K.A.K.; Writing—Review and Editing, Ł.K., Ł.M., K.G., P.P.L., A.M.M.-M. and K.A.K.; Visualization, M.C. (Magdalena Chlabicz); Supervision, K.A.K.; Project Administration, K.A.K.; Funding Acquisition, K.A.K. All authors have read and agreed to the published version of the manuscript.

Funding: This research was funded by Medical University of Bialystok, Poland for Bialystok PLUS study (grant number SUB/1/00/19/001/1201), the analysis was supported by the National Science Centre, Poland grant within the program OPUS-19 (grant number 2020/37/B/NZ7/03380).

Institutional Review Board Statement: The study was conducted in accordance with the Declaration of Helsinki. Ethical approval for Bialystok Plus study was provided by the Ethics Committee of the Medical University of Bialystok (Poland) on 31 March 2016 (approval number: R-I-002/108/2016).

Informed Consent Statement: Informed consent was obtained from all subjects involved in the study.

Data Availability Statement: The datasets are not publicly available because the individual privacy of the participants should be protected. Data are however available from the corresponding author on reasonable request.

Conflicts of Interest: The authors declare no conflict of interest.

References

1. Elling, J.M.; Crutzen, R.; Talhout, R.; de Vries, H. Tobacco smoking and smoking cessation in times of COVID-19. *Tob. Prev. Cessat.* **2020**, *6*, 39. [CrossRef] [PubMed]
2. Clerkin, K.J.; Fried, J.A.; Raikhelkar, J.; Sayer, G.; Griffin, J.M.; Masoumi, A.; Jain, S.S.; Burkhoff, D.; Kumaraiah, D.; Rabbani, L.; et al. COVID-19 and Cardiovascular Disease. *Circulation* **2020**, *141*, 1648–1655. [CrossRef] [PubMed]
3. Cevik, M.; Bamford, C.G.G.; Ho, A. COVID-19 pandemic-a focused review for clinicians. *Clin. Microbiol. Infect.* **2020**, *26*, 842–847. [CrossRef] [PubMed]
4. WHO. Coronavirus (COVID-19) Statistics. Available online: https://covid19.who.int/region/euro/country/pl (accessed on 28 December 2022).
5. Postawy Polaków Wobec Palenia Tytoniu—Raport 2019. Available online: https://www.gov.pl/web/gis/postawy-polakow-wobec-palenia-tytoniu{-}{-}raport-2017 (accessed on 3 January 2023).
6. Schuckit, M.A. Alcohol-use disorders. *Lancet* **2009**, *373*, 492–501. [CrossRef] [PubMed]
7. OECD. Data Alcohol Consumption. Available online: https://data.oecd.org/healthrisk/alcohol-consumption.htm (accessed on 3 January 2023).
8. Chlabicz, M.; Jamiolkowski, J.; Laguna, W.; Sowa, P.; Paniczko, M.; Lapinska, M.; Szpakowicz, M.; Drobek, N.; Raczkowski, A.; Kaminski, K.A. A Similar Lifetime CV Risk and a Similar Cardiometabolic Profile in the Moderate and High Cardiovascular Risk Populations: A Population-Based Study. *J. Clin. Med.* **2021**, *10*, 1584. [CrossRef]
9. Chlabicz, M.; Jamiolkowski, J.; Laguna, W.; Dubatowka, M.; Sowa, P.; Lapinska, M.; Szpakowicz, A.; Zieleniewska, N.; Zalewska, M.; Raczkowski, A.; et al. Effectiveness of Lifestyle Modification vs. Therapeutic, Preventative Strategies for Reducing Cardiovascular Risk in Primary Prevention-A Cohort Study. *J. Clin. Med.* **2022**, *11*, 688. [CrossRef]
10. Saunders, J.B.; Aasland, O.G. WHO Collaborative Project on Identification and Treatment of Persons with Harmful Alcohol Consumption. Report on Phase I. In *Development of a Screening Instrument*; WHO: Geneva, Switzerland, 1987.
11. Higgins-Biddle, J.C.; Babor, T.F. A review of the Alcohol Use Disorders Identification Test (AUDIT), AUDIT-C, and USAUDIT for screening in the United States: Past issues and future directions. *Am. J. Drug Alcohol. Abuse* **2018**, *44*, 578–586. [CrossRef]
12. Heatherton, T.F.; Kozlowski, L.T.; Frecker, R.C.; Fagerstrom, K.O. The Fagerstrom Test for Nicotine Dependence: A revision of the Fagerstrom Tolerance Questionnaire. *Br. J. Addict.* **1991**, *86*, 1119–1127. [CrossRef]
13. Diener, E.; Emmons, R.A.; Larsen, R.J.; Griffin, S. The Satisfaction With Life Scale. *J. Pers. Assess.* **1985**, *49*, 71–75. [CrossRef]
14. Le Foll, B.; Piper, M.E.; Fowler, C.D.; Tonstad, S.; Bierut, L.; Lu, L.; Jha, P.; Hall, W.D. Tobacco and nicotine use. *Nat. Rev. Dis. Primers* **2022**, *8*, 19. [CrossRef]
15. Kayhan Tetik, B.; Gedik Tekinemre, I.; Tas, S. The Effect of the COVID-19 Pandemic on Smoking Cessation Success. *J. Community Health* **2021**, *46*, 471–475. [CrossRef] [PubMed]
16. Nyman, A.L.; Spears, C.A.; Churchill, V.; Do, V.V.; Henderson, K.C.; Massey, Z.B.; Reynolds, R.M.; Huang, J. Associations between COVID-19 risk perceptions and smoking and quitting behavior among U.S. adults. *Addict. Behav. Rep.* **2021**, *14*, 100394. [CrossRef] [PubMed]
17. Celik, F.G.N.; Demirel, G. Impact of a Coronavirus Pandemic on Smoking Behavior in University Students: An Online Survey in Turkiye. *Turk. J. Pharm. Sci.* **2022**, *19*, 416–421. [CrossRef] [PubMed]
18. Roberts, A.; Rogers, J.; Mason, R.; Siriwardena, A.N.; Hogue, T.; Whitley, G.A.; Law, G.R. Alcohol and other substance use during the COVID-19 pandemic: A systematic review. *Drug Alcohol. Depend.* **2021**, *229*, 109150. [CrossRef]
19. Killgore, W.D.S.; Cloonan, S.A.; Taylor, E.C.; Lucas, D.A.; Dailey, N.S. Alcohol dependence during COVID-19 lockdowns. *Psychiatry Res.* **2021**, *296*, 113676. [CrossRef]
20. Nalbandian, A.; Sehgal, K.; Gupta, A.; Madhavan, M.V.; McGroder, C.; Stevens, J.S.; Cook, J.R.; Nordvig, A.S.; Shalev, D.; Sehrawat, T.S.; et al. Post-acute COVID-19 syndrome. *Nat. Med.* **2021**, *27*, 601–615. [CrossRef]
21. Choi, H.G.; Kim, S.Y.; Joo, Y.H.; Cho, H.J.; Kim, S.W.; Jeon, Y.J. Incidence of Asthma, Atopic Dermatitis, and Allergic Rhinitis in Korean Adults before and during the COVID-19 Pandemic Using Data from the Korea National Health and Nutrition Examination Survey. *Int. J. Environ. Res. Public. Health* **2022**, *19*, 4274. [CrossRef]
22. Loewenthal, L.; Menzies-Gow, A. FeNO in Asthma. *Semin. Respir. Crit. Care Med.* **2022**, *43*, 635–645. [CrossRef]
23. Barnes, P.J.; Dweik, R.A.; Gelb, A.F.; Gibson, P.G.; George, S.C.; Grasemann, H.; Pavord, I.D.; Ratjen, F.; Silkoff, P.E.; Taylor, D.R.; et al. Exhaled nitric oxide in pulmonary diseases: A comprehensive review. *Chest* **2010**, *138*, 682–692. [CrossRef]
24. Gewurz, H. Biology of C-reactive protein and the acute phase response. *Hosp. Pract.* **1982**, *17*, 67–81. [CrossRef]
25. McFadyen, J.D.; Kiefer, J.; Braig, D.; Loseff-Silver, J.; Potempa, L.A.; Eisenhardt, S.U.; Peter, K. Dissociation of C-Reactive Protein Localizes and Amplifies Inflammation: Evidence for a Direct Biological Role of C-Reactive Protein and Its Conformational Changes. *Front. Immunol.* **2018**, *9*, 1351. [CrossRef] [PubMed]
26. Maamar, M.; Artime, A.; Pariente, E.; Fierro, P.; Ruiz, Y.; Gutierrez, S.; Tobalina, M.; Diaz-Salazar, S.; Ramos, C.; Olmos, J.M.; et al. Post-COVID-19 syndrome, low-grade inflammation and inflammatory markers: A cross-sectional study. *Curr. Med. Res. Opin.* **2022**, *38*, 901–909. [CrossRef] [PubMed]

27. Gul, M.; Ozyilmaz, S.; Bastug Gul, Z.; Kacmaz, C.; Satilmisoglu, M.H. Evaluation of cardiac injury with biomarkers and echocardiography after COVID-19 infection. *J. Physiol. Pharmacol.* **2022**, *73*, 89–95. [CrossRef]
28. Wang, W.; Zhu, L.; Zheng, S.; Ji, Y.; Xiang, Y.; Lv, B.; Xiong, L.; Li, Z.; Yi, S.; Huang, H.; et al. Survey on the Progression of Myopia in Children and Adolescents in Chongqing During COVID-19 Pandemic. *Front. Public Health* **2021**, *9*, 646770. [CrossRef] [PubMed]

Disclaimer/Publisher's Note: The statements, opinions and data contained in all publications are solely those of the individual author(s) and contributor(s) and not of MDPI and/or the editor(s). MDPI and/or the editor(s) disclaim responsibility for any injury to people or property resulting from any ideas, methods, instructions or products referred to in the content.

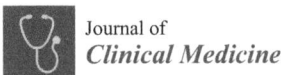

Article

Reduced Reliability of Procalcitonin (PCT) as a Biomarker of Bacterial Superinfection: Concerns about PCT-Driven Antibiotic Stewardship in Critically Ill COVID-19 Patients—Results from a Retrospective Observational Study in Intensive Care Units

Giancarlo Ceccarelli [1,2,†], Francesco Alessandri [1,2,3,*,†], Giuseppe Migliara [1,2], Valentina Baccolini [1,2], Giovanni Giordano [1,2,3], Gioacchino Galardo [1], Carolina Marzuillo [2], Corrado De Vito [2], Alessandro Russo [4], Massimo Ciccozzi [5], Paolo Villari [2], Mario Venditti [1,2], Claudio M. Mastroianni [1,2], Francesco Pugliese [1,2,3] and Gabriella d'Ettorre [1,2]

1 Hospital Policlinico Umberto I, 00161 Rome, Italy; giancarlo.ceccarelli@uniroma1.it (G.C.); giordano.gj@gmail.com (G.G.); giuseppe.migliara@uniroma1.it (G.M.); valentina.baccolini@uniroma1.it (V.B.); gioacchino.galardo@gmail.com (G.G.); mario.venditti@uniroma1.it (M.V.); claudio.mastroianni@uniroma1.it (C.M.M.); f.pugliese@uniroma1.it (F.P.); gabriella.dettorre@uniroma1.it (G.d.)
2 Department of Public Health and Infectious Diseases, University of Rome Sapienza, 00185 Rome, Italy; carolina.marzuillo@uniroma1.it (C.M.); paolo.villari@uniroma1.it (P.V.)
3 Intensive Care Unit, Department of General, Specialistic Surgery, University of Rome Sapienza, 00185 Rome, Italy
4 Infectious and Tropical Disease Unit, Department of Medical and Surgical Sciences, 'Magna Graecia' University of Catanzaro, 88100 Catanzaro, Italy; a.russo@unicz.it
5 Unit of Medical Statistics and Molecular Epidemiology, University Campus Bio-Medico of Rome, 00128 Rome, Italy; massimo.ciccozzi@unicampus.it
* Correspondence: francesco.alessandri@uniroma1.it
† These authors contributed equally to this work.

Abstract: Background: The aim of this study was to assess whether procalcitonin levels is a diagnostic tool capable of accurately identifying sepsis and ventilator-associated pneumonia (VAP) even in critically ill COVID-19 patients. Methods: In this retrospective, observational study, all critically ill COVID-19 patients who survived for ≥2 days in a single university hospital and had at least one serum procalcitonin (PCT) value and associated blood culture and/or culture from a lower respiratory tract specimen available were eligible for the study. Results: Over the research period, 184 patients were recruited; 67 VAP/BSI occurred, with an incidence rate of 21.82 episodes of VAP/BSI (95% CI: 17.18–27.73) per 1000 patient-days among patients who were included. At the time of a positive microbiological culture, an average PCT level of 1.25–3.2 ng/mL was found. Moreover, also in subjects without positive cultures, PCT was altered in 21.7% of determinations, with an average value of 1.04–5.5 ng/mL. Both PCT and PCT-72 h were not linked to a diagnosis of VAP/BSI in COVID-19 patients, according to the multivariable GEE models (aOR 1.13, 95% CI 0.51–2.52 for PCT; aOR 1.32, 95% CI 0.66–2.64 for PCT-72 h). Conclusion: Elevated PCT levels might not always indicate bacterial superinfections or coinfections in a severe COVID-19 setting.

Keywords: procalcitonin; PCT; biomarker; SARS-CoV-2; COVID-19; ICU; intensive care unit; critically ill

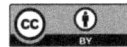

1. Introduction

The management of superinfections was one of the key issues in Intensive Care Units (ICUs) throughout the pandemic. In particular, bacterial secondary infections have been reported to have a variable incidence depending on the local epidemiology and clinical setting, and to severely affect morbidity and mortality in critically ill COVID-19 patients [1–4]. The challenge for clinicians was to identify superinfections early, quickly, and correctly due to the possible syndromic overlap between bacterial and SARS-CoV-2-related sepsis. In this sense, monitoring procalcitonin (PCT) levels has been widely adopted in clinical practice even during COVID-19, considering that, in the pre-pandemic era, it represented a reliable laboratory tool in diagnosing and managing bacterial infections, as well as guiding antibiotic therapy [5,6]. In fact, PCT is a peptide precursor of the hormone calcitonin, which is primarily produced by the C-cells of the thyroid gland. Its blood levels selectively increase in response to systemic bacterial infections in COVID-19-negative patients, and, for this reason, is used as a biomarker for differentiating between bacterial and viral infections, as viral infections typically do not lead to significant increases in procalcitonin levels [6]. In fact, its utilization relies on two fundamental assumptions: first, that viruses indirectly inhibit PCT production by inducing inhibitory interferons, primarily interferon-γ (IFN-γ) [7–11], and, second, that bacteria directly stimulate the expression of PCT through lipopolysaccharide and indirectly via the induction of proinflammatory cytokines such as interleukin-1β (IL-1β), IL-6, and tumor necrosis factor α (TNF-α) [12–15]. Moreover, PCT can also assist clinicians in determining the severity of the infection and monitoring the response to treatment [6]. In the clinical practice, the use of PCT was approved by the Food and Drug Administration (FDA) to guide antibiotic treatment in sepsis and lower respiratory tract infections for SARS-CoV-2-uninfected patients [16]. Moreover, PCT-guided antibiotic stewardship has been shown to be useful in optimizing antibiotic prescription with an improvement in clinical outcomes, a reduction in potential side-effects, and better control over the emergence of antibiotic resistance [5]. The sudden appearance of the SARS-CoV-2 pandemic at the end of 2019 put health services under great pressure, requiring maximum clinical effort in the absence of sufficient scientific evidence for the effective management of patients with COVID-19. Especially in the early pandemic phases, patient management was based on the use of already existing diagnostic, clinical monitoring, and therapeutic approaches brought about by settings different from that of SARS-CoV-2 infection. The validation of such approaches in the COVID-19 setting necessarily took place on the pandemic battlefield, as there was no time for validation in clinical studies.

The purpose of this study was to evaluate whether procalcitonin levels could be a diagnostic tool capable of correctly marking sepsis and ventilator-associated pneumonia (VAP) even in the setting of critically ill COVID-19 patients.

2. Materials and Methods

2.1. Design of the Study, Population, Settings, Data Collection, and Outcomes

This study is a "real-life" retrospective, observational study conducted on data from the healthcare-associated infection (HAI) surveillance system active in the ICUs of the Umberto I University Hospital of Rome (Italy). The study design was based on matching the available PCT values to blood culture and cultures *of* bronchoalveolar lavage (BAL) collected at the same time in critically ill COVID-19 patients, to evaluate whether PCT values increased due to synchronous clinically significant bacteremia and/or VAP, as expected in no-COVID-19 setting (Figure 1). All critically ill COVID-19 patients who recovered for more than 2 days in the 2 ICUs of the Umberto I University Hospital of Rome (Italy) from March 2020 to February 2021 with at least one serum PCT value and related blood culture/BAL culture available were eligible for the analysis.

The sources for patient data were medical records stored in the electronic information system of the ICU involved. The variables considered included: past clinical history (co-morbidities), current clinical history, treatment, ventilation parameters, and laboratory and microbiological data. The study's primary endpoint was to evaluate positive and negative predictive values (PPV and NPV) of PCT test in identifying an underlying VAP/BSI on the same date of the test. The secondary endpoint was the same evaluations using a model that takes into consideration a 72 h window (i.e., considering as positive the PCT test in the 24 h preceding or following a positive PCT test) (Figure 1).

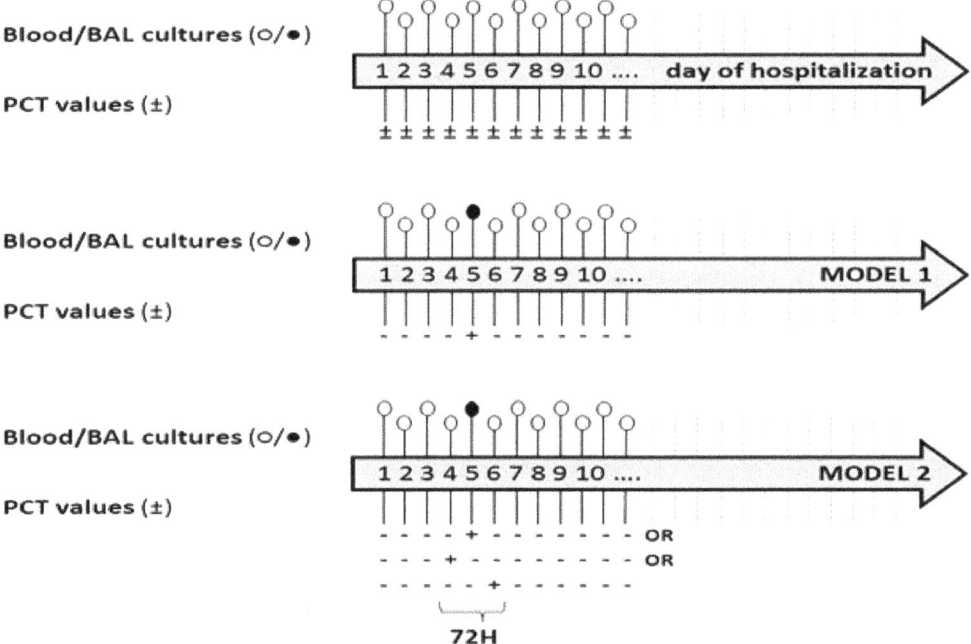

Figure 1. Design of the study and models of analysis. Legend—PCT: (+) positive, (−) negative. Blood cultures: ○ normal value, ● pathological value.

2.2. Diagnosis of SARS-CoV-2 Infection and COVID-19-Related Pneumonia, and COVID-19 Treatments

The diagnosis of SARS-CoV-2 infection was defined as at least one positive oronasopharyngeal swab or bronchoalveolar liquid for SARS-CoV-2 E and S gene by a RT-PCR. Stratification of SARS-CoV-2 infection severity was based on World Health Organization (WHO) criteria [17]. COVID-19-related pneumonia was diagnosed by high-resolution CT/non-contrast enhanced chest CT. The patients were treated with ad interim routinely used therapy as suggested by the provisional guidelines of the Italian Society of Infectious and Tropical Diseases (SIMIT) and the Italian Medicine Agency (AIFA) [18]. All patients included in the study were supported by oxygen therapy delivered via invasive mechanical ventilation.

2.3. Clinical Evaluation, PCT Dosage, and Microbiological Analysis

Multiparametric monitoring and clinical evaluations of critically ill patients were carried out continuously: subjects who developed clinical signs suggestive of sepsis or persistent fevers, or deteriorated clinically, without other plausible explanations, were also subjected to microbiological examination and PCT dosage, as part of an overall evaluation for the differential diagnosis.

Quantitative analysis of serum PCT was performed routinely at least every 72 h, and every 24 h in case of suspected superinfection, using BRAHMSTM PCT sensitive KRYPTOR® immunoassay (ThermoFisher, Hennigsdorf, Germany). Plasma levels of >0.5 ng/mL were interpreted as abnormal and suggested a possible bacterial superinfection. The half-lifetime of PCT was considered to be 22.3–28.9 h (25–50 percentiles) with no significant difference due to gender, age, and renal dysfunction [6,19].

Three sets of blood cultures (fill volume 10 mL/bottle) and a semiquantitative culture from a lower respiratory tract specimen (such as distal protected aspirate) were drawn at admission from every critical COVID-19 patient transferred to the ICU from the isolation ward. Blood and respiratory tract specimen were also retaken for cultures if the patient developed clinical signs of sepsis, had persistent fever, or deteriorated clinically, without other plausible explanations.

Bacterial identification was performed by a matrix-assisted laser desorption/ionization time-of-flight mass spectrometry (MALDI-TOF MS) system (Bruker Daltonik GmbH, Bremen, Germany).

The guidelines of the European Committee on Antimicrobial Susceptibility Testing (EUCAST) were used for the interpretations of isolate susceptibility. [20]

2.4. Definition

VAP was defined according to the criteria proposed by the European Center for Disease Control [21]. Sepsis was defined according to SEPSIS-3 criteria and ARDS was identified according to the 2012 Berlin criteria [22,23]. Single cultures positive for coagulase-negative staphylococci were only considered as environmental contaminations and, therefore, considered as negative in terms of infectious events (BSI).

2.5. Statistical Analysis

Descriptive statistics were calculated using median and interquartile range (IQR) for non-normal continuous variables and frequencies and proportions for dichotomous and categorical variables. Normality of continuous variables was checked through the Shapiro–Wilk test. To avoid any potential increase of PCT values that could occur during a confirmed VAP/BSI, the seven days following a VAP/BSI diagnosis were excluded from the analysis. At first, PCT values were considered positive for values greater than 0.5 ng/mL. Then, to take into account the repeated PCT measurements for each patient, a multivariable generalized estimating equation (GEE) regression model with a logit link, a binomial error structure, and exchangeable correlation structure (Model 1) was built to explore the association of the exposure of interest (PCT positivity) to the outcome of interest (positive blood culture) through the estimation of its adjusted odds ratio (aOR) and the associated 95% confidence intervals (CI). Variables were included in the model based on expert opinion. The final model included the following variables: sex (dichotomous); age (continuous); comorbidity (dichotomous); and Simplified Acute Physiology Score (SAPS) II (continuous). To also account for possible delays between the PCT blood peak and the blood culture positivity, a second statistical model (Model 2) was built considering as positive the PCT test in the 24 h preceding and following the identification of the PCT positivity (PCT-72 h) (Figure 1). Sensitivity and specificity of PCT and PCT-72 h test in predicting an underlying VAP/BSI were calculated using the GEE regression method for clustered data [24]. In addition, we also estimated adjusted sensitivities and specificities for PCT and PCT-72 h, accounting for the imperfect accuracy of hemoculture to detect micro-organisms in the blood during sepsis as the gold standard [24–26]. Given that this adjustment method is unable to account for repeated measures, the adjustment was performed on the standard sensitivity and specificity of PCT, calculated without any further adjustment as a way to study the effect of the imperfect accuracy of the gold standard.

Positive and negative predicted values were calculated using Bayes Theorem, considering the period prevalence of VAP/BSI that registered in our study sample (i.e., 36.41%).

Lastly, as a sensibility analysis, PPVs and NPVs were estimated for increasing PCT and PCT-72 h cut-off values, using an interval of 0.1 ng/mL from 0.1 to 15.0 ng/mL.

All statistical analyses were performed using Stata (StataCorp LLC, 4905 Lakeway Drive, College Station, TX, USA) version 17.0. A two-sided p-value < 0.05 was considered statistically significant.

2.6. Ethics Committee Approval

The Ethics Committee of Policlinico Umberto I approved the study with number 109/2020. This study follows the relevant EQUATOR network reporting guidelines and STROBE reporting guidelines for observational studies.

3. Results

Demographic and clinical characteristics of the patients enrolled were reported in Table 1.

Table 1. Characteristics of the COVID-19 patients who recovered in the ICU from March 2020 to February 2021.

		COVID-19 Patients n (%)
Patients		184
Gender		
	Female	48 (26.1)
	Male	136 (73.9)
Age, years		
	Median (IQR)	66 (55.5, 73)
SAPS II ($n = 162$)		
	Median (IQR)	35 (27, 43)
Comorbidities (yes)		146 (79.4)
	Diabetes mellitus (yes)	40 (21.7)
	Obesity (yes)	22 (12.0)
	Hypertension (yes)	86 (46.7)
	Cardiopathy (yes)	35 (19.0)
	Renal failure (yes)	12 (6.5)
	COPD (yes)	26 (14.1)
	Hepatopathy (yes)	4 (2.2)
	Neurological disorders (yes)	28 (15.2)
	Other disorders (yes)	63 (34.3)
Outcome		
	Discharge	115 (62.5)
	Death	69 (37.5)

SAPS: Simplified Acute Physiology Score.

In the study period, 67 instances of VAP/BSI occurred, and an incidence rate of 21.82 episodes of VAP/BSI (95% CI: 17.18–27.73) per 1000 patient-days was observed among patients enrolled. The most frequently isolated strain was *Acinetobacter baumannii* (55.2%), followed by *Klebsiella pneumoniae* (20.9%), Enterococci (13.4%), *Staphylococcus aureus* (9.0%), Enterobacteriaceae other than *K.pneumoniae* (7.5%), and other micro-organisms (4.5%).

Overall, 2044 determinations of PCT were collected over 3070 cumulative days of hospitalization (66.6%): pathological values were reported in 21.7% of cases. In particular, a median of 9 PCT determinations (IQR 5–15) and a median time of 13 days of follow-up (IQR 8–22) was available for each patient enrolled. The average PCT level reported at the moment of a positive culture was 1.25 ± 3.4 ng/mL. On the other hand, PCT was found to be altered in 21.7% of the determinations in subjects without positive cultures, with an average value of 1.04 ± 5.5 ng/mL. Finally, 19 of the 67 VAP/BSI (28.4%) occurred without a PCT evaluation, 15 of which were not even in the previous and following 24 h.

3.1. Predictors of VAP/BSI

The multivariable GEE models showed that neither PCT nor PCT-72 h were associated with a diagnosis of VAP/BSI in COVID-19 patients (aOR 1.13, 95% CI 0.51–2.52 for PCT; aOR 1.32, 95% CI 0.66–2.64 for PCT-72 h) (Table 2). No other factor showed any association with the outcome.

Table 2. Multivariable models predicting VAP/BSI in COVID-19 patients hospitalized in the intensive care unit from March 2020 to February 2021.

	Model 1 [a] (n = 162, Observations = 1702)			Model 2 [b] (n = 162, Observations = 1810)		
	aOR	95% CI	p-Value	aOR	95% CI	p-Value
Positive PCT (yes)	1.13	0.51–2.52	0.764	--	--	--
Positive PCT-72 h (yes)	--	--	--	1.32	0.66–2.64	0.427
Age in years	1.02	1.00–1.05	0.099	1.02	1.00–1.05	0.099
Gender (male)	1.00	0.57–1.05	0.993	0.98	0.58–1.67	0.939
SAPS II	0.98	0.95–1.01	0.202	0.98	0.95–1.01	0.129
Comorbidity (yes)	1.13	0.55–2.39	0.623	1.25	0.62–2.51	0.536

[a] Multivariable generalized estimating equation regression model (logit link, binomial error structure, exchangeable correlation structure) [b] Multivariable generalized estimating equation regression model (logit link, binomial error structure, exchangeable correlation structure) considering the PCT as positive 24 h before and after the PCR positive test. aOR: adjusted odds ratio; CI: confidence interval; PCT: procalcitonin; SAPS: Simplified Acute Physiology Score.

3.2. Diagnostic Accuracy of PCT and PCT-72 h

The estimation of the accuracy of PCT in discriminating positive cultures had a sensibility of 19.2% (95% CI: 10.1–33.3%) and a specificity of 81.6% (95% CI: 76.4–85.9%). Using the less stringent PCT-72 h as a marker for positive cultures, the sensibility increased to 30.8% (95% CI: 19.7–44.7%), while the specificity remained high (77.0%; 95% CI: 71.3–82.0%). Accordingly, PPVs and NPVs increased from 37.4% (95% CI: 25.9–51.8%) to 43.5% (95% CI: 33.3–54.2%) and from 63.8% (60.5–67.0%) to 66.0% (95% CI: 61.7–70.2%), respectively.

Given the high sensibility of hemocultures in triplicates (97%) and their virtually perfect specificity [20], the adjusted sensitivity and specificity remained virtually identical to the unadjusted ones for both PCT (18.7% and 79.0%, respectively; PPV: 33.9%; PNV: 62.9%) and PCT-72 h (35.7% and 69.3%, respectively; PPV: 30.7%; PNV: 70.2%).

3.3. Sensitivity Analysis

Supplementary Table S1 shows the diagnostic accuracy of PCT and PCT-72 h values in predicting an underlying VAP/BSI, considering different cut-off values. For PCT, the highest sensibility was reached for a cut-off value of 0.10 ng/mL (82.5%; 95% CI: 69.5–90.7%), whereas the highest specificity was reached using a cut-off value of 13.90 ng/mL (98.9%; 95% CI: 97.5–99.5); for PCT-72 h, the maximum sensitivity was 86.2% (95% CI: 69.5–90.7; cut-off value: 0.10 ng/mL) and the maximum specificity was 98.0% (95% CI: 95.8–99.1; cut-off value: 15.60 ng/mL).

Lastly, the highest PPVs were reached using cut-off values of PCT (67.9%, 95% CI: 34.0–89.7) and PCT-72 h (58.8%, 95% CI: 31.5–81.6) of 13.90 ng/mL and 10.40 ng/mL, respectively, while the highest NPVs values were obtained for cut-off values of PCT (66.6%; 95% CI: 60.8–71.9) and PCT-72 h (69.4%; 95% CI: 58.1–78.8) of 0.30 ng/mL and 0.20 ng/mL, respectively.

4. Discussion

Bacterial superinfections, including VAP and BSI, are a dangerous complication in COVID-19 patients admitted to the ICU [1–4,27–30]. The prompt recognition and appropriate treatment of superinfections are crucial in managing these cases effectively. The diagnosis of superinfections in COVID-19 patients typically involves clinical evaluation, microbiological tests, and imaging studies. In this context, a biomarker such as PCT, a widely used clinical practice to rapidly detect severe bacterial infections in the period before the pandemic, was thought to play a key role in early diagnosis and the modulation of antibiotic therapy even in the superinfected COVID-19 patients [5–16,31].

In any case, the SARS-CoV-2 pandemic was a severe test for many of the diagnostic resources designed for contexts other than COVID-19: our results showed that abnormal procalcitonin levels in critically ill COVID-19 patients do not necessarily indicate the presence of a bacterial coinfection or superinfection. In particular, the adjusted sensitivity and specificity for the PCT test in COVID-19 patients were 18.7% and 79.0%, respectively; the PPV was 33.9% and PNV 62.9%. Similarly, also, PCT-72 h model analysis confirmed the limits of PCT as a biomarker of superinfection in SARS-CoV-2-infected patients (35.7% and 69.3%, respectively; PPV: 30.7%; PNV: 70.2%).

Similarly to our experience, a recent review and meta-analysis on the topic that encompassed five large studies involving a total of 2775 patients has shown that the predictive ability of PCT for the diagnosis of coinfections in COVID-19 patients was limited, with an AUC of 0.72, sensitivity of 0.60, and specificity of 0.71 [32]. Additionally, three of the included studies indicated that PCT was an effective tool for ruling out bacterial coinfections, boasting a negative predictive value of over 93% when its concentration was below 0.50 μg/L [33–35].

As previously reported, PCT blood levels selectively increase in response to systemic bacterial infections in COVID-19-negative patients and, for this reason, is used as a biomarker for differentiating between bacterial and viral infections. Recently, however, concerns about the appropriateness of PCT in the management of SARS-CoV-2-infected patients arose. In fact, several studies observed that elevated PCT levels may not reflect bacterial coinfections or superinfections in a severe COVID-19 setting [36–38]. In this case, the increase of PCT levels, even in the absence of bacterial coinfection, has been hypothesized to be a part of the human immunological response to SARS-CoV-2 infection [39,40]. In particular, a biological model has been proposed in which the increase in PCT production could be related to SARS-CoV-2 ORF6 and NSP1. These SARS-CoV-2 proteins inhibit host STAT1 phosphorylation and increase STAT3-dependent transcriptional pathways. The resulting increase of STAT3 signaling enhances an unexpected PCT production in monocytes in COVID-19 infection not linked to concomitant bacteremia [39].

This hypothesis was indirectly corroborated by a cohort study conducted in the pre-pandemic period: the authors reported that PCT levels increased during pure non-COVID viral infections in correlation with the severity of the disease, and severe respiratory viral infection induces a PCT increase also in the absence of concomitant bacterial pneumonia [11]. Moreover, they demonstrated that PCT synthesis was not suppressed by interferon signaling; PCT concentration was elevated despite bacteriologic sterility and its levels correlated with markers of disease severity in murine and cellular models of influenza infection [11].

In the clinical practice, these pieces of evidence were recently confirmed in a retrospective study involving hospitalized patients with severe COVID-19 and designed to evaluate the effectiveness of PCT in diagnosing respiratory superinfection. The results indicated that PCT levels measured at the time of lower respiratory culture were not able to distinguish patients with a bacterial infection and its diagnostic accuracy was not influenced by factors such as the timing of the procalcitonin measurement, exposure to antibiotics, or treatment with immunomodulatory agents [41].

Our research diverges from several previous reports supporting the utility of PCT and does not endorse the extensive use of this biomarker in the setting of critically ill COVID-19 patients for the management of bacterial superinfections [42–44]. The multivariable GEE models conducted on the cohort confirmed that neither PCT nor PCT-72 h were associated with a diagnosis of VAP/BSI.

However, the results obtained from our study may be of support in identifying new PCT operating values that can more precisely support the clinical diagnosis of superinfection even in the setting of critically ill COVID-19 patients. In fact, we observed that the diagnostic accuracy of PCT in predicting an underlying VAP/BSI in COVID-19 was recovered when considering different cut-off values. In particular, the highest sensibility was reached for a cut-off value of 0.10 ng/mL whereas the highest specificity was reached using a cut-off value of 13.90 ng/mL; similarly, for PCT-72 h, the maximum sensitivity available was 86.2% with a cut-off value of 0.10 ng/mL, and the maximum specificity was 98.0% for a cut-off value of 15.60 ng/mL. These new cut-offs should be kept in mind by clinicians when redesigning the risk management of superinfections and for developing new antibiotic stewardship strategies in the context of COVID-19.

Unlike many other studies on the topic, the main strength of the study is that it is based on a homogeneous cohort for clinical severity: the feature significantly reduces the risk of bias, minimizing the effect of this potential confounder. Notwithstanding this, the study has several limitations. First of all, the retrospective nature of the data could reduce the quality of the results and restrict their interpretation. Secondarily, the study was restricted to critically ill patients managed in ICUs and supported with mechanical ventilation. Moreover, the design of the study evaluates the PCT in relation to chronologically synchronous superinfections marked by the simultaneous microbiological isolation of the causal bacterial pathogen in blood or in BAL cultures. Consequently, the results obtained can be related to the diagnostic accuracy of microbiological cultures. For this reason, we performed an adjusted analysis. Moreover, we underline that the limitation of poor blood culture sensitivity could also be overcome by increasing the number of blood culture sets taken, ensuring a blood culture sensitivity of at least 95%. [25] Another important aspect to consider is that our study was conducted in the early stages of the pandemic, before the emergence of the Omicron variant and the availability of vaccines, both of which have led to a change in the severity of the disease towards milder cases. Finally, in this study, we evaluated PCT as a "static" value; in any case, it is used also as a "dynamic" marker and its variation could possibly better describe a bacterial superinfection.

5. Conclusions

The validation of diagnostic tools in contexts other than those in which they were previously tested and approved is one of the most significant concerns in clinical practice. Monitoring procalcitonin levels could help healthcare providers to assess the likelihood of a bacterial infection and guide decisions regarding the use of antibiotics in the pre-pandemic period, but it can mislead clinicians in the setting of severe COVID-19. It is worth noting that procalcitonin levels alone can be not sufficient for use in differentiating between viral SARS-CoV-2 infection and bacterial infections. Additional clinical evaluations, including other laboratory tests and imaging studies, are required in order to make an accurate diagnosis of superinfection in critically ill COVID-19 patients.

Supplementary Materials: The following supporting information can be downloaded at: https://www.mdpi.com/article/10.3390/jcm12196171/s1, Table S1: The diagnostic accuracy of PCT and PCT-72 h values in predicting an underlying VAP/BSI, considering different cut-off values.

Author Contributions: Conceptualization, G.C. and F.A.; methodology, G.C., F.A. and M.C.; software, G.M. and V.B.; formal analysis, G.M. and V.B.; investigation, G.G. (Giovanni Giordano), G.G. (Gioacchino Galardo), and C.M.; resources, F.P. and G.d.; data curation, G.G. (Giovanni Giordano), G.G. (Gioacchino Galardo), A.R. and C.M.; writing—original draft preparation, G.C.; writing—review and editing, G.C., F.A. and G.d.; visualization, C.D.V., P.V., M.V., C.M.M. and F.P.; supervision, C.D.V., P.V., M.V., M.C., A.R., C.M.M., F.P. and G.d.; project administration, G.C., F.A. and G.d. All authors have read and agreed to the published version of the manuscript.

Funding: This research was supported by EU funding within the MUR PNRR Extended Partnership initiative on Emerging Infectious Diseases (Project no. PE00000007, INF-ACT).

Institutional Review Board Statement: The Ethics Committee of Policlinico Umberto I approved the study with number 109/2020. Ethical approval for this study was in accordance with the ethical standards in the 1964 Declaration of Helsinki and US Health Insurance Portability and Accountability Act (HIPAA), and, furthermore, informed consent was obtained from participants.

Informed Consent Statement: Informed consent was obtained from all subjects involved in the study.

Acknowledgments: The authors want to thank all those who, at any level, made this project possible.

Conflicts of Interest: The authors declare no conflict of interest.

References

1. Falcone, M.; Suardi, L.R.; Tiseo, G.; Galfo, V.; Occhineri, S.; Verdenelli, S.; Ceccarelli, G.; Poli, M.; Merli, M.; Bavaro, D.; et al. Superinfections caused by carbapenem-resistant Enterobacterales in hospitalized patients with COVID-19, a multicentre observational study from Italy (CREVID Study). *JAC Antimicrob. Resist.* **2022**, *4*, dlac064. [CrossRef] [PubMed]
2. Polly, M.; de Almeida, B.L.; Lennon, R.P.; Cortês, M.F.; Costa, S.F.; Guimarães, T. Impact of the COVID-19 pandemic on the incidence of multidrug-resistant bacterial infections in an acute care hospital in Brazil. *Am. J. Infect. Control* **2022**, *50*, 32–38. [CrossRef] [PubMed]
3. Grasselli, G.; Scaravilli, V.; Mangioni, D.; Scudeller, L.; Alagna, L.; Bartoletti, M.; Bellani, G.; Biagioni, E.; Bonfanti, P.; Bottino, N.; et al. Hospital-Acquired Infections in Critically Ill Patients with COVID-19. *Chest* **2021**, *160*, 454–465. [CrossRef] [PubMed]
4. Alshrefy, A.J.; Alwohaibi, R.N.; Alhazzaa, S.A.; Almaimoni, R.A.; AlMusailet, L.I.; Al Qahtani, S.Y.; Alshahrani, M.S. Incidence of Bacterial and Fungal Secondary Infections in COVID-19 Patients Admitted to the ICU. *Int. J. Gen. Med.* **2022**, *15*, 7475–7485. [CrossRef] [PubMed]
5. Schuetz, P.; Beishuizen, A.; Broyles, M.; Ferrer, R.; Gavazzi, G.; Gluck, E.H.; González Del Castillo, J.; Jensen, J.U.; Kanizsai, P.L.; Kwa, A.L.H.; et al. Procalcitonin (PCT)-guided antibiotic stewardship: An international experts consensus on optimized clinical use. *Clin. Chem. Lab. Med.* **2019**, *57*, 1308–1318. [CrossRef]
6. Meisner, M. Update on procalcitonin measurements. *Ann. Lab. Med.* **2014**, *34*, 263–273. [CrossRef]
7. Linscheid, P.; Seboek, D.; Nylen, E.S.; Langer, I.; Schlatter, M.; Becker, K.L.; Keller, U.; Müller, B. In vitro and in vivo calcitonin I gene expression in parenchymal cells: A novel product of human adipose tissue. *Endocrinology* **2003**, *144*, 5578–5584. [CrossRef] [PubMed]
8. Linscheid, P.; Seboek, D.; Zulewski, H.; Keller, U.; Müller, B. Autocrine/paracrine role of inflammation mediated calcitonin gene-related peptide and adrenomedullin expression in human adipose tissue. *Endocrinology* **2005**, *146*, 2699–2708. [CrossRef] [PubMed]
9. Gilbert, D.N. Role of procalcitonin in the management of infected patients in the intensive care unit. *Infect. Dis. Clin. N. Am.* **2017**, *31*, 435–453. [CrossRef]
10. Bergin, S.P.; Tsalik, E.L. Procalcitonin: The right answer but to which question? *Clin. Infect. Dis.* **2017**, *65*, 191–193. [CrossRef]
11. Gautam, S.; Cohen, A.J.; Stahl, Y.; Valda Toro, P.; Young, G.M.; Datta, R.; Yan, X.; Ristic, N.T.; Bermejo, S.D.; Sharma, L.; et al. Severe respiratory viral infection induces procalcitonin in the absence of bacterial pneumonia. *Thorax* **2020**, *75*, 974–981. [CrossRef]
12. Linscheid, P.; Seboek, D.; Schaer, D.J.; Zulewski, H.; Keller, U.; Müller, B. Expression and secretion of procalcitonin and calcitonin gene-related peptide by adherent monocytes and by macrophage-activated adipocytes. *Crit. Care Med.* **2004**, *32*, 1715–1721. [CrossRef]
13. Whang, K.T.; Vath, S.D.; Becker, K.L.; Snider, R.H.; Nylen, E.S.; Muller, B.; Li, Q.; Tamarkin, L.; White, J.C. Procalcitonin and proinflammatory cytokine in interactions in sepsis. *Shock* **2000**, *14*, 73–78. [CrossRef]
14. Nijsten, M.W.; Olinga, P.; The, T.H.; de Vries, E.G.; Koops, H.S.; Groothuis, G.M.; Limburg, P.C.; ten Duis, H.J.; Moshage, H.; Hoekstra, H.J.; et al. Procalcitonin behaves as a fast responding acute phase protein in vivo and in vitro. *Crit. Care Med.* **2000**, *28*, 458–461. [CrossRef] [PubMed]
15. Preas, H.L., 2nd; Nylen, E.S.; Snider, R.H.; Becker, K.L.; White, J.C.; Agosti, J.M.; Suffredini, A.F. Effects of anti-inflammatory agents on serum levels of calcitonin precursors during human experimental endotoxemia. *J. Infect. Dis.* **2001**, *184*, 373–376. [CrossRef] [PubMed]
16. Kim, J.H. Clinical Utility of Procalcitonin on Antibiotic Stewardship: A Narrative Review. *Infect. Chemother.* **2022**, *54*, 610–620. [CrossRef] [PubMed]
17. World Health Organization. Clinical Management of COVID-19, Interim Guidance. *World Health Organization 2020*. Available online: https://apps.who.int/iris/handle/10665/332196 (accessed on 27 December 2022).
18. Mussini, C.; Falcone, M.; Nozza, S.; Sagnelli, C.; Parrella, R.; Meschiari, M.; Petrosillo, N.; Mastroianni, C.; Cascio, A.; Iaria, C.; et al. Italian Society of Infectious and Tropical Diseases. Therapeutic strategies for severe COVID-19, A position paper from the Italian Society of Infectious and Tropical Diseases (SIMIT). *Clin. Microbiol. Infect.* **2021**, *27*, 389–395. [CrossRef]
19. Meisner, M.; Schmidt, J.; Hüttner, H.; Tschaikowsky, K. The natural elimination rate of procalcitonin in patients with normal and impaired renal function. *Intensive Care Med.* **2000**, *26* (Suppl. 2), S212–S216. [CrossRef]
20. Eucast: EUCAST. Available online: https://www.eucast.org (accessed on 24 December 2022).
21. Plachouras, D.; Lepape, A.; Suetens, C. ECDC definitions and methods for the surveillance of healthcare-associated infections in intensive care units. *Intensive Care Med.* **2018**, *44*, 2216–2218. [CrossRef]
22. Singer, M.; Deutschman, C.S.; Seymour, C.W.; Shankar-Hari, M.; Annane, D.; Bauer, M.; Bellomo, R.; Bernard, G.R.; Chiche, J.D.; Coopersmith, C.M. The Third International Consensus Definitions for Sepsis and Septic Shock (Sepsis-3). *JAMA* **2016**, *315*, 801–810. [CrossRef] [PubMed]
23. ARDS Definition Task Force; Ranieri, V.M.; Rubenfeld, G.D.; Thompson, B.T.; Ferguson, N.D.; Caldwell, E.; Fan, E.; Camporota, L.; Slutsky, A.S. Acute respiratory distress syndrome: The Berlin Definition. *JAMA* **2012**, *307*, 2526–2533. [CrossRef]
24. Staquet, M.; Rozencweig, M.; Lee, Y.J.; Muggia, F.M. Methodology for the assessment of new dichotomous diagnostic tests. *J. Chronic Dis.* **1981**, *34*, 599–610. [CrossRef] [PubMed]

25. Laupland, K.B.; Church, D.L. Population-based epidemiology and microbiology of community-onset bloodstream infections. *Clin. Microbiol. Rev.* **2014**, *27*, 647–664. [CrossRef]
26. Genders, T.S.; Spronk, S.; Stijnen, T.; Steyerberg, E.W.; Lesaffre, E.; Hunink, M.G. Methods for calculating sensitivity and specificity of clustered data: A tutorial. *Radiology* **2012**, *265*, 910–916. [CrossRef] [PubMed]
27. Omoush, S.A.; Alzyoud, J.A.M. The Prevalence and Impact of Coinfection and Superinfection on the Severity and Outcome of COVID-19 Infection: An Updated Literature Review. *Pathogens* **2022**, *11*, 445. [CrossRef] [PubMed]
28. De Marignan, D.; Vacheron, C.H.; Ader, F.; Lecocq, M.; Richard, J.C.; Frobert, E.; Casalegno, J.S.; Couray-Targe, S.; Argaud, L.; Rimmele, T.; et al. A retrospective comparison of COVID-19 and seasonal influenza mortality and outcomes in the ICUs of a French university hospital. *Eur. J. Anaesthesiol.* **2022**, *39*, 427–435. [CrossRef]
29. Giacobbe, D.R.; Battaglini, D.; Ball, L.; Brunetti, I.; Bruzzone, B.; Codda, G.; Crea, F.; De Maria, A.; Dentone, C.; Di Biagio, A.; et al. Bloodstream infections in critically ill patients with COVID-19. *Eur. J. Clin. Invest.* **2020**, *50*, e13319. [CrossRef] [PubMed]
30. Alessandri, F.; Ceccarelli, G.; Migliara, G.; Baccolini, V.; Russo, A.; Marzuillo, C.; Ceparano, M.; Giordano, G.; Tozzi, P.; Galardo, G.; et al. High Incidence of Candidemia in Critically Ill COVID-19 Patients Supported by Veno-Venous Extracorporeal Membrane Oxygenation: A Retrospective Study. *J. Fungi* **2023**, *9*, 119. [CrossRef]
31. Russo, A.; Venditti, M.; Ceccarelli, G.; Mastroianni, C.M.; d'Ettorre, G. Procalcitonin in daily clinical practice: An evergreen tool also during a pandemic. *Intern. Emerg. Med.* **2021**, *16*, 541–543. [CrossRef] [PubMed]
32. Wei, S.; Wang, L.; Lin, L.; Liu, X. Predictive values of procalcitonin for coinfections in patients with COVID-19, a systematic review and meta-analysis. *Virol. J.* **2023**, *20*, 92. [CrossRef] [PubMed]
33. Pink, I.; Raupach, D.; Fuge, J.; Vonberg, R.P.; Hoeper, M.M.; Welte, T.; Rademacher, J. C-reactive protein and procalcitonin for antimicrobial stewardship in COVID-19. *Infection* **2021**, *49*, 935–943. [CrossRef] [PubMed]
34. May, M.; Chang, M.; Dietz, D.; Shoucri, S.; Laracy, J.; Sobieszczyk, M.E.; Uhlemann, A.C.; Zucker, J.; Kubin, C.J. Limited Utility of Procalcitonin in Identifying Community-Associated Bacterial Infections in Patients Presenting with Coronavirus Disease 2019. *Antimicrob. Agents Chemother.* **2021**, *65*, e02167-20. [CrossRef]
35. Vanhomwegen, C.; Veliziotis, I.; Malinverni, S.; Konopnicki, D.; Dechamps, P.; Claus, M.; Roman, A.; Cotton, F.; Dauby, N. Procalcitonin accurately predicts mortality but not bacterial infection in COVID-19 patients admitted to intensive care unit. *Ir. J. Med. Sci.* **2021**, *190*, 1649–1652. [CrossRef]
36. Heer, R.S.; Mandal, A.K.; Kho, J.; Szawarski, P.; Csabi, P.; Grenshaw, D.; Walker, I.A.; Missouris, C.G. Elevated procalcitonin concentrations in severe Covid-19 may not reflect bacterial co-infection. *Ann. Clin. Biochem.* **2021**, *58*, 520–527. [CrossRef] [PubMed]
37. Dolci, A.; Robbiano, C.; Aloisio, E.; Chibireva, M.; Serafini, L.; Falvella, F.S.; Pasqualetti, S.; Panteghini, M. Searching for a role of procalcitonin determination in COVID-19, a study on a selected cohort of hospitalized patients. *Clin. Chem. Lab. Med.* **2020**, *59*, 433–440. [CrossRef] [PubMed]
38. Patel, N.; Adams, C.; Brunetti, L.; Bargoud, C.; Teichman, A.L.; Choron, R.L. Evaluation of Procalcitonin's Utility to Predict Concomitant Bacterial Pneumonia in Critically Ill COVID-19 Patients. *J. Intensive Care Med.* **2022**, *37*, 1486–1492. [CrossRef]
39. Lugito, N.P.H. Is procalcitonin a part of human immunological response to SARS-CoV-2 infection or "just" a marker of bacterial coinfection? *Curr. Res. Transl. Med.* **2021**, *69*, 103289. [CrossRef]
40. Martinez, F.O.; Combes, T.W.; Orsenigo, F.; Siamon Gordon, S. Monocyte activation in systemic Covid-19 infection: Assay and rationale. *EBioMedicine* **2020**, *59*, 102964. [CrossRef]
41. Daubin, C.; Fournel, F.; Thiollière, F.; Daviaud, F.; Ramakers, M.; Polito, A.; Flocard, B.; Valette, X.; Du Cheyron, D.; Terzi, N.; et al. Ability of procalcitonin to distinguish between bacterial and nonbacterial infection in severe acute exacerbation of chronic obstructive pulmonary syndrome in the ICU. *Ann. Intensive Care* **2021**, *11*, 39. [CrossRef]
42. Cohen, A.J.; Glick, L.R.; Lee, S.; Kunitomo, Y.; Tsang, D.A.; Pitafi, S.; Valda Toro, P.; Ristic, N.R.; Zhang, E.; Carey, G.B.; et al. Nonutility of procalcitonin for diagnosing bacterial pneumonia in patients with severe COVID-19. *Eur. Clin. Respir. J.* **2023**, *10*, 2174640. [CrossRef]
43. Hughes, S.; Mughal, N.; Moore, L.S.P. Procalcitonin to Guide Antibacterial Prescribing in Patients Hospitalised with COVID-19. *Antibiotics* **2021**, *10*, 1119. [CrossRef] [PubMed]
44. Atallah, N.J.; Warren, H.M.; Roberts, M.B.; Elshaboury, R.H.; Bidell, M.R.; Gandhi, R.G.; Adamsick, M.; Ibrahim, M.K.; Sood, R.; Bou Zein Eddine, S.; et al. Baseline procalcitonin as a predictor of bacterial infection and clinical outcomes in COVID-19, A case-control study. *PLoS ONE* **2022**, *17*, e0262342. [CrossRef] [PubMed]

Disclaimer/Publisher's Note: The statements, opinions and data contained in all publications are solely those of the individual author(s) and contributor(s) and not of MDPI and/or the editor(s). MDPI and/or the editor(s) disclaim responsibility for any injury to people or property resulting from any ideas, methods, instructions or products referred to in the content.

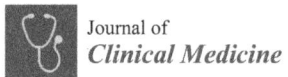

Article

Long-Term Consequences of COVID-19 in Predominantly Immunonaive Patients: A Canadian Prospective Population-Based Study

Justine Benoit-Piau [1], Karine Tremblay [2], Alain Piché [3], Frédéric Dallaire [4], Mathieu Bélanger [5], Marc-André d'Entremont [6,7], Jean-Charles Pasquier [8], Martin Fortin [5], Catherine Bourque [6], Fanny Lapointe [2], Jean-François Betala-Belinga [9], Geneviève Petit [10], Guillaume Jourdan [3], Renata Bahous [11], Camilo Maya [11], Amira Benzina [11], Muhammad Faiyaz Hossain [11], Marie-Audrey Peel [11], Olivier Houle [11], Marie-Sandrine Auger [11], Antoine Rioux [11] and Paul Farand [6,*]

1. Research Center of the Centre Hospitalier Universitaire de Sherbrooke (CHUS), University of Sherbrooke, Sherbrooke, QC J1H 5N4, Canada; justine.benoit-piau@usherbrooke.ca
2. Pharmacology and Physiology Department, Faculty of Medicine and Health Sciences, University of Sherbrooke, Sherbrooke, QC J1H 5N4, Canada; karine.tremblay@usherbrooke.ca (K.T.); fanny.lapointe@usherbrooke.ca (F.L.)
3. Department of Microbiology and Infectiology, University of Sherbrooke, Sherbrooke, QC J1H 5N4, Canada; alain.piche@usherbrooke.ca (A.P.); guillaume.jourdan@usherbrooke.ca (G.J.)
4. Department of Pediatrics, University of Sherbrooke, Sherbrooke, QC J1H 5N4, Canada; frederic.a.dallaire@usherbrooke.ca
5. Department of Family and Emergency Medicine, University of Sherbrooke, Sherbrooke, QC J1H 5N4, Canada; mathieu.belanger@usherbrooke.ca (M.B.); martin.fortin@usherbrooke.ca (M.F.)
6. Division of Cardiology, Department of Medicine, Faculty of Medicine and Health Sciences, University of Sherbrooke, Sherbrooke, QC J1H 5N4, Canada; marc-andre.dentremont@usherbrooke.ca (M.-A.d.); catherine.bourque@usherbrooke.ca (C.B.)
7. Population Health Research Institute, Hamilton, ON L8L 2X2, Canada
8. Department of Obstetrics and Gynecology, University of Sherbrooke, Sherbrooke, QC J1H 5N4, Canada; jean-charles.pasquier@usherbrooke.ca
9. Direction of Saguenay-Lac-Saint-Jean Public Health Department, Saguenay, QC J1H 5N4, Canada; jean-francois.betala-belinga@usherbrooke.ca
10. Department of Community Health Sciences, Faculty of Medicine and Health Sciences, University of Sherbrooke, Sherbrooke, QC J1H 5N4, Canada; genevieve.petit@usherbrooke.ca
11. Faculty of Medicine and Health Sciences, University of Sherbrooke, Sherbrooke, QC J1H 5N4, Canada; renata.bahous@usherbrooke.ca (R.B.); camilo.maya@usherbrooke.ca (C.M.); amira.benzina@usherbrooke.ca (A.B.); muhammad.faiyaz.hossain@usherbrooke.ca (M.F.H.); marie-audrey.peel@usherbrooke.ca (M.-A.P.); olivier.houle3@usherbrooke.ca (O.H.); marie-sandrine.auger@usherbrooke.ca (M.-S.A.); antoine.rioux3@usherbrooke.ca (A.R.)
* Correspondence: paul.farand@usherbrooke.ca; Tel.: +1-819-821-8000 (ext. 70324)

Abstract: Background: Lingering symptoms are frequently reported after acute SARS-CoV-2 infection, a condition known as post-COVID-19 condition (PCC). The duration and severity of PCC in immunologically naïve persons remain unclear. Furthermore, the long-term consequences of these chronic symptoms on work and mental health are poorly documented. **Objective**: To determine the outcome, the risk factors, and the impact on work and mental health associated with post-COVID-19 symptoms. **Methods**: This prospective population-based study assessed acute COVID-19 symptoms and their evolution for up to nine months following infection. Individuals aged 18 years and older with COVID-19 in three Canadian regions between 1 November 2020 and 31 May 2021 were recruited. Participants completed a questionnaire that was either administered by trained student investigators over the phone or self-administered online. **Results**: A total of 1349 participants with a mean age of 46.6 ± 16.0 years completed the questionnaire. Participants were mostly unvaccinated at the time of their COVID-19 episode (86.9%). Six hundred and twenty-two participants (48.0%) exhibited one symptom or more, at least three months post-COVID-19. Among participants with PCC, 23.0% to 37.8% experienced fatigue at the time of survey. Moreover, 6.1% expressed psychological distress. Risk factors for PCC and fatigue included female sex (OR = 1.996), higher number of symptoms

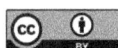

(OR = 1.292), higher severity of episode (OR = 3.831), and having a mental health condition prior to the COVID-19 episode (OR = 5.155). **Conclusions**: In this multicenter cohort study, almost half (47%) of the participants reported persistent symptoms >3 months after acute infection. Baseline risk factors for PCC include female sex, number and severity of symptoms during acute infection, and a previous diagnosis of mental health disorder. Having PCC negatively impacted health-related quality of life and these patients were more likely to exhibit psychological distress, as well as fatigue.

Keywords: COVID-19; post-acute COVID-19 syndrome; health-related quality of life; risk factors

1. Introduction

SARS-CoV-2 is a single-stranded RNA virus responsible for the coronavirus disease (COVID-19). COVID-19 has caused over 4.3 million infections and 46 thousand deaths in Canada thus far [1]. The disease was first thought to mainly affect the respiratory system. However, various studies rapidly showed that it affects multiple other systems [2–4]. In order to reduce mortality, healthcare resources were at first overwhelmingly focused on acutely ill patients and those exhibiting greater severity in symptoms [5]. Growing evidence suggests that a number of COVID-19 survivors exhibit long-term sequelae, also known as post-COVID-19 conditions (PCC). Common symptoms associated with PCC include fatigue, post-exertional fatigue, cognitive impairments, headaches, insomnia, and cardiopulmonary problems [6]. Due to the heterogenous severity of lingering symptoms, these people do not always seek medical attention [4,5]. Thus, a majority of experts agree that PCC should be managed by an interdisciplinary team [7].

Multiple cohort studies have investigated PCC in various populations [8–10]. These studies allowed for identifying common symptoms suffered through PCC and a number of risk factors. However, many of these studies had limitations including small sample size; inclusion of hospitalized individuals only, not limited to polymerase chain reaction (PCR) proven infections; and inclusion of specific groups, such as only healthcare workers. Moreover, few studies investigated the impact of PCC on quality of life. There remain significant gaps in our understanding of PCC, and our healthcare systems are still struggling to accommodate all of the specific needs of these patients [11]. Indeed, care trajectories have yet to be completely established [11].

To help improve our understanding of PCC, we recruited participants with documented SARS-CoV-2 infection, irrespective of disease severity. The primary objective was to document the prevalence of PCC after SARS-CoV-2 infection. Our secondary objectives were (1) to compare characteristics of PCC between three Canadian regions, (2) to compare characteristics of patients with PCC to those without PCC, and (3) to identify risk factors of PCC.

2. Methods

2.1. Setting and Design

This prospective population-based study was conducted in close collaboration with the Public Health Departments of three administrative regions in Canada: Estrie, Saguenay-Lac-Saint-Jean, and New Brunswick. A stratified block randomization was used to select a sample of individuals with SARS-CoV-2-proven infection from each of the study regions. The random selection was completed in multiple steps. Briefly, all subjects with a positive PCR test between 1 November 2020 and 31 May 2021 were first divided by region and age range. The second step was to determine how many participants per region and age range were needed. A number was assigned to every participant and randomly reorganized. The first participants corresponding to the required number per region and age range were selected. The details of sample size calculation and randomization are provided in Supplementary S1. The questionnaires were either administered by a trained third-year medical student investigator over the phone or self-administered by the participant online. This study was registered with ClinicalTrials (NCT03928509).

2.2. Participants and Ethics

Participants were randomly sampled among persons diagnosed with COVID-19 (SARS-CoV-2 PCR positive) residing in one of the study regions between November 2020 and May 2021. The study protocol was approved by the appropriate institutional research ethics boards (MP-31-2019-3172). Public Health Departments of Saguenay-Lac-Saint-Jean and New Brunswick provided a list of patients having consented to be contacted for research purposes. The Public Health Department of Estrie, in its framework of population monitoring, identified people that could be reached for the study purposes. Informed consent was obtained from all study participants prior to study participation.

Eligibility criteria included (1) a COVID-19 diagnosis confirmed using a SARS-CoV-2 PCR test, with or without symptoms; (2) being reachable by phone or e-mail for the duration of the study, and (3) being aged 18 years or older. Participants were excluded if they were deceased at the time of study, if their health would not allow the questionnaire to be completed, if they were unfit, or could not provide informed consent. All participants were at least 12 weeks post-COVID-19.

2.3. Data Collection

Data collection was carried out by third-year students of the undergraduate medical program at Université de Sherbrooke. Participants were invited to respond to the study questionnaire over the phone or online, at their convenience. Student investigators were trained and standardized to administer the survey questionnaire by the study principal investigator (PF) and the study coordinator (JBP).

Data were collected during the months of August and September of 2021. All data entry was carried out in REDCap (Research Electronic Data Capture, Vanderbilt University, Nashville, TN, USA) by either student investigators or participants [12].

2.4. Questionnaires and Data

Participants' sociodemographic profiles were established from responses to study questions relating to language preference, year of birth, sex at birth, gender, education level, socioeconomic level, occupation, time off occupation due to confinement, and time off occupation due to COVID-19 episode.

Data collected on COVID-19 included self-reported information on episode severity (asymptomatic, symptomatic, hospitalized), access to a physician or a nurse practitioner, and vaccination status. The list of symptoms investigated was based on a 25-symptom list established by the Quebec COVID-19 Biobank ("Biobanque Québécoise de la COVID-19") [13]. Fatigue in adult participants was examined using the Fatigue Severity Scale (FSS) and the Schedule of Fatigue and Anergia/General Practice (SOFA/GP) [14,15].

Participants were asked whether they had the following long-term health conditions: cancer, pulmonary diseases, cardiovascular diseases, digestive, endocrine and urinary diseases, musculoskeletal conditions, and mental health conditions. In addition, they were asked about their cardiovascular capacities using selected questions from the Duke Activity Scale Index (M-DASI-4Q) [16].

Participants' lifestyle information addressed their fruit and vegetable consumption, height, and weight. Participants 18 years and older were also asked about tobacco, alcohol, and cannabis consumption [17].

Participants' mental health status was evaluated using the 6-item Kessler Psychological Distress Scale [18].

The World Health Organization (WHO) defines PCC as the persistence of at least one symptom of COVID-19 three months after the initial episode, lasting for at least 2 months, and not being better explained by another diagnosis [19]. This definition was used in the current study. Since all participants were at least three months post-COVID-19, symptoms had been lingering for at least 2 months. The questions were designed in such a way that the symptoms were asked in relation to their COVID-19 episode to ensure that they could not be explained by another pathology. The clinical severity of the initial infection was defined according to WHO severity scale [20].

The complete English and French questionnaires administered are available in Supplementary S2.

2.5. Data Analysis

All analyses were performed using SPSS 28.0 (Statistical Package for the Social Sciences, IBM, Armonk, NY, USA). Descriptive analyses were used to characterize participants. For exploratory comparisons between regions, chi-squared tests and ANOVAs were used with Bonferroni corrections. A classification tree analysis was also performed to identify what combination of factors best differentiates between individuals with and without PCC.

3. Results

3.1. Participation Rate

During the study period, 9048 adults ≥ 18 years received a positive PCR COVID-19 result in Estrie. Of these, 4400 were randomly selected and prorated based on relative population age group size. Out of the 5526 individuals diagnosed with COVID-19 in Saguenay-Lac-Saint-Jean, 1200 agreed to be contacted for research purposes. Of these, 400 adults were randomly selected and prorated based on relative population age group size. In New Brunswick, between November 2020 and May 2021, out of 1857 individuals diagnosed with COVID-19, a total of 698 agreed to be contacted for research on COVID-19.

Figure 1 shows the participant flow chart. During the 2021 data collection, out of a total of 6884 selected eligible individuals, we attempted to contact 6741 (97.9%) participants at least once. Among the 4266 individuals reached, a total of 3318 (77.8%) agreed to participate. A total of 592 (17.8%) responded to the survey questionnaire administered over the phone. Of the 2398 who agreed to self-administer the questionnaire online, 969 (40.4%) eventually completed it. Overall, 1349 respondents completed the questionnaire, yielding an overall response rate of 43.8% (1367/3124).

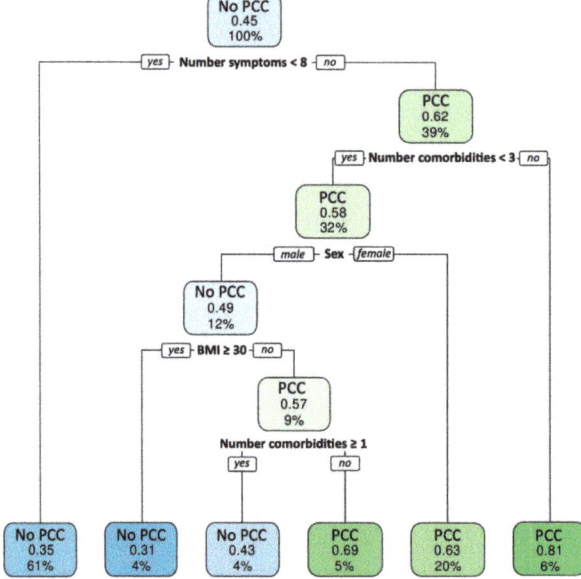

Figure 1. PCC classification tree.

3.2. Clinical Characteristics of the Study Cohort

As shown in Table 1, mean age was 46.7 ± 16.1 years old. Most participants were women (58.2%), spoke French (91.9%), and were full-time workers (55.0%). Most participants had a college or university diploma (53.0%). Of 1376 participants, 311 (27.3%) were healthcare workers. Most participants reported eating between two and four portions of fruits or vegetables daily (62.5%), never smoked tobacco (58.2%), never participated in binge drinking (49.0%), and never used recreational cannabis (86.0%).

Most common comorbidities included musculoskeletal conditions (22.4%), mental health conditions (21.9%), and cardiovascular diseases (20.6%) (Table 1). Interestingly, while 67.5% of participants reported having a stable mental health condition prior to their COVID-19 episode, 22.7% reported that their mental health condition had worsened, 4.0% reported that the condition had improved, and 5.8% had a new diagnosis of mental health condition since their COVID-19 episode.

Table 1. Characteristics of COVID-19-positive study participants.

	Total [a] N = 1349	Estrie N = 824	SLSJ N = 434	New-Brunswick N = 91	p-Value [b]
	Anthropometry and demographics				
Age in years (mean ± SD)	46.6 ± 16.0	46.6 ± 16.5	46.0 ± 15.1	49.5 ± 15.7	0.163
Sex (n of men (%))	522 (41.9)	327 (43.7)	156 (38.0)	39 (44.3)	0.160
BMI in kg/m^2 (mean ± SD)	27.8 ± 5.6	27.7 ± 5.7	27.7 ± 5.5	28.7 ± 5.8	0.515
Language (n (%))					<0.001
French	1239 (91.8)	762 (92.7)	430 (99.1)	47 (51.6) [†]	
English	78 (5.8)	34 (4.1)	3 (0.7) [†]	41 (45.1) [†]	
Others	30 (2.2)	26 (3.2) [‡]	1 (0.2) [†]	3 (3.3)	
Environment (n (%))					<0.001
Private household	1012 (75.1)	582 (70.6) [†]	362 (83.6)	68 (74.7)	
Apartment	296 (22.0)	217 (26.3)	60 (13.9) [†]	19 (20.9)	
Private residence for seniors or CHSLD	24 (1.8)	17 (2.1)	5 (1.2)	2 (2.2)	
Others	16 (1.2)	8 (1.0)	6 (1.4)	2 (2.2)	
Main occupation (n (%))					0.452
Self-employed	111 (8.3)	69 (8.4)	36 (8.4)	6 (6.7)	
Full-time worker	741 (55.2)	439 (53.5)	253 (58.7)	49 (54.4)	
Part-time worker	82 (6.1)	52 (6.3)	23 (5.3)	7 (7.8)	
Student	98 (7.3)	68 (8.3)	27 (6.3)	3 (3.3)	
Retired	194 (14.5)	125 (15.2)	52 (12.1)	17 (18.9)	
Others	116 (8.6)	68 (8.3)	40 (9.3)	8 (8.9)	
Education (n (%))					<0.001
No certificate	91 (7.4)	68 (9.2)	18 (4.4) [†]	5 (5.7)	
High school diploma	278 (22.5)	196 (26.4)	60 (14.7) [†]	22 (25.3)	
Apprenticeship or trade school diploma or other	209 (16.9)	115 (15.5)	80 (19.7)	14 (16.1)	
College diploma	349 (28.2)	189 (25.4)	142 (34.9) [†]	18 (20.7)	
University diploma	310 (25.1)	175 (23.6)	107 (26.3)	28 (32.2)	
Income (n (%))					0.007
<CAD 19,999 to CAD 29,999	151 (13.9)	100 (15.8)	42 (11.2)	9 (12.2)	
CAD 30,000 to CAD 89,999	514 (47.5)	317 (50.0)	162 (43.2)	35 (47.3)	
>CAD 90,000	418 (38.6)	217 (34.2) [‡]	171 (45.6) [†]	30 (40.5) [‡†]	
Health and social services worker (n (%))	308 (27.3)	194 (28.6)	83 (22.3)	31 (39.7)	0.003
	Lifestyle (in consumption)				
Fruits and vegetables in portions (n (%))					0.948
Five or more	266 (21.4)	164 (21.9)	82 (20.1)	20 (23.3)	
Between 2 and 4	778 (62.7)	467 (62.4)	259 (63.6)	52 (60.5)	
Less than 2	197 (15.9)	117 (15.6)	66 (16.2)	14 (16.3)	

Table 1. Cont.

	Total [a] N = 1349	Estrie N = 824	SLSJ N = 434	New-Brunswick N = 91	p-Value [b]
Tobacco in smoking (n (%))					
Current	152 (12.2)	84 (11.2)	62 (15.0)	6 (6.9)	
Former	370 (29.6)	214 (28.5)	126 (30.5)	30 (34.5)	0.091
Never	739 (58.3)	453 (60.3)	225 (54.5)	51 (58.6)	
Alcohol in terms of binge drinking (n (%))					
Less than once a month	217 (17.3)	128 (17.0)	75 (18.3)	14 (15.7)	
At least once a month	239 (19.1)	138 (18.4)	86 (21.0)	15 (16.9)	0.011
At least once a week	185 (14.8)	94 (12.5)	79 (19.3) †	12 (13.5)	
Never	610 (48.8)	392 (52.1)	170 (41.5) †	48 (53.9)	
Recreational cannabis (n (%))					
Less than once a month	86 (6.9)	50 (6.6)	26 (6.3)	10 (11.2)	
At least once a month	26 (2.1)	15 (2.0)	11 (2.7)	0 (0.0)	0.389
At least once a week	65 (5.2)	36 (4.8)	23 (5.6)	6 (6.7)	
Never	1077 (85.9)	653 (86.6)	351 (85.4)	73 (82.0)	
Long-term health problems (n (%))					
Cancers [c]	31 (2.4)	22 (2.9)	7 (1.7)	2 (2.2)	0.456
Pulmonary diseases [d]	177 (13.9)	94 (12.2)	70 (16.9)	13 (14.6)	0.082
Cardiovascular diseases [e]	261 (20.6)	150 (19.7)	85 (20.5)	26 (29.2)	0.108
Digestive, endocrine, and urinary diseases [f]	159 (12.6)	97 (12.8)	52 (12.7)	10 (11.2)	0.919
Musculoskeletal conditions [g]	264 (22.4)	157 (22.2)	82 (21.4)	25 (29.1)	0.293
Mental health conditions [h]	276 (21.9)	165 (21.7)	89 (21.5)	22 (24.7)	0.795

Abbreviations used: N/n = number; SD = standard deviation; SLSJ = Saguenay-Lac-Saint-Jean; BMI = body mass index; CHSLD = Centre d'hébergement et de soins longue durée. [a] Proportion was calculated on available data for each variable. [b] Post-hoc comparison: symbols (‡ and †) indicate a subset of categories whose column proportions differ significantly from each other at the 0.5 level. [c] Includes all cancers and melanoma, excludes other types of skin cancer in the last 5 years. [d] Includes asthma, chronic bronchitis, emphysema, chronic obstructive pulmonary disease (COPD). [e] Includes stroke, angina, heart attack, auricular fibrillation, heart failure. [f] Includes bowel disease, liver disease, diabetes, renal failure. [g] Includes musculoskeletal disorders, arthritis or rheumatoid arthritis. [h] Includes mood and anxiety disorders.

3.3. Acute COVID-19 Characteristics

As shown in Table 2, most participants had a mild episode of COVID-19 (159 asymptomatic (12.0%) and 1100 symptomatic (82.8%)). Few had moderate (4.0%) or severe (1.2%) episodes based on WHO severity scale [20]. The most reported symptoms included constitutional (73.6%), neurological (69.0%), and otorhinolaryngology manifestations (64.9%). The majority of participants (86.9%) were immunonaive, that is, unvaccinated against COVID-19, or had received one dose (11.0%), and only 2.1% were considered fully vaccinated (received at least two doses).

Participants showed very few functional disabilities three to nine months after their COVID-19 episode. The majority returned to work within four weeks (87.8%). Other participants returned to work one to three months after their episode (7.2%), more than three months after their episode (2.9%) or did not return to work at all (1.9%). Regarding access to healthcare professionals, 17.0% of participants did not have a practitioner or nurse practitioner. Additionally, 17.3% had difficulties with the appointment system and 17.4% had limited access due to the unavailability of professionals.

Table 2. COVID-19 episode.

	At Onset	Total N = 1349
Severity (n (%))		
Mild		1259 (94.8)
Moderate		53 (4.0)
Severe		16 (1.2)

Table 2. *Cont.*

At Onset	Total N = 1349
Symptoms (n (%))	
Asymptomatic	159 (12.0)
Respiratory [a]	718 (55.4)
Gastrointestinal [b]	592 (45.8)
Musculoskeletal [c]	568 (44.0)
Neurologic [d]	890 (69.0)
Constitutional [e]	946 (73.6)
ORL [f]	837 (64.9)
Other assessed [g]	285 (22.2)
Vaccination at episode (number of doses) (n (%))	
None	1131 (86.9)
One	143 (11.0)
Two	27 (2.1)
At time of survey	
Post-COVID-19 conditions	622 (48.0)
Fatigue	
FSS (mean ± SD)	3.3 ± 1.6
FSS (n (%) of ≥5)	234 (19.6)
SOFA (mean ± SD)	1.6 ± 0.6
SOFA (n (%) of ≥2)	266 (22.6)
FSS ≥ 5 and SOFA ≥ 2 (n (%))	158 (13.0)
Psychological distress (mean ± SD)	4.0 ± 4.0
Psychological distress (n (%) of ≥14)	44 (3.5)
Daily function (n (%) of no)	
DASI1	134 (10.7)
DASI2	108 (8.6)
DASI3	97 (7.9)
DASI4	354 (33.3)
Function (EQ-5D) (n (%) of no or slight problems)	
Ability to walk	1228 (95.0)
Ability to bathe and dress	1281 (99.0)
Ability to complete activities of daily life	1227 (94.9)
Having pain or discomfort	1151 (89.6)
Being anxious or depressive	1093 (85.0)
Being short of breath (n (%))	
Out of breath with intense exercise	889 (71.2)
Out of breath when rushing or climbing a slight incline	265 (21.2)
Slower than most people of the same age on flat ground	55 (4.4)
Stop to breathe when walking 100 m on flat ground	34 (2.7)
Too out of breath to leave the house	5 (0.4)
Ceased occupation (n (%))	
Two weeks	766 (62.0)
Three to four weeks	321 (26.0)
One to three months	89 (7.2)
More than three months	36 (2.9)
Ceased occupation	24 (1.9)
Changes to occupation (n (%))	
Same occupation, more demanding	118 (10.7)
Same occupation, same conditions	863 (77.8)
Same occupation, less demanding	43 (3.9)
Different occupation, more demanding	24 (2.2)
Different occupation, same conditions	30 (2.7)
Different occupation, less demanding	31 (2.8)
Practitioner or nurse practitioner (n (%))	
Practitioner	1047 (78.5)
Nurse practitioner	34 (2.6)
Both	24 (1.8)
None	228 (17.1)
Access to health professionals (n (%))	
Difficulties with appointment system	122 (17.4)
Professionals not available	118 (17.6)
Transportation problems	20 (3.0)

Abbreviations used: N/n = number, SD = standard deviation, FSS = Fatigue Severity Scale, SOFA = Schedule of Fatigue and Anergia/General Practice, DASI = Duke Activity Status Index, EQ-5D = EuroQol-5D. [a] Includes cough, sibilance, hissing, stridor. [b] Includes nausea/vomiting, dysphagia, diarrhea, abdominal pain. [c] Includes joint pain and lower limb edema. [d] Includes aphasia, dysarthria, confusion, convulsions, ageusia, dysgeusia, anosmia, paresthesia of the lower or upper limbs. [e] Includes fever, dizziness, inappetence. [f] Includes earache, sore throat, hemoptysis, nasal discharge or congestion. [g] Includes eye infection, chest pain, rash.

3.4. Post-COVID-19 Conditions

As shown in Table 3, among participants with PCC (n = 622, 48.0%), symptoms at onset were most often neurological (83.5%) or constitutional (80.9%). The symptoms most often reported at the time of survey 3 to 9 months (median of 6 months) after their COVID-19 episode were neurological (59.3%) and musculoskeletal (43.9%). As for fatigue, there were 31.9% of participants who had a score higher or equal to five for the FSS and 37.8% who had a score higher or equal to two for the SOFA. When combined, 23.0% of participants met both criteria for fatigue. Psychological distress was reported by 6.1% of participants with PCC compared to 1.2% by those without PCC.

As shown in Table 4, participants with PCC were older and had a higher BMI than participants who did not have PCC ($p \leq 0.010$). Moreover, they were predominantly female ($p < 0.001$). They also showed a higher prevalence of comorbidities ($p < 0.001$) and number of symptoms ($p < 0.001$), and a higher proportion of moderate or severe episode ($p < 0.001$).

Risk factors at baseline regarding the onset of PCC and PCC with fatigue are shown in Table 5. Baseline risk factors for developing PCC included age (OR = 1.010), being a female (OR = 1.383), and a higher BMI (OR = 1.029). All comorbidities were associated with an increased risk of having PCC without fatigue (OR $\geq$ 1.340). The severity of episode (OR = 1.764) and number of symptoms (OR = 1.136) were also risk factors of PCC. Being a health professional also increased this likelihood (OR = 1.038). Risk factors were similar for PCC with fatigue. Age (OR = 1.012), being a female (OR = 1.996), and higher BMI (OR = 1.056) were risk factors. Again, all comorbidities were linked to a higher risk of PCC (OR $\geq$ 2.421). The severity of episode (OR = 3.831) and number of symptoms at onset (OR = 1.292) were also risk factors for PCC and fatigue. Being a health professional also put participants at risk of PCC with fatigue (OR = 1.525).

Figure 1 presents the classification tree analysis showing that the number of symptoms at the initial presentation (with a cutoff of 8) is the main discriminant factor to determine who will have PCC or not. Other factors determined by the algorithm, but with less weight, are number of comorbidities, sex, and BMI.

Table 3. Post-COVID-19 conditions.

	At the Time of Survey
	PCC N = 622 (48.0%)
Symptoms at onset (n (%))	
Respiratory [a]	389 (62.9)
Gastrointestinal [b]	353 (57.5)
Musculoskeletal [c]	319 (52.0)
Neurologic [d]	512 (83.5)
Constitutional [e]	494 (80.9)
ORL [f]	451 (73.7)
Other assessed [g]	189 (31.2)
Symptoms at time of survey (n (%))	
Respiratory [a]	176 (28.6)
Gastrointestinal [b]	161 (26.2)
Musculoskeletal [c]	270 (43.9)
Neurologic [d]	366 (59.3)
Constitutional [e]	176 (28.6)
ORL [f]	195 (31.9)
Other assessed [g]	128 (21.1)
Fatigue at the time of survey	
FSS (n (%) of $\geq$5)	181 (31.9)
SOFA (n (%) of $\geq$2)	205 (37.8)
FSS $\geq$ 5 and SOFA $\geq$ 2 (n (%))	131 (23.0)
Psychological distress at the time of survey (n (%) of $\geq$14)	36 (6.1)

Abbreviations used: N/n = number, FSS = Fatigue Severity Scale, SOFA = Schedule of Fatigue and Anergia/General Practice. [a] Includes cough, sibilance, hissing, stridor. [b] Includes nausea/vomiting, dysphagia, diarrhea, abdominal pain. [c] Includes joint pain and lower limb edema. [d] Includes aphasia, dysarthria, confusion, convulsions, ageusia, dysgeusia, anosmia, paresthesia of the lower or upper limbs. [e] Includes fever, dizziness, inappetence. [f] Includes earache, sore throat, hemoptysis, nasal discharge or congestion. [g] Includes eye infection, chest pain, rash.

Table 4. Post-COVID-19 condition characteristics.

	At Time of Onset				
	No PCC and FSS < 5 N = 571 (47.9)	PCC and FSS < 5 N = 387 (32.5)	No PCC and FSS ≥ 5 N = 53 (4.4)	PCC and FSS ≥ 5 N = 181 (15.2)	p-Value
Age	45.8 ± 15.1	48.2 ± 16.9	43.0 ± 16.3	48.7 ± 15.0	0.010
Sex (Female)	288 (51.8)	226 (59.8)	34 (66.7)	120 (68.2)	<0.001
BMI	27.1 ± 5.5	28.1 ± 5.6	27.4 ± 5.4	29.0 ± 6.3	0.004
Pulmonary diseases	48 (8.5)	59 (15.4)	6 (11.8)	48 (26.8)	<0.001
Cardiovascular diseases	92 (16.3)	79 (20.7)	13 (24.5)	57 (32.0)	<0.001
Musculoskeletal conditions	74 (14.3)	94 (25.9)	12 (26.7)	69 (40.4)	<0.001
Mental health conditions	77 (13.7)	82 (21.4)	21 (40.4)	80 (44.9)	<0.001
Severity of episode Mild Moderate or severe	551 (96.7) 19 (3.3)	362 (94.3) 22 (5.7)	51 (98.1) 1 (1.9)	159 (88.3) 21 (11.7)	<0.001
Number of symptoms at onset	4.9 ± 3.9	7.1 ± 4.3	6.5 ± 4.9	9.6 ± 4.2	<0.001

Table 5. Post-COVID-19 condition risk factors.

	At Time of Onset		
	PCC and FSS < 5 N = 387 (32.5)		
	OR	95% CI	p-Value
Age	1.010	1.002–1.018	0.020
Sex (Female)	1.383	1.062–1.802	0.016
BMI	1.029	1.003–1.058	0.028
Pulmonary diseases	1.965	1.308–2.941	0.001
Cardiovascular diseases	1.340	0.961–1.873	0.085
Musculoskeletal conditions	2.100	1.495–2.950	<0.001
Mental health conditions	1.715	1.218–2.415	0.002
Severity of episode	1.764	0.941–3.300	0.077
Number of symptoms	1.136	1.098–1.176	<0.001
Being a health professional	1.038	0.752–1.434	0.819
	PCC and FSS ≥ 5 N = 181 (15.2)		
	OR	95% CI	p-Value
Age	1.012	1.001–1.023	0.029
Sex (Female)	1.996	1.395–2.849	<0.001
BMI	1.056	1.024–1.090	<0.001
Pulmonary diseases	3.968	2.545–6.173	<0.001
Cardiovascular diseases	2.421	1.647–3.559	<0.001
Musculoskeletal conditions	4.065	2.747–6.024	<0.001
Mental health conditions	5.155	3.509–7.519	<0.001
Severity of episode	3.831	2.008–7.299	<0.001
Number of symptoms	1.292	1.234–1.352	<0.001
Being a health professional	1.525	1.024–2.270	0.038

4. Discussion

4.1. Main Observations

To our knowledge, this study is the largest to date to describe long-term functional impairments of COVID-19 in a Canadian population. Most patients included in our study had a mild episode of COVID-19 and were not hospitalized. This is consistent with reported distribution of symptom severity in the population [8,10]. Another strength of this study is the high number of participants with functional data and extensive characterization of fatigue. Also, all participants included in the study had a PCR test confirming the infection.

The prevalence of PCC in our study population was 48%. That proportion is congruent with other studies [10,21–24]. Describing functional impacts in patients with PCC is essential since it could affect the burden of their condition. Patients who experience one minor symptom more than 3 months post-infection could be different than patients experiencing PCC who also reported fatigue or other functional impairments. Fatigue was reported by more than 30% of participants with PCC, making it a major manifestation of this condition. Prevalence of post-COVID-19 fatigue has been reported for other countries [25]. This study adds to our understanding of the prevalence of fatigue post-COVID-19 in a Canadian population. We also used a well-known fatigue score to identify the 15.2% of patients with PCC who also experience fatigue.

Among participants with functional impairments, being slower than most people of the same age on flat ground or being short of breath was described by only 7.6% of participants with PCC. Although COVID-19 and PCC can severely affect cardiovascular capacities for some people, the populational burden seems to be mild for that aspect. In a similar way, in our study, very few patients (1.9%) completely ceased their occupation in the long term. It should however be noted that 12.7% of patients who continued an occupation found it more demanding. Among the symptoms reported by patients with PCC at the time of the survey, the most frequently reported were neurological symptoms, including fatigue and cognitive and functional impairments. These symptoms could be linked to other long-term functional impacts of COVID-19 [26,27]. These symptoms could limit functional capacities and aptitude to be active and work.

We also explored factors that can predict the occurrence of PCC. Consistent with other studies, we found that the numbers of symptoms at onset is the main predictor of PCC [22,23]. We also observed that participants with PCC without fatigue showed a higher prevalence of comorbidities and higher number of symptoms at onset. When we look at participants with PCC and fatigue, we see that the odds ratios were even higher for being female and for the presence of comorbidities. Among them, mental health condition was the comorbidity with the higher odds ratio. These patients showed a higher prevalence of comorbidities that could be linked with less efficient coping mechanisms and lesser physical reserves [28].

All lingering symptoms and functional impacts reported in the current study should be interpreted considering the absence of a control group. The negative background effect brought by the pandemic could be a confounder [29]. Indeed, studies have found that psychological impacts were present in the overall population in the wake of the pandemic, not only in people who were infected with COVID-19 [30]. Moreover, the pandemic has had an impact on the workforce of the general population.

With regard to the timeframe of the study, patients included in this cohort were mainly unvaccinated or partially vaccinated related to the prevalence of vaccination at the time of recruitment. The exact proportion of COVID-19 variants among our study population is unknown. However, based on epidemiological data, we know that there was not a predominant variant at the beginning of our study period and that Alpha was the predominant variant at the end of the study period [31]. These epidemiological observations and the low vaccination coverage at the time of the study could explain the high rate of PCC observed. The proportion of patients who will experience PCC and the burden of fatigue as well as functional impacts with different variants and with the increased vaccination coverage is unknown. This will be documented in a follow-up study. This future study will also describe the evolution of patients who suffered from PCC in the 2021 survey.

4.2. Limitations

This study has inherent selection and information biases in its design that were considered in the data collection process by the application of preventive measures or in the interpretation of the results that were carefully made.

With regard to the selection bias, the subjects were selected randomly among the COVID-19-positive patients of the public health records, but only those who could be reached by phone participated in this study. This, as well as the timing of call periods, may have biased participants' characteristics. We explored data about the COVID-19-positive patients of the Estrie region who did not complete the survey. They have the same sex distribution (women 56.4% for patients included in the study vs. 53.7% for patients who did not complete the questionnaire), but less patients who participated in the study were over 70 years old (9.0% of the sample vs. 20.0% of the COVID-19-positive patients). This later finding can be explained by many of the screening tests for patients over 70 years old occurring among patients residing in nursing homes with health conditions, making participation in this kind of study difficult. We do not think that this difference interfered significantly with our results.

In addition, the volunteer bias of the study sampling limits our generalization of the results to the whole population. However, since we did not collect the reasons of refusal to participate or the retrospective data on COVID-19 patients having died from the disease or other causes, we cannot stipulate that our sample is representative of all SARS-CoV-2-infected individuals. Since the primary objective of this study was to compile data on PCC, absence of retrospective data from deceased COVID-19 patients should not bias interpretation of the results.

Another limitation of this study may result from possible information biases. Firstly, a chronological bias in recruitment of the subjects may have introduced a misclassification of the PCC conditions. Indeed, some of the subjects were 3 months post-infection at the time of recruitment while others were at 6 months post-infection. Such delay may underestimate the PCC status (as per the WHO definition) in this sample. Moreover, it should be considered that although questions were designed to identify lingering symptoms from the participants' COVID-19 episode, it cannot be entirely ruled out that symptoms may be due to other causes. Secondly, the self-reported retrospective data are submitted to the recall bias for which we have no way to verify the veracity (no data collected from medical records). This bias may affect measured frequencies of the data such as symptoms or other health conditions at COVID-19 diagnosis given the time lapse between diagnosis and questionnaire administration. To mitigate this, most questions were formulated to gather information regarding symptoms in the week or month prior to the survey's administration. Thirdly, although the majority of participants were unvaccinated, some were partially or fully vaccinated. This could have impacted the prevalence of PCC among participants [24,32]. Finally, the large number of student investigator interviewers could be viewed as an observer bias. However, all of those involved in data collection were trained on and standardized to the questionnaire used in this study and trained on how to record information.

5. Conclusions

This study describes the long-term functional impacts of the COVID-19 pandemic among a Canadian population. It was found that having comorbidities prior to the COVID-19 episode, particularly mental health conditions, is the main predictor of PCC. Participants with PCC and fatigue were predominantly women and had more symptoms at onset and a higher severity of episode. This research contributes to our understanding of the intricate pathophysiology of PCC.

Supplementary Materials: The following supplementary information can be downloaded at: https://www.mdpi.com/article/10.3390/jcm12185939/s1. Supplementary S1 details sample size calculation and randomization. Supplementary S2 presents the complete questionnaires in English and French.

Author Contributions: Conceptualization, P.F., K.T., A.P., F.D., M.B., M.-A.d., J.-C.P., M.F., C.B., J.-F.B.-B., G.P., G.J.; methodology, J.B.-P., K.T., A.P., F.D., M.B., J.-C.P., M.F., C.B., J.-F.B.-B., G.P., G.J., R.B., C.M., A.B., M.F.H., M.-A.P., O.H., M.-S.A., A.R., P.F.; software, F.L.; formal analysis, J.B.-P.; investigation, J.B.-P., R.B., C.M., A.B., M.F.H., M.-A.P., O.H., M.-S.A., A.R.; resources, P.F.; data curation, J.B.-P., F.L.; writing—original draft preparation, J.B.-P., K.T., A.P., P.F.; writing—review and editing, J.B.-P., K.T., A.P., F.D., M.B., J.-C.P., M.F., M.-A.d., C.B., J.-F.B.-B., G.P., G.J., R.B., C.M., A.B., M.F.H., M.-A.P., O.H., M.-S.A., A.R., P.F.; supervision, K.T., M.B., P.F.; project administration, J.B.-P., F.L.; funding acquisition, P.F. All authors have read and agreed to the published version of the manuscript.

Funding: This study was funded by the faculty of medicine and health sciences, as well as the Department of Medicine of Université de Sherbrooke.

Institutional Review Board Statement: The study was conducted in accordance with the Declaration of Helsinkin, and approved by the Ethis Committee of the Research Center of CIUSSS de l'Estrie—CHUS (MP31-2019-3172).

Informed Consent Statement: Informed consent was obtained from all subjects involved in the study.

Data Availability Statement: The data presented in this study are available on request from the corresponding author. The data are not publicly available due to ethical and privacy issues.

Conflicts of Interest: The authors declare no conflict of interest.

References

1. Canada, A. de la Santé Publique du Maladie à Coronavirus (COVID-19): Mise à Jour Sur L'éclosion, Symptômes, Prévention, Voyage, Préparations. Available online: https://www.canada.ca/fr/sante-publique/services/maladies/maladie-coronavirus-covid-19.html (accessed on 17 June 2022).
2. Gupta, A.; Madhavan, M.V.; Sehgal, K.; Nair, N.; Mahajan, S.; Sehrawat, T.S.; Bikdeli, B.; Ahluwalia, N.; Ausiello, J.C.; Wan, E.Y.; et al. Extrapulmonary manifestations of COVID-19. *Nat. Med.* **2020**, *26*, 1017–1032. [CrossRef] [PubMed]
3. Wadman, M.; Couzin-Frankel, J.; Kaiser, J.; Matacic, C. A rampage through the body. *Science* **2020**, *368*, 356–360. [CrossRef]
4. Higgins, V.; Sohaei, D.; Diamandis, E.P.; Prassas, I. COVID-19: From an acute to chronic disease? Potential long-term health consequences. *Crit. Rev. Clin. Lab. Sci.* **2021**, *58*, 297–310. [CrossRef] [PubMed]
5. Wang, F.; Kream, R.M.; Stefano, G.B. Long-Term Respiratory and Neurological Sequelae of COVID-19. *Med. Sci. Monit.* **2020**, *26*, e928996. [CrossRef]
6. Burke, M.J.; Del Rio, C. Long COVID has exposed medicine's blind-spot. *Lancet Infect. Dis.* **2021**, *21*, 1062–1064. [CrossRef]
7. Norton, A.; Olliaro, P.; Sigfrid, L.; Carson, G.; Paparella, G.; Hastie, C.; Kaushic, C.; Boily-Larouche, G.; Suett, J.C.; O'Hara, M.; et al. Long COVID: Tackling a multifaceted condition requires a multidisciplinary approach. *Lancet Infect. Dis.* **2021**, *21*, 601–602. [CrossRef]
8. Menges, D.; Ballouz, T.; Anagnostopoulos, A.; Aschmann, H.E.; Domenghino, A.; Fehr, J.S.; Puhan, M.A. Burden of post-COVID-19 syndrome and implications for healthcare service planning: A population-based cohort study. *PLoS ONE* **2021**, *16*, e0254523. [CrossRef] [PubMed]
9. Premraj, L.; Kannapadi, N.V.; Briggs, J.; Seal, S.M.; Battaglini, D.; Fanning, J.; Suen, J.; Robba, C.; Fraser, J.; Cho, S.-M. Mid and long-term neurological and neuropsychiatric manifestations of post-COVID-19 syndrome: A meta-analysis. *J. Neurol. Sci.* **2022**, *434*, 120162. [CrossRef]
10. Davis, H.E.; Assaf, G.S.; McCorkell, L.; Wei, H.; Low, R.J.; Re'em, Y.; Redfield, S.; Austin, J.P.; Akrami, A. Characterizing long COVID in an international cohort: 7 months of symptoms and their impact. *EClinicalMedicine* **2021**, *38*, 101019. [CrossRef]
11. Krausz, M.; Westenberg, J.N.; Vigo, D.; Spence, R.T.; Ramsey, D. Emergency Response to COVID-19 in Canada: Platform Development and Implementation for eHealth in Crisis Management. *JMIR Public Health Surveill.* **2020**, *6*, e18995. [CrossRef]
12. Harris, P.A.; Taylor, R.; Minor, B.L.; Elliott, V.; Fernandez, M.; O'Neal, L.; McLeod, L.; Delacqua, G.; Delacqua, F.; Kirby, J.; et al. The REDCap consortium: Building an international community of software platform partners. *J. Biomed. Inform.* **2019**, *95*, 103208. [CrossRef]
13. Tremblay, K.; Rousseau, S.; Zawati, M.H.; Auld, D.; Chassé, M.; Coderre, D.; Falcone, E.L.; Gauthier, N.; Grandvaux, N.; Gros-Louis, F.; et al. The Biobanque québécoise de la COVID-19 (BQC19)-A cohort to prospectively study the clinical and biological determinants of COVID-19 clinical trajectories. *PLoS ONE* **2021**, *16*, e0245031. [CrossRef]

14. Cohen, E.T.; Matsuda, P.N.; Fritz, N.E.; Allen, D.D.; Yorke, A.M.; Widener, G.L.; Jewell, S.T.; Potter, K. Self-Report Measures of Fatigue for People With Multiple Sclerosis: A Systematic Review. *J. Neurol. Phys. Ther.* **2023**. [CrossRef]
15. Hadzi-Pavlovic, D.; Hickie, I.B.; Wilson, A.J.; Davenport, T.A.; Lloyd, A.R.; Wakefield, D. Screening for prolonged fatigue syndromes: Validation of the SOFA scale. *Soc. Psychiatry Psychiatr. Epidemiol.* **2000**, *35*, 471–479. [CrossRef]
16. Riedel, B.; Li, M.H.; Lee, C.A.; Ismail, H.; Cuthbertson, B.H.; Wijeysundera, D.N.; Ho, K.M.; Wallace, S.; Thompson, B.; Ellis, M.; et al. A simplified (modified) Duke Activity Status Index (M-DASI) to characterise functional capacity: A secondary analysis of the Measurement of Exercise Tolerance before Surgery (METS) study. *Br. J. Anaesth.* **2021**, *126*, 181–190. [CrossRef]
17. Stronach, N.; Des Roches, M.; Perreault, G.; Poirier, B.; Martin, B.; Grégoire, A. Tableau de Bord Santé Publique Estrie—Définitions, Notes Méthodologiques et Sources de Données. 2018. Available online: https://www.santeestrie.qc.ca/clients/SanteEstrie/Publications/Sante-publique/Portrait-population/Outils-tableaux-de-bord/notes_methos_TdB-SPEstrie_fevrier2018.pdf (accessed on 17 June 2022).
18. Cornelius, B.L.; Groothoff, J.W.; van der Klink, J.J.; Brouwer, S. The performance of the K10, K6 and GHQ-12 to screen for present state DSM-IV disorders among disability claimants. *BMC Public Health* **2013**, *13*, 128. [CrossRef] [PubMed]
19. A Clinical Case Definition of Post COVID-19 Condition by a Delphi Consensus. 2021. Available online: https://www.who.int/publications-detail-redirect/WHO-2019-nCoV-Post_COVID-19_condition-Clinical_case_definition-2021.1 (accessed on 7 November 2022).
20. de Terwangne, C.; Laouni, J.; Jouffe, L.; Lechien, J.R.; Bouillon, V.; Place, S.; Capulzini, L.; Machayekhi, S.; Ceccarelli, A.; Saussez, S.; et al. Predictive Accuracy of COVID-19 World Health Organization (WHO) Severity Classification and Comparison with a Bayesian-Method-Based Severity Score (EPI-SCORE). *Pathogens* **2020**, *9*, 880. [CrossRef] [PubMed]
21. Alkodaymi, M.S.; Omrani, O.A.; Fawzy, N.A.; Shaar, B.A.; Almamlouk, R.; Riaz, M.; Obeidat, M.; Obeidat, Y.; Gerberi, D.; Taha, R.M.; et al. Prevalence of post-acute COVID-19 syndrome symptoms at different follow-up periods: A systematic review and meta-analysis. *Clin. Microbiol. Infect.* **2022**, *28*, 657–666. [CrossRef]
22. Gallant, M.; Rioux-Perreault, C.; Lemaire-Paquette, S.; Piché, A. SARS-CoV-2 infection outcomes associated with the Delta variant: A prospective cohort study. *J. Assoc. Med. Microbiol. Infect. Dis. Can.* **2022**, *8*, 49–56. [CrossRef]
23. Gallant, M.; Mercier, K.; Rioux-Perreault, C.; Lemaire-Paquette, S.; Piché, A. Prevalence of persistent symptoms at least 1 month after SARS-CoV-2 Omicron infection in adults. *J. Assoc. Med. Microbiol. Infect. Dis. Can.* **2022**, *8*, 57–63. [CrossRef] [PubMed]
24. Sadat Larijani, M.; Ashrafian, F.; Bagheri Amiri, F.; Banifazl, M.; Bavand, A.; Karami, A.; Asgari Shokooh, F.; Ramezani, A. Characterization of long COVID-19 manifestations and its associated factors: A prospective cohort study from Iran. *Microb. Pathog.* **2022**, *169*, 105618. [CrossRef]
25. Ceban, F.; Ling, S.; Lui, L.M.W.; Lee, Y.; Gill, H.; Teopiz, K.M.; Rodrigues, N.B.; Subramaniapillai, M.; Di Vincenzo, J.D.; Cao, B.; et al. Fatigue and cognitive impairment in Post-COVID-19 Syndrome: A systematic review and meta-analysis. *Brain Behav. Immun.* **2022**, *101*, 93–135. [CrossRef] [PubMed]
26. Calabria, M.; García-Sánchez, C.; Grunden, N.; Pons, C.; Arroyo, J.A.; Gómez-Anson, B.; Estévez García, M.D.C.; Belvís, R.; Morollón, N.; Vera Igual, J.; et al. Post-COVID-19 fatigue: The contribution of cognitive and neuropsychiatric symptoms. *J. Neurol.* **2022**, *269*, 3990–3999. [CrossRef] [PubMed]
27. Lamontagne, S.J.; Winters, M.F.; Pizzagalli, D.A.; Olmstead, M.C. Post-acute sequelae of COVID-19: Evidence of mood & cognitive impairment. *Brain Behav. Immun. Health* **2021**, *17*, 100347. [CrossRef]
28. Fluharty, M.; Fancourt, D. How have people been coping during the COVID-19 pandemic? Patterns and predictors of coping strategies amongst 26,016 UK adults. *BMC Psychol.* **2021**, *9*, 107. [CrossRef]
29. Shields, M.; Tonmyr, L.; Gonzalez, A.; Weeks, M.; Park, S.-B.; Robert, A.-M.; Blair, D.-L.; MacMillan, H.L. Symptoms of major depressive disorder during the COVID-19 pandemic: Results from a representative sample of the Canadian population. *Health Promot. Chronic Dis. Prev. Can. Res. Policy Pract.* **2021**, *41*, 340–358. [CrossRef]
30. Généreux, M.; Schluter, P.J.; Landaverde, E.; Hung, K.K.; Wong, C.S.; Mok, C.P.Y.; Blouin-Genest, G.; O'Sullivan, T.; David, M.D.; Carignan, M.-E.; et al. The Evolution in Anxiety and Depression with the Progression of the Pandemic in Adult Populations from Eight Countries and Four Continents. *Int. J. Environ. Res. Public Health* **2021**, *18*, 4845. [CrossRef] [PubMed]
31. National Collaborating Centre for Infectious Diseases. Updates on COVID-19 Variants of Concern (VOC). 2022. Available online: https://nccid.ca/covid-19-variants/ (accessed on 8 June 2022).
32. Mumtaz, A.; Sheikh, A.A.E.; Khan, A.M.; Khalid, S.N.; Khan, J.; Nasrullah, A.; Sagheer, S.; Sheikh, A.B. COVID-19 Vaccine and Long COVID: A Scoping Review. *Life* **2022**, *12*, 1066. [CrossRef]

Disclaimer/Publisher's Note: The statements, opinions and data contained in all publications are solely those of the individual author(s) and contributor(s) and not of MDPI and/or the editor(s). MDPI and/or the editor(s) disclaim responsibility for any injury to people or property resulting from any ideas, methods, instructions or products referred to in the content.

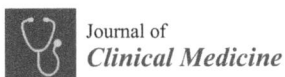

Article

Quality of Life 6 Months after COVID-19 Hospitalisation: A Single-Centre Polish Registry

Maciej Koźlik [1,*], Maciej Kaźmierski [1], Wojciech Kaźmierski [2], Paulina Lis [3], Anna Lis [3], Weronika Łowicka [3], Marta Chamera [3], Barbara Romanowska [3], Jakub Kufel [4], Maciej Cebula [5] and Marek Jędrzejek [1]

[1] Division of Cardiology and Structural Heart Disease, Medical University of Silesia, 40-635 Katowice, Poland; kazmierski.maciej@gmail.com (M.K.); jedrzejekmarek@gmail.com (M.J.)
[2] Faculty of Medicine and Health Sciences, Andrzej Frycz Modrzewski Krakow University, 30-705 Krakow, Poland; wkazmierski97@gmail.com
[3] Cardiology Students' Scientific Association, Department of Cardiology, SHS, Medical University of Silesia, 40-635 Katowice, Poland; lispaulinab@gmail.com (P.L.); lis.anna9898@gmail.com (A.L.); weronikalowicka22@gmail.com (W.Ł.); marta.chamera@op.pl (M.C.); barbara.romanowska@gmail.com (B.R.)
[4] Department of Biophysics, Faculty of Medical Sciences in Zabrze, Medical University of Silesia, 41-808 Zabrze, Poland; jakubkufel92@gmail.com
[5] Individual Medical Practice Maciej Cebula, 40-754 Katowice, Poland; maciejmichalcebula@gmail.com
* Correspondence: kozlik.maciej@gmail.com

Abstract: Background: The COVID-19 pandemic, which affected the entire global population, had an impact on our health and quality of life. Many people had complications, were hospitalised or even died due to SARS-CoV-2 infection. The health systems of many countries had to radically change their way of functioning and scientists around the world worked intensively to develop a vaccine for the SARS-CoV-2 virus. Aim: The aim of this work is to assess the quality of life of patients who were hospitalised for COVID-19, using the SF-36 questionnaire. Methods: Between May and August 2022, we conducted a telephone assessment of quality of life in patients who were hospitalised for COVID-19 at the Temporary Hospital in Pyrzowice (Silesia, Poland), between November 2021 and January 2022. Results: Quality of life was significantly lower in women ($p = 0.040$), those with DM2 ($p = 0.013$), CKD ($p = 0.041$) and the vaccinated ($p = 0.015$). Conclusions: People with chronic kidney disease, diabetes mellitus and women had a lower quality of life after COVID-19 disease. However, people who were vaccinated for SARS-CoV-2 had a lower quality of life than non-vaccinated people did. This is possibly due to the higher mean age, and probably the higher disease burden, in the vaccinated group.

Keywords: SARS-CoV-2 infection; COVID-19; quality of life; SF-36

1. Introduction

At the turn of 2019/2020, the COVID-19 pandemic, caused by severe acute respiratory syndrome coronavirus 2 (SARS-CoV-2) became a global concern. As of 16 March 2023, there have been 6,462,369 confirmed cases of the disease in Poland and 760,360,956 globally [1]. The predominant symptoms include shortness of breath, fever, fatigue, cough, diarrhoea, loss of smell or headache, but in some cases the disease can lead to more serious complications such as acute respiratory distress syndrome (ARDS), myocardial damage or thrombotic symptoms [2–4]. Regardless of the severity of the course of infection, distant consequences have also been observed with varying frequency, including long-COVID-19 syndrome [5,6]. Long COVID includes symptoms such as shortness of breath, fatigue and cognitive impairment occurring continuously since the initial infection or appearing after three months and lasting a minimum of two months [7]. All these factors significantly affect the quality of life of patients who have experienced SARS-CoV-2 infection.

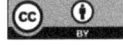

The intensive work of scientists from all over the world has led to the invention and introduction of vaccines with different mechanisms of action. Of these, the highest efficacy of 94.29% is demonstrated by vaccines based on RNA [8]. In Poland, 57,935,715 distributed doses of vaccine and 22,643,631 fully vaccinated persons were registered by 21 March 2023. One dose was received by 22,871,721 persons, two doses were received by 19,757,415 persons, three doses were by 192,285 persons and a booster dose was received by 15,114,294 persons [9].

In Poland, since the beginning of the pandemic, more than a dozen so-called 'temporary hospitals' (COVID-19 hospitals) have been set up to receive only patients with confirmed SARS-CoV-2 infection [10]. The majority of patients were in a severe general condition, with increased dyspnoea and reduced saturation.

With the length of the pandemic and the emergence of new data, increasing attention has been paid to the impact of surviving SARS-CoV-2 infection on patients' quality of life. Various forms can be used for this purpose, including The Medical Outcomes Study 36-item Short-Form Health Survey (SF-36) in the Polish-language version. Interest in short-form health questionnaires arose when the relatively frequent refusal to complete long forms during the Health Insurance Experiment was noted, resulting in a loss of patients from follow-up [11]. Through this, a method has been developed that should take a few minutes of a telephone call. The form comprehensively assesses the patient's perceived health status across broad domains of physical and emotional health. It focuses on evaluating eight quality of life indicators: physical functioning, role limitations due to physical health, pain complaints, a general sense of health, vitality, social functioning, role limitations due to emotional problems and a sense of mental health [12]. SF-36 has been used in a number of studies published in prestigious scientific journals on a variety of conditions, including rheumatoid arthritis, brain tumours, endometriosis and type 2 diabetes [13–16]. During the COVID-19 pandemic, it has also become useful for assessing quality of life after surviving this infection, examining, for example, the benefits of pulmonary rehabilitation [17]. The majority of previous studies focused on the assessment of quality of life among COVID-19 patients using different questionnaires such as EQ-5D-5L or WHOQOL-BREF.

The aim of our single-centre study is to evaluate the quality of life of patients who underwent SARS-CoV-2 infection and were hospitalised at the Pyrzowice Temporary Hospital for patients with COVID-19 at the multi-profile unit. We focused on a later period of time, 6 months after hospitalisation, to emphasise the long-term consequences on patients' overall well-being after this infection, specifically in the Polish population of internal medicine patients.

2. Materials and Methods

2.1. Study Population

Between November 2021 and January 2022, 598 patients were hospitalised at the Temporary Hospital in Katowice-Pyrzowice, Poland, due to SARS-CoV-2 infection and required urgent hospitalisation in a specialised internal medicine unit for acute respiratory failure. In total, 354 patients (159 women and 195 men) who survived the hospitalisation were invited to participate in the study. Ultimately, 125 patients (54 women and 71 men) who met all inclusion criteria and did not meet the exclusion criteria were included in the study (Figure 1).

Telephone interviews were conducted between May and August 2022, during which questions from the SF-36 questionnaire were asked to subjectively assess quality of life 6 months after hospitalisation for SARS-CoV-2 infection. At the beginning of the telephone call, each patient was asked for consent to the survey. All procedures performed in the studies were in accordance with the 1964 Helsinki declaration and its later amendments or comparable ethical standards. Respondents were also asked about receiving a SARS-CoV-2 vaccine before and after hospitalisation and the number of doses taken.

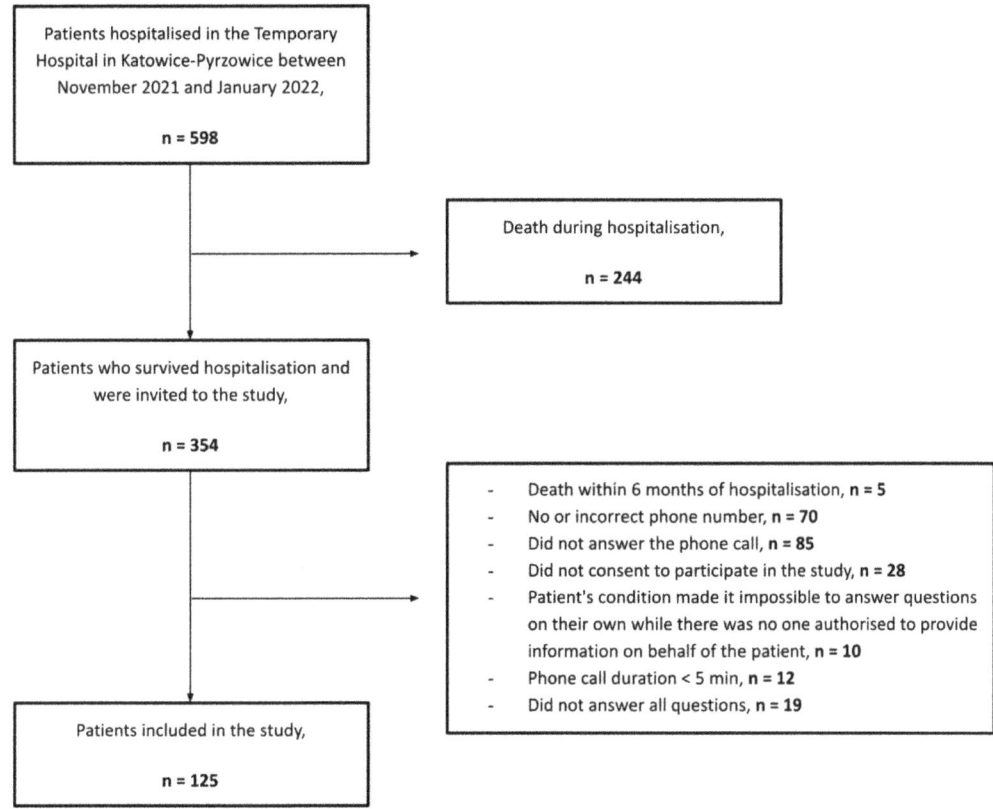

Figure 1. Study flowchart.

The protocol for this study was approved by the Bioethics Committee of the Medical University of Silesia in Katowice (consent nr. PCN/CBN/0052/KB/103/22). Inclusion and exclusion criteria are presented in Table 1.

Table 1. Inclusion and exclusion criteria.

Inclusion Criteria	Exclusion Criteria
Patient age ≥ 18 years old	Death of a patient within 6 months from the end of hospitalisation in the Temporary Hospital in Katowice-Pyrzowice
Call duration ≥ 5 min	Missing or incorrect contact telephone number of the patient
Verbal consent of the patient to a telephone interview	Failure to answer the phone by the patient (after 3 attempts, with an interval of 5 days between each attempt)
Obtaining answers to all questions in the SF-36 questionnaire during a telephone interview	Patient's condition not allowing him/her to answer the SF-36 questionnaire on his/her own during the telephone interview (dementia; mental disorder) while there was no authorized person to provide information on behalf of the patient

2.2. SF-36 Questionnaire and Score Calculations

The Polish version of the SF-36 (Short Form Health Survey) questionnaire [12], which was based on the English version [18], was used to assess quality of life (QOL). In the Polish version, the wording of 4 from 36 items was changed in 4 different questions. The SF-36 questionnaire is a subjective tool that allows a simple and quick assessment of QOL. It was designed so that the questions are understandable to the respondent and measure different aspects of quality of life. It allows for the study of both the general population and different groups of patients and is designed to meet the psychometric standards necessary for group comparison [19]. The SF-36 questionnaire and its Polish version are well-researched methods with proven reliability and validity [20–22].

The questionnaire consists of 11 questions with 36 statements that assess 8 quality of life indicators: physical functioning (PF; 10 items), role—physical (RP; 4 items), bodily pain (BP; 2 items), general health (GH; 5 items), vitality (VT; 4 items), social functioning (SF; 2 items), role—emotional (RE; 3 items), and mental health (MH; 5 items). The questionnaire contains two subscales, one assessing physical health based on PF, RP, BP and GH, and a subscale assessing mental health based on VT, SF, RE and PW. The respondent evaluates the statements based on the last 4 weeks. In addition, question 2 assesses current health status compared to that one year ago.

In the Polish version of the questionnaire, points are given when a dysfunction or limitation is present when assessing a statement. Questions 4 and 5 are answered in a dichotomous yes/no manner, and the remaining questions (1–3, 6–11) are rated on a 3-, 5-, or 6-point Likert scale. The Likert scale is a psychometric scale commonly used in questionnaire studies and allows for the differentiation of respondents' attitudes. The respondent selects the answer on the scale that most closely matches how they feel. It is usually an unpaired scale in which the extreme values correspond to the most positive and negative responses and the middle response is neutral [23].

The total quality of life index is the sum of the scores for all 11 questions and ranges from 0 to 171 in the Polish version of the questionnaire. This provides an overall assessment of health status, where the highest scores indicate the lowest subjective level of quality of life. Questionnaires, complete scoring instructions and differences between the Polish SF-36 questionnaire and English SF-36 questionnaire are specified in the supplementary (Supplementary File S1).

2.3. Statistical Analysis

Quantitative and qualitative data were collected using Excel (version 16.75.2, Microsoft, Redmond, WA, USA), and statistical analysis was performed in Statistica 13.3 (StatSoft, Kraków, Poland). An initial, automatic analysis was performed to search for missing data and anomalous values. The assessment of the normality of the distribution of quantitative variables was performed with the Shapiro–Wilk test. In the absence of a normal distribution, the analysis of quantitative variables in relation to two-state grouping variables was performed using the Mann–Whitney U test. An attempt was made to evaluate the correlation of quantitative variables using the Spearman test and multi-parameter evaluation using the stepwise regression method without obtaining reliable results. The level of significance was $p < 0.05$.

3. Results

3.1. Characteristic of the Study Group

A total of 125 patients, including 71 men (56.8%), were qualified for the study on the basis of criteria defined by the SF-36 questionnaire. Among the patients who were in the study group, hospitalised at the Temporary Hospital in Katowice-Pyrzowice, many had a positive medical history. Sixty patients were confirmed to have hypertension (HA), which accounted for 48% of the study group. There was also a significant proportion of patients with ischaemic heart disease (IHD), numbered at 26, accounting for 20.8% of the total. A similar proportion comprised obese patients, with 27 patients (21.6%). There were 22 patients with chronic kidney disease (CKD), corresponding to 17.6% of patients in the study group. There were 20 patients with diabetes mellitus (DM), representing 16% of the study group. A positive oncological history was confirmed in 12 subjects (9.6%). Similarly, a history of stroke was frequently found in the study group, with 10 patients (8%). A smaller group of patients consisted of those with a positive pulmonary history, i.e., 11 patients with bronchial asthma, 4 patients with chronic obstructive pulmonary disease (COPD) and 3 patients with obstructive sleep apnoea (OBS), corresponding to 8.8%, 3.2% and 2.4% of the study group, respectively. The number of post-pulmonary embolism (PE) patients was 4 (3.2%). Nicotinism was reported by 12 patients (9.6%). The full list of characteristics of the study group is presented in the table below (Table 2).

Table 2. Characteristics of the study group.

Parameter	Value
Females	54 (43.2%)
Males	71 (56.8%)
Age	62.22 ± 14.61
Body Mass Index (kg/m^2)	29.64 ± 12.62
Obesity	27 (21.6%)
Smoking	12 (9.6%)
Chronic obstructive pulmonary disease	4 (3.2%)
Asthma	11 (8.8%)
Pulmonary embolism	4 (3.2%)
Organic brain syndrome	3 (2.4%)
Chronic kidney disease	22 (17.6%)
Diabetes mellitus	20 (16.0%)
Hypertension	60 (48.0%)
Ischaemic heart disease	26 (20.8%)
Ischaemic stroke	10 (8.0%)
Cancer	12 (9.6%)
Vaccinated	39 (31.2%)
Vaccinated—1 dose	3 (2.4%)
Vaccinated—2 doses	33 (26.4%)
Vaccinated—3 doses	3 (2.4%)

Among all patients included in the study, 39 patients were vaccinated against COVID-19, representing 31.2% of the total, of whom 3 patients (2.4%) received a baseline dose and 2 booster doses, 33 patients (26.4%) received a baseline dose and 1 booster dose, and 3 patients (2.4%) received only the baseline dose of the vaccine. No patients received a third booster dose because there was still no opportunity to be vaccinated with a third booster dose during the period before and during hospitalisation and during the follow-up (Table 2).

The mean age of all patients vaccinated against COVID-19 was 67.15 ± 13.06 years. The mean age of patients vaccinated against COVID-19 before hospitalisation was 68.60 ± 11.35 years, and that of patients vaccinated against COVID-19 after hospitalisation was 67.31 ± 12.92 years. In comparison, the mean age of all patients not vaccinated against COVID-19 was 60.35 ± 14.62 years. The mean age of patients not vaccinated against COVID-19 before hospitalisation was 64.57 ± 15.81 years, and that of patients vaccinated against COVID-19 after hospitalisation was 66.85 ± 13.86 years.

3.2. Main Findings

Statistical analysis was performed. The female:male gender ratio in the study group was 1:1.31. The study showed that women had significantly higher SF-36 scores ($p = 0.040$) compared to men, i.e., women received an average of 69.50 ± 35.63 points and men received an average of 56.65 ± 32.02 points on the SF-36 questionnaire. The study also found that patients with a history of CKD had significantly higher SF-36 scores ($p = 0.041$) compared to those without a history of CKD. Patients with CKD had an average score of 74.18 ± 29.10, while patients without CKD had an average score of 50.96 ± 34.66. This research indicated that patients with DM had significantly higher SF-36 scores ($p = 0.013$) compared to patients without known DM. Those with a history of DM had a mean score of 77.15 ± 26.68 and those without a history of DM had a mean score of 59.35 ± 34.71. The study revealed that COVID-19-vaccinated patients had significantly higher SF-36 values ($p = 0.015$) compared to COVID-19-non-vaccinated patients. COVID-19-vaccinated patients had an average score of 73.05 ± 30.92, and COVID-19-non-vaccinated patients had an average score of 56.23 ± 34.34. Median values for statistically significant variables are presented in the form of diagrams in the supplementary (Supplementary File S2). While analysing the data, some disease entities and burdens turned out not to be statistically significant. All independent variables are presented below (Table 3).

Table 3. Analysed independent variables in the study group of patients.

Parameter	*p*-Value
General	
Sex	0.04
Obesity	0.838
Smoking	0.746
Vaccinated	0.015
Diseases	
Chronic obstructive pulmonary disease	0.581
Asthma	0.8
Pulmonary embolism	0.555
Organic brain syndrome	0.162
Chronic kidney disease	0.041
Diabetes mellitus	0.013
Hypertension	0.429
Ischemic heart disease	0.098
Ischemic stroke	0.458
Cancer	0.11

4. Discussion

The study showed that COVID-19 vaccination does not improve quality of life after SARS-CoV-2 virus infection compared to that of non-vaccinated individuals. The study showed that people with CKD have significantly higher SF-36 scores, meaning that their QOL scores are worse than those without CKD. The study also found that people with DM have higher values on the questionnaire, which translates into a worse assessment of quality of life than that of people without DM. In the study, women's quality of life scores are significantly lower than men's.

Taboada et al. investigated quality of life in patients who underwent hospitalisation in an intensive care unit for SARS-CoV-2 infection. Patients assessed their quality of life and functional status 3–6 months before COVID-19 using the EuroQol Group Association's five-domain, three-level questionnaire (EQ-5D-3L), which consists of two sections: a descriptive system and a visual analogue scale. They obtained results showing that 67% of the patients studied had a significantly lower quality of life after hospital discharge, mainly due to reduced mobility and pain or discomfort [24]. In our study, we examined patients who were hospitalised in the internal medicine ward and did not end up in the intensive care unit. The difference in the study group (patients hospitalised in the ICU vs. patients hospitalised in the internal medicine ward) may have influenced the difference in the patients' quality of life scores as we suspect a more severe course of the disease in those who had to go to the ICU for this reason. In addition, these patients may have had an initially higher burden of concomitant diseases and may have been of older age than those hospitalised in an internal medicine ward. The EQ-5D-3L questionnaire was also used by Taboada et al. in their study, comparing quality of life and persistent symptoms after hospitalisation for COVID-19 among patients who required hospitalisation in an intensive care unit for COVID-19 and those who did not require intensive care hospitalisation. More ICU patients showed a worsening of their QOL compared to patients who were not hospitalised in an ICU ward (71.9% vs. 43.7%, $p = 0.004$). In total, 52.4% of all patients reported a worsening of at least one of the five dimensions analysed in the EQ-5D-3L, and 24% of all patients reported a worsening of two or more dimensions. More women than men reported problems with usual activities (25.0% vs. 12.1%, $p = 0.024$), pain or discomfort (45.2% vs. 26.3%, $p = 0.007$) and anxiety or depression (53.6% vs. 24.2%, $p < 0.001$) [25]. Similarly, in our study, women had significantly higher scores on the SF-36 and therefore had a lower quality of life than men did. As with the previous study, the differences in scores may have been due to the different study groups.

The EQ-5D-5L questionnaire was used by Tarazona et al. to assess quality of life in outpatients who had survived COVID-19. COVID-19 outpatients ($n = 96$) had significantly lower health-related quality of life than controls ($n = 81$) did one year after SARS-CoV-2 infection; the EQ-5D-5L index averaged 0.87 in examined cases and 0.95 in controls ($p = 0.002$) [26]. This work compared outpatients who developed COVID-19 to patients who were not diagnosed with COVID-19 disease. The difference in results between this work and those of Tarazona et al. can also be explained by the different selection of the study group—in our work, we only considered patients diagnosed with COVID-19 and investigated the impact of the disease on their quality of life after the disease. We did not compare this with a control group that had not contracted COVID-19 or had not been hospitalised for COVID-19 disease. Qu et al. also used the SF-36 questionnaire to assess the quality of life of patients after hospitalisation for COVID-19, in a version with scores ranging from 0 to 100 points. Apart from the 'general health' category, in all other categories included in the questionnaire, the study participants scored significantly lower ($p < 0.001$). Quality of life was assessed 3 months after discharge and compared to norms for the general Chinese population. In addition, men relative to women had a better quality of physical and mental health after hospital discharge [27]. Despite the similar timing of the QOL assessment in patients in this study, the QOL scores obtained were compared to the overall norms for the general population and not to quality of life before the disease, as in our study. This may have influenced the difference in results between the papers.

Navarro et al., who also used the EQ-5D-5L scale, observed a reduction in the quality of life of up to 56% in patients hospitalised with moderate to severe SARS-CoV-2 infection. In contrast to this work, Navarro et al. included patients as early as 30 days after the onset of first symptoms, whereas in our study, patients were not interviewed until approximately three months after hospitalisation at the earliest. Bearing in mind that COVID-19 disease is an acute viraemic infection, this may have influenced the final results of the study, as the severity of COVID-19 disease symptoms may be greater (and thus quality of life in such individuals may be visibly lower) in those newly recovered from the disease compared to those who have already undergone some convalescence [28]. Van der Sar-van der Brugge et al. used the SF-36 to assess HRQoL in 101 patients with SARS-CoV-2 pneumonia, classified as moderate or severe pneumonia according to WHO definitions. Six weeks after hospital discharge, significant deterioration was found in all SF-36 domains except pain ($p = 0.0001$). The domains with the greatest reductions were physical role limitation, physical functioning and vitality [29]. Similar to the work of Navarro et al. the timing of the QOL assessment occurred earlier than that in our study (6 weeks after discharge vs. 3 months after hospitalisation) which may have influenced the difference in results. Howlader et al. used the WHOQOL-BREF questionnaire to assess quality of life in 3244 randomly selected patients in Bangladesh. The study found significantly lower QoL in women, those with chronic concomitant diseases, the unemployed and the elderly. However, symptoms decreased each day after diagnosis [30]. Similarly, in our study, women and people with chronic diseases (such as DM2 or CKD) had a lower quality of life. It can also be hypothesised that the later the QOL assessment is carried out, the less it will be influenced by COVID-19-related symptoms and more by the patient's current illnesses and situation, such as age, gender or chronic diseases. The EQ-5D-5L questionnaire was also used in Giao et al.'s study, with the addition of the EuroQoL-Visual Analogue Scale (EQ-VAS) score to determine self-assessed health status. Lower scores were reported among those aged 60 years and older, women, those with comorbidities, those with persistent symptoms, those who were living alone and those who were experiencing stress (all $p < 0.001$) [31]. Ayuso Garcia et al. also used the EQ-5D in combination with the EQ-VAS and EQ-Health. Both the EQ-VAS and EQ-Health Index were lower in women, patients older than 65 years, patients with comorbidities and those who required hospitalisation during acute SARS-CoV-2 infection [32]. In our study, similarly lower scores were obtained for people with diabetes, chronic kidney disease, women and vaccinated people who initially had more comorbidities and were older. In the study by d'Ettorre et al. using the EQ-5D-5L and EQ-VAS scales, female gender, unemployment status and chronic comorbidities were the most common predictors of having any problems in each EQ-5D-5L domain, and an older age and higher body mass index (BMI) were also found to be associated with lower EQ-VAS scores [33]. As in our study, lower quality of life was shown here among patients with pre-existing chronic diseases, including type 2 diabetes.

It should be noted that the study analysed survivors of life-threatening conditions associated with severe respiratory failure due to SARS-CoV-2 virus infection. A large number of patients were ultimately not included in the study group due to death during hospitalisation itself and after the hospitalisation period. The status of having been vaccinated of this population was not assessed in this work.

Those vaccinated against COVID-19 who were included in the study described their health status by assessing their quality of life as worse than those who were not vaccinated. However, the mean age of the unvaccinated patients was visibly lower than that of the vaccinated patients (60.35 ± 14.62 vs. 67.15 ± 13.06). Additionally, the number of concomitant diseases was higher in the vaccinated than in the unvaccinated group (2.44 ± 1733 vs. 1.13 ± 1170). We can therefore suspect that vaccinated persons present a lower quality of life than unvaccinated persons do due to a higher burden of concomitant diseases and an older age. In this study, the quality of life assessed by women was lower compared to that of men, which is confirmed by other studies. In the work by Lee, K.H. et al. and Badr, H.E. et al. that assessed quality of life, women also scored lower than men did [34,35]. In this work, patients with CKD and DM reported worse quality of life than did those who did not have the aforementioned disease entities.

In summary, other studies present similar findings of reduced quality of life after SARS-CoV-2 infection; however, they used either a different questionnaire or focused on another time point than those in our study. We concentrated on a specific period of time, 6 months after hospitalisation, to highlight the long-term implications on patients' general condition after this disease. Moreover, most of the existing studies presented the results obtained from specific populations, such as the Chinese population in Qu et al.'s study or the Bangladeshi population in Howlander et al.'s study. We strongly believe that our results can be a valuable source of information about the QOL of COVID-19 survivors 6 months after hospitalisation in the Polish population.

5. Limitations

Several limitations of this study should be highlighted. Firstly, the study involved a small group of patients and all patients were treated at a single centre, so the results of this study should not be generalised. There were more unvaccinated patients in the study group than there were vaccinated patients, which may have influenced the QOL results obtained. Another limitation is that the QOL of patients was examined only once after 6 months of hospitalisation, so the data obtained do not describe the long-term status of patients and make it impossible to compare patients' status over time. A very important problem is the lack of SF-36 norms for the Polish population, which makes it impossible to compare the results obtained to those of the general Polish population. In addition, conducting the survey by telephone resulted in the elimination of many patients from the study due to problems with correct contact details, availability or ability to respond. Finally, a disadvantage of surveying by telephone questionnaire is the inability to verify the veracity of patients' answers and the lack of use of objective methods such as laboratory tests. A multicentre study including more follow-ups over several years would allow a more complete assessment of the QOL of patients after hospitalisation for COVID-19.

6. Conclusions

Our study showed that people with persistent diseases, such as chronic kidney disease or diabetes mellitus, had lower quality of life after SARS-CoV-2 infection. Moreover, women complained about a lower quality of life than that of men. However, people who were vaccinated for COVID-19 had a lower quality of life than did non-vaccinated people. This is possibly due to the higher mean age, and probably the higher disease burden, in the vaccinated group. More research is needed to further investigate this matter.

Supplementary Materials: The following supporting information can be downloaded at https://www.mdpi.com/article/10.3390/jcm12165327/s1, File S1: Differences between Polish and English version of SF-36 questionnaire; File S2: Diagrams with median values for statistically significant variables.

Author Contributions: Conceptualisation, M.C. (Marta Chamera), M.J., M.K. (Maciej Kaźmierski), P.L. and W.Ł.; methodology, J.K. and M.C. (Marta Chamera); software, B.R. and M.C. (Maciej Cebula); validation, A.L., M.K. (Maciej Koźlik), M.K. (Maciej Kaźmierski)., M.C. (Maciej Cebula) and W.K.; formal analysis, M.C. (Marta Chamera), W.K. and W.Ł.; investigation, W.Ł., B.R. and W.K.; resources, P.L., M.J. and M.K. (Maciej Koźlik); data curation, B.R., M.K. (Maciej Koźlik), J.K. and P.L.; writing—original draft preparation, A.L., M.K. (Maciej Koźlik), P.L. and W.K.; writing—review and editing, A.L and B.R.; visualisation, M.C. (Marta Chamera) and W.Ł.; supervision, M.K. (Maciej Koźlik) and M.K. (Maciej Kaźmierski); project administration, A.L. and M.K. (Maciej Koźlik). All authors have read and agreed to the published version of the manuscript.

Funding: This research received no external funding.

Institutional Review Board Statement: The study was conducted in accordance with the Declaration of Helsinki, and approved by the Institutional Review Board (or Ethics Committee) of Medical University of Silesia (CN/CBN/0052/KB/103/22).

Informed Consent Statement: Informed consent was obtained from all subjects involved in the study.

Data Availability Statement: The data presented in this study are available on request from the corresponding author. The data are not publicly available due to privacy reasons.

Conflicts of Interest: The authors declare no conflict of interest.

References

1. WHO Coronavirus (COVID-19) Dashboard | WHO Coronavirus (COVID-19) Dashboard with Vaccination Data. Available online: https://covid19.who.int/ (accessed on 14 June 2023).
2. Kaur, N.; Gupta, I.; Singh, H.; Karia, R.; Ashraf, A.; Habib, A.; Patel, U.K.; Malik, P. Epidemiological and Clinical Characteristics of 6635 COVID-19 Patients: A Pooled Analysis. *SN Compr. Clin. Med.* **2020**, *2*, 1048–1052. [CrossRef] [PubMed]

3. Patel, U.; Malik, P.; Usman, M.S.; Mehta, D.; Sharma, A.; Malik, F.A.; Khan, N.; Siddiqi, T.J.; Ahmed, J.; Patel, A.; et al. Age-Adjusted Risk Factors Associated with Mortality and Mechanical Ventilation Utilization Amongst COVID-19 Hospitalizations—A Systematic Review and Meta-Analysis. *SN Compr. Clin. Med.* **2020**, *2*, 1740–1749. [CrossRef]
4. Gavriatopoulou, M.; Ntanasis-Stathopoulos, I.; Korompoki, E.; Fotiou, D.; Migkou, M.; Tzanninis, I.-G.; Psaltopoulou, T.; Kastritis, E.; Terpos, E.; Dimopoulos, M.A. Emerging Treatment Strategies for COVID-19 Infection. *Clin. Exp. Med.* **2021**, *21*, 167–179. [CrossRef] [PubMed]
5. Crook, H.; Raza, S.; Nowell, J.; Young, M.; Edison, P. Long COVID—Mechanisms, Risk Factors, and Management. *BMJ* **2021**, *374*, n1648. [CrossRef] [PubMed]
6. Malik, P.; Patel, K.; Pinto, C.; Jaiswal, R.; Tirupathi, R.; Pillai, S.; Patel, U. Post-acute COVID-19 Syndrome (PCS) and Health-related Quality of Life (HRQoL)—A Systematic Review and Meta-analysis. *J. Med. Virol.* **2022**, *94*, 253–262. [CrossRef]
7. Post COVID-19 Condition (Long COVID). Available online: https://www.who.int/europe/news-room/fact-sheets/item/post-covid-19-condition (accessed on 14 June 2023).
8. Cai, C.; Peng, Y.; Shen, E.; Huang, Q.; Chen, Y.; Liu, P.; Guo, C.; Feng, Z.; Gao, L.; Zhang, X.; et al. A Comprehensive Analysis of the Efficacy and Safety of COVID-19 Vaccines. *Mol. Ther.* **2021**, *29*, 2794–2805. [CrossRef]
9. Raport Szczepień Przeciwko COVID-19—Szczepienie Przeciwko COVID-19—Portal Gov.pl (COVID-19 Vaccination Report—COVID-19 Vaccination—Portal Gov.pl). Available online: https://www.gov.pl/web/szczepimysie/raport-szczepien-przeciwko-covid-19 (accessed on 14 June 2023).
10. Interpelacja Nr 22352—Tekst—Sejm Rzeczypospolitej Polskiej (Interpellation No 22352—Text—Parliament of the Republic of Poland). Available online: https://sejm.gov.pl/Sejm9.nsf/InterpelacjaTresc.xsp?key=BZZFXZ (accessed on 14 June 2023).
11. Ware, J.; Snoww, K.; Ma, K.; Bg, G. *SF36 Health Survey: Manual and Interpretation Guide*; Quality Metric, Inc.: Lincoln, RI, USA, 1993; Volume 1, p. 30.
12. Tylka, J.; Piotrowicz, R. Cardiac Rehabilitation Quality of Life SF-36 Questionnaire-the Polish Version. *Kardiol. Pol. (Pol. Heart J.)* **2009**, *67*, 1166–1169.
13. Matcham, F.; Scott, I.C.; Rayner, L.; Hotopf, M.; Kingsley, G.H.; Norton, S.; Scott, D.L.; Steer, S. The Impact of Rheumatoid Arthritis on Quality-of-Life Assessed Using the SF-36: A Systematic Review and Meta-Analysis. *Semin. Arthritis Rheum.* **2014**, *44*, 123–130. [CrossRef]
14. Bunevicius, A. Reliability and Validity of the SF-36 Health Survey Questionnaire in Patients with Brain Tumors: A Cross-Sectional Study. *Health Qual. Life Outcomes* **2017**, *15*, 92. [CrossRef]
15. Sima, R.-M.; Pleş, L.; Socea, B.; Sklavounos, P.; Negoi, I.; Stănescu, A.-D.; Iordache, I.-I.; Hamoud, B.H.; Radosa, M.P.; Juhasz-Boess, I.; et al. Evaluation of the SF-36 Questionnaire for Assessment of the Quality of Life of Endometriosis Patients Undergoing Treatment: A Systematic Review and Meta-Analysis. *Exp. Ther. Med.* **2021**, *22*, 1283. [CrossRef]
16. Abbasi-Ghahramanloo, A.; Soltani-Kermanshahi, M.; Mansori, K.; Khazaei-Pool, M.; Sohrabi, M.; Baradaran, H.R.; Talebloo, Z.; Gholami, A. Comparison of SF-36 and WHOQoL-BREF in Measuring Quality of Life in Patients with Type 2 Diabetes. *Int. J. Gen. Med.* **2020**, *13*, 497–506. [CrossRef]
17. Gloeckl, R.; Leitl, D.; Jarosch, I.; Schneeberger, T.; Nell, C.; Stenzel, N.; Vogelmeier, C.F.; Kenn, K.; Koczulla, A.R. Benefits of Pulmonary Rehabilitation in COVID-19: A Prospective Observational Cohort Study. *ERJ Open Res.* **2021**, *7*, 00108–02021. [CrossRef]
18. Ware, J.E.J.; Sherbourne, C.D. The MOS 36-Ltem Short-Form Health Survey (SF-36): I. Conceptual Framework and Item Selection. *Med. Care* **1992**, *30*, 473. [CrossRef]
19. Ware, J.E. SF-36 Health Survey Update. *Spine* **2000**, *25*, 3130–3139. [CrossRef]
20. Ware, J.E.; Gandek, B. Overview of the SF-36 Health Survey and the International Quality of Life Assessment (IQOLA) Project. *J. Clin. Epidemiol.* **1998**, *51*, 903–912. [CrossRef] [PubMed]
21. Żołnierczyk-Zreda, D. The Polish version of the SF-36v2 questionnaire for the quality of life assessment. *Przegląd Lek.* **2010**, *67*, 1302–1307.
22. Marcinowicz, L.; Sienkiewicz, J. Assessment of the Validity and Reliability of the Polish Version of the SF-36 Questionnaire—Preliminary Findings. *Przegląd Lek.* **2003**, *60* (Suppl. S6), 103–106.
23. Joshi, A.; Kale, S.; Chandel, S.; Pal, D. Likert Scale: Explored and Explained. *Br. J. Appl. Sci. Technol.* **2015**, *7*, 396–403. [CrossRef]
24. Taboada, M.; Moreno, E.; Cariñena, A.; Rey, T.; Pita-Romero, R.; Leal, S.; Sanduende, Y.; Rodríguez, A.; Nieto, C.; Vilas, E.; et al. Quality of Life, Functional Status, and Persistent Symptoms after Intensive Care of COVID-19 Patients. *Br. J. Anaesth.* **2021**, *126*, e110–e113. [CrossRef] [PubMed]
25. Taboada, M.; Rodríguez, N.; Diaz-Vieito, M.; Domínguez, M.J.; Casal, A.; Riveiro, V.; Cariñena, A.; Moreno, E.; Pose, A.; Valdés, L.; et al. Quality of life and persistent symptoms after hospitalization for COVID-19. A prospective observational study comparing ICU with non-ICU patients. *Rev. Esp. Anestesiol. Reanim. (Engl. Ed.)* **2022**, *69*, 326–335. [CrossRef] [PubMed]
26. Tarazona, V.; Kirouchena, D.; Clerc, P.; Pinsard-Laventure, F.; Bourrion, B. Quality of Life in COVID-19 Outpatients: A Long-Term Follow-Up Study. *J. Clin. Med.* **2022**, *11*, 6478. [CrossRef]
27. Qu, G.; Zhen, Q.; Wang, W.; Fan, S.; Wu, Q.; Zhang, C.; Li, B.; Liu, G.; Yu, Y.; Li, Y.; et al. Health-related Quality of Life of COVID-19 Patients after Discharge: A Multicenter Follow-up Study. *J. Clin. Nurs.* **2021**, *30*, 1742–1750. [CrossRef] [PubMed]

28. Ordinola Navarro, A.; Cervantes-Bojalil, J.; Cobos Quevedo, O.d.J.; Avila Martínez, A.; Hernández-Jiménez, C.A.; Pérez Álvarez, E.; González Gil, A.; Peralta Amaro, A.L.; Vera-Lastra, O.; Lopez Luis, B.A. Decreased Quality of Life and Spirometric Alterations Even after Mild-Moderate COVID-19. *Respir. Med.* **2021**, *181*, 106391. [CrossRef]
29. van der Sar-van der Brugge, S.; Talman, S.; Boonman-de Winter, L.; de Mol, M.; Hoefman, E.; van Etten, R.W.; De Backer, I.C. Pulmonary Function and Health-Related Quality of Life after COVID-19 Pneumonia. *Respir. Med.* **2021**, *176*, 106272. [CrossRef] [PubMed]
30. Hawlader, M.D.H.; Rashid, M.U.; Khan, M.A.S.; Ara, T.; Nabi, M.H.; Haque, M.M.A.; Matin, K.F.; Hossain, M.A.; Rahman, M.A.; Hossian, M.; et al. Quality of Life of COVID-19 Recovered Patients in Bangladesh. *PLoS ONE* **2021**, *16*, e0257421. [CrossRef]
31. Huynh, G.; Nguyen, B.T.; Nguyen, H.T.N.; Le, N.T.; An, P.L.; Tran, T.D. Health-Related Quality of Life Among Patients Recovered From COVID-19. *Inquiry* **2022**, *59*, 469580221143630. [CrossRef]
32. Ayuso García, B.; Pérez López, A.; Besteiro Balado, Y.; Romay Lema, E.; García País, M.J.; Marchán-López, Á.; Rodríguez Álvarez, A.; Corredoira Sánchez, J.; Rabuñal Rey, R. Health-related quality of life in patients recovered from COVID-19. *J. Healthc. Qual. Res.* **2022**, *37*, 208–215. [CrossRef]
33. d'Ettorre, G.; Vassalini, P.; Coppolelli, V.; Gentilini Cacciola, E.; Sanitinelli, L.; Maddaloni, L.; Fabris, S.; Mastroianni, C.M.; d'Ettorre, G.; Ceccarelli, G. Health-Related Quality of Life in Survivors of Severe COVID-19 Infection. *Pharmacol. Rep.* **2022**, *74*, 1286–1295. [CrossRef]
34. Lee, K.H.; Xu, H.; Wu, B. Gender Differences in Quality of Life among Community-Dwelling Older Adults in Low- and Middle-Income Countries: Results from the Study on Global AGEing and Adult Health (SAGE). *BMC Public Health* **2020**, *20*, 114. [CrossRef] [PubMed]
35. Badr, H.E.; Rao, S.; Manee, F. Gender Differences in Quality of Life, Physical Activity, and Risk of Hypertension among Sedentary Occupation Workers. *Qual. Life Res.* **2021**, *30*, 1365–1377. [CrossRef]

Disclaimer/Publisher's Note: The statements, opinions and data contained in all publications are solely those of the individual author(s) and contributor(s) and not of MDPI and/or the editor(s). MDPI and/or the editor(s) disclaim responsibility for any injury to people or property resulting from any ideas, methods, instructions or products referred to in the content.

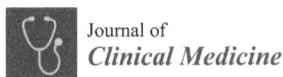

Article

Indirect Effects of the COVID-19 Pandemic on In-Hospital Outcomes among Internal Medicine Departments: A Double-Center Retrospective Study

Maurizio Di Marco [†], Nicoletta Miano [†], Simona Marchisello, Giuseppe Coppolino, Giuseppe L'Episcopo, Sabrina Scilletta, Concetta Spichetti, Serena Torre, Roberto Scicali, Luca Zanoli, Agostino Gaudio, Pietro Castellino, Salvatore Piro, Francesco Purrello and Antonino Di Pino *

Department of Clinical and Experimental Medicine, University of Catania, 95122 Catania, Italy; maurizio.dimarco@studium.unict.it (M.D.M.); nicoletta.miano@gmail.com (N.M.); simomarchi91@hotmail.it (S.M.); giuseppecoppolino93@gmail.com (G.C.); peppe94@gmail.com (G.L.); sabrinascilletta@gmail.com (S.S.); ketty1985@virgilio.it (C.S.); serenatorre@tiscali.it (S.T.); roberto.scicali@unict.it (R.S.); luca.zanoli@unict.it (L.Z.); agostino.gaudio@unict.it (A.G.); pcastell@unict.it (P.C.); salvatore.piro@unict.it (S.P.); francesco.purrello@unict.it (F.P.)
* Correspondence: antonino.dipino@unict.it; Tel.: +39-0957595453
[†] These authors contributed equally to this work.

Abstract: The coronavirus disease 19 (COVID-19) emergency led to rearrangements of healthcare systems with a significant impact on those internal medicine departments that had not been converted to COVID-19 wards. A reduced number of departments, indeed, had to cope with the same number of patients along with a lack of management of patients' chronic diseases. We conducted a retrospective study aimed at examining the consequences of the COVID-19 pandemic on internal medicine departments that were not directly managing COVID-19 patients. Data from 619 patients were collected: 247 subjects hospitalized in 2019 (pre-COVID-19 era), 178 in 2020 (COVID-19 outbreak era) and 194 in 2021 (COVID-19 ongoing era). We found that in 2020 in-hospital mortality was significantly higher than in 2019 (17.4% vs. 5.3%, $p = 0.009$) as well as length of in-hospital stay (LOS) (12.7 ± 6.8 vs. 11 ± 6.2, $p = 0.04$). Finally, we performed a logistic regression analysis of the major determinants of mortality in the entire study population, which highlighted an association between mortality, being bedridden ($\beta = 1.4$, $p = 0.004$), respiratory failure ($\beta = 1.5$, $p = 0.001$), glomerular filtration rate ($\beta = -0.16$, $p = 0.03$) and hospitalization in the COVID-19 outbreak era ($\beta = 1.6$, $p = 0.005$). Our study highlights how the COVID-19 epidemic may have caused an increase in mortality and LOS even in patients not directly suffering from this infection.

Keywords: COVID-19; internal medicine departments; in-hospital outcomes; length of in-hospital stay; in-hospital mortality; sepsis

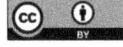

1. Introduction

The coronavirus disease 19 (COVID-19) pandemic has been an ongoing global emergency since the first case was detected in December 2019; accordingly, from 1 January 2020 to 31 December 2021, a total of 5.94 million COVID-19 deaths were reported worldwide [1] and seroprevalence studies showed that the real prevalence of severe acute respiratory syndrome coronavirus 2 (SARS-CoV-2) infection could be 10 times more than recorded [2,3]. This led many governments around the world to modify population lifestyle through social distancing and lockdown measures to limit the spread of infection. The SARS-CoV-2 pandemic led to several devastating effects not only on directly affected patients, but also on the general population in terms of healthcare, economic and social damage [4]. Regarding mortality, a recent study published in The Lancet demonstrated that the global all-age rate of excess deaths related to COVID-19 was 120.3 deaths per 100,000 people [5]. These data reflect not only deaths due to COVID-19 alone, but also the mortality indirectly caused by the SARS-CoV-2 pandemic. Specifically, the COVID-19 emergency led to rearrangements of healthcare systems including a reduction in outpatient visits, an increased use of telemedicine, a redistribution of healthcare professionals and a different organization of resources in an emergency setting [6–9]. Among the several arrangements implemented to tackle this burden, hospital wards of almost all medical and surgical specialties were closed or converted into wards for the sub-intensive care of COVID-19 patients, and in many cases entire hospitals were converted into COVID-19 hospitals. Moreover, the number of emergency hospital admissions significantly dropped during the COVID-19 epidemic, with the exception of admissions for falls and fragility fractures that continued at comparable rates [10]. These indirectly COVID-19-related changes were the result of a variety of factors, including societal disruptions, psychological disorders in families of patients severely affected by COVID-19, decreased social interaction, which mitigated the transmission of endemic pathogens, and diminished air pollution [11]. The COVID-19 pandemic had significant indirect effects on the elderly population, including social isolation, malnutrition, and physical inactivity, with a consequent negative impact on their mobility and respiratory function, which provoked a frailty condition [12].

The above-mentioned changes had a significant impact on internal medicine departments that had not been converted to COVID-19 wards. A reduced number of departments had to cope with the same number of patients as before the pandemic and also with a lack of management of patients' chronic diseases, which had a negative influence on the acute events for which they were admitted. Furthermore, this situation led to increased pressure on internal medicine departments from emergency departments (EDs) due to a lack of beds [13,14].

Based on these considerations, we conducted a retrospective study, which aimed to examine the indirect consequences of the COVID-19 pandemic on internal medicine departments that were not directly managing SARS-CoV-2 patients. In particular, we examined different clinical outcomes during these period to investigate whether COVID-19 influenced the morbidity and mortality of non-SARS-CoV-2 infected patients and whether, after more than one year since the beginning of the pandemic, these data underwent modifications.

2. Materials and Methods

2.1. Patients and Calculations

We collected clinical-pathological data from the medical records of patients hospitalized in two internal medicine departments of Catania (Azienda Ospedaliera di Alta Specializzazione Garibaldi Nesima, and Azienda Ospedaliera Universitaria—Policlinico/San Marco Gaspare Rodolico) from September to November in the years 2019, 2020 and 2021. These data were collected to obtain a retrospective evaluation of the clinical characteristics of patients hospitalized in internal medicine departments in the pre-COVID-19 (2019), COVID-19 outbreak (2020), and COVID-19 ongoing (2021) eras. According to hospital protocol, all the patients underwent a double negative PCR swab test for SARS-CoV-2 before admission to exclude the possibility of SARS-CoV-2 infection. Moreover, in patients with radiological or clinical elements suspected to be COVID-19, research using a PCR to detect SARS-CoV-2 from a sample of bronchus alveolar lavage was performed.

The data included: (1) age, gender, comorbidities (hypertension, diabetes mellitus, chronic heart failure, chronic kidney disease, previous myocardial infarction, previous stroke, chronic obstructive pulmonary disease [COPD], chronic liver diseases, solid tumors, onco-hematological diseases, and being bedridden), home-therapy drugs; (2) the department from which the patient was transferred to the internal medicine department; (3) clinical events that occurred during hospitalization (death, length of in-hospital stay [LOS], diagnosis of sepsis, the need for blood transfusion, multidrug-resistant [MDR] germ isolation, and respiratory failure); (3) clinical and biochemical characteristics of the patients on admission to internal medicine departments (systolic, diastolic and mean blood pressure

[SBP, DBP and MBP], fasting glucose, creatinine, estimated glomerular filtration rate [eGFR], total cholesterol, high-density lipoprotein cholesterol [HDL], low-density lipoprotein cholesterol [LDL], triglycerides, total proteins, albumin, aspartate aminotransferase [AST], alanine aminotransferase [ALT], N-terminal pro-brain natriuretic peptide [NT-proBNP], procalcitonin, high-sensitivity C-reactive protein [hs-CRP], erythrocyte sedimentation rate [ESR], complete blood count, hemoglobin, hematocrit, international normalized ratio [INR], and venous thromboembolism [VTE] risk).

We considered the high/low cut-off of NT-proBNP, procalcitonin, AST, ALT and hs-CRP according to upper laboratory limits as follows: NT-proBNP, 260 pg/mL; procalcitonin, 0.5 µg/L; AST, 34 UI/L; ALT, 55 UI/L; hs-CRP, 0.5 mg/dL.

eGFR was assessed using the chronic kidney disease epidemiology collaboration (CKD-EPI) equation [15]; and VTE risk was estimated using the Padua score [16].

2.2. Statistical Analysis

Statistical comparisons of clinical and biomedical parameters were performed using Stat View 6.0 for Windows. Data are given as means SD or median (IQR). Each variable's distributional characteristics including normality were assessed using the Kolmogorov–Smirnov test. Statistical analysis included ANOVA for continuous variables and the chi-square test for non-continuous variables. A p-value less than 0.05 was considered statistically significant. When necessary, numerical variables were logarithmically transformed to reduce skewness, and values are expressed as median and interquartile range.

Furthermore, a logistic regression analysis using a stepwise approach was performed to investigate the association of clinical and biochemical variables with in-hospital mortality. This analysis was performed for each group (pre-COVID-19 era, COVID-19 outbreak era and post-COVID-19 era) separately and also considering the entire population.

2.3. Ethics

This retrospective study was approved by the Ethical Board of Catania 2 (N° prot. 370/2021). All procedures performed in studies involving human participants were in accordance with the ethical standards of institutional and/or national research committees and with the Declaration of Helsinki. The requirement for informed consent was waived because of the retrospective design of the data collection.

3. Results

Data from 619 patients were collected: 247 subjects were hospitalized in 2019 (pre-COVID-19 era), 178 in 2020 (COVID-19 outbreak era) and 194 in 2021 (COVID-19 ongoing era).

The clinical characteristics of the subjects are presented in Table 1 and the biochemical parameters at admission to the internal medicine departments are shown in Table 2.

3.1. Comparison between COVID-19 Outbreak Era, Pre-COVID-19 Era, and COVID-19 Ongoing Era

No differences were found regarding age, number of bedridden patients, number of home-therapy drugs, SBP, DBP or MBP between the COVID-19 outbreak era (2020) and the pre-COVID-19 era (2019) patients. In the COVID-19 outbreak era, patients were mainly admitted from the ED short stay unit (SSU) (58.4%), whereas in 2019, patients were admitted directly from the ED (60.7%). Furthermore, the number of elective admissions was significantly lower in 2020 than in 2019 (1.7% vs. 9.3%, $p = 0.001$) and the number of patients transferred from other departments was significantly higher (19.7% in 2020 vs. 0.8% in 2019, $p < 0.001$). The percentage of subjects with chronic kidney disease (CKD) was significantly higher in 2020 than in 2019 (26.4% vs. 13.4% respectively; $p < 0.001$) and the Padua score was higher in 2020 than in 2019 (3.74 ± 1.95 vs. 3.14 ± 1.8 respectively, $p = 0.006$) (Table 1).

In the COVID-19 outbreak era, patients showed a significantly lower eGFR than in the pre-COVID-19 era (69.8 ± 34.6 vs. 82.7 ± 31.2 mL/min/1.63 m^2, p = 0.001) and INR was higher without reaching statistical significance (1.3 ± 0.5 vs. 1.2 ± 0.33, p = 0.12) (Table 2).

Table 1. Clinical characteristics of the study population.

	Pre-COVID-19 Era (2019) (n = 247)	COVID-19 Outbreak Era (2020) (n = 178)	COVID-19 Ongoing Era (2021) (n = 194)
Age—years	65 ± 18.3	67.6 ± 17.8	68.6 ± 16.2
Sex—female n. (%)	120 (48.6%)	58 (32.6%) *	82 (42.3%)
DEPARTMENT OF PROVENANCE—n. (%)			
Emergency department	150 (60.7%)	36 (20.2%) *	35 (18.2%) *
ED SSU	72 (29.1%)	104 (58.4%) *	143 (73.7%) *
Elective admissions	23 (9.3%)	3 (1.7%) *	0 (0%) *
Transferred from other departments	2 (0.8%)	35 (19.7%) *	16 (8.1%)
Bedridden subjects—n. (%)	67 (27.3%)	65 (36.5%)	67 (34.5%)
COMORBIDITIES—n. (%)			
Hypertension	138 (55.9%)	107 (60.1%)	114 (58.8%)
Myocardial infarction history	38 (15.4%)	27 (15.2%)	30 (15.4%)
Chronic heart failure	48 (19.4%)	31 (17.4%)	68 (35.1%) * †
COPD	56 (22.7%)	37 (20.8%)	41 (21.1%)
Chronic liver diseases	28 (11.3%)	27 (15.1%)	22 (11.3%)
Diabetes mellitus	86 (34.8%)	53 (29.8%)	57 (29.4%)
CKD	33 (13.4%)	47 (26.4%) *	43 (22.2%)
Solid tumors	67 (27.1%)	47 (26.4%)	43 (22.2%)
Onco-hematological diseases	28 (11.3%)	16 (9.0%)	21 (10.8%)
Number of drugs in home-therapy	5.7 ± 4	5.7 ± 4	5.8 ± 4
VTE risk (Padua Score)	3.14 ± 1.8	3.74 ± 1.95 *	3.53 ± 1.63
SBP—mmHg	122.9 ± 17.1	127.0 ± 21.3	128.3 ± 20.1 *
DBP—mmHg	70.1 ± 10.6	71.1 ± 10.9	74.7 ± 11.1 * †
MBP—mmHg	87.1 ± 13.4	89.9 ± 13.2	92.5 ± 12.6 *

Data are presented as percentage or mean ± SD. ED SSU: emergency department short stay unit; COPD: chronic obstructive pulmonary disease; CKD: chronic kidney disease; VTE: venous thromboembolism; SBP: systolic blood pressure; DBP: diastolic blood pressure; MBP: mean blood pressure. * p < 0.05 vs. 2019; † p < 0.05 vs. 2020.

Table 2. Blood test parameters at admission to internal medicine departments.

	Pre-COVID-19 Era (2019) (n = 247)	COVID-19 Outbreak Era (2020) (n = 178)	COVID-19 Ongoing Era (2021) (n = 194)
Fasting glucose—mg/dL	110.14 ± 47	114.87 ± 53.9	102.35 ± 53.4
Urea—mg/dL	47.83 ± 32.9	63 ± 53.5 *	49.73 ± 40.6 †
Creatinine—mg/dL	1 ± 1.05	1.43 ± 1.56 *	1.35 ± 1.78
eGFR—mL/min/1.73 m^2	82.7 ± 31.2	69.8 ± 34.6 *	75.7 ± 33.5
Albumin—g/dL	3.15 ± 0.6	3.07 ± 0.6	3.4 ± 2.9
Total bilirubin—mg/dL	1.29 ± 2.14	1.26 ± 2.02	1.92 ± 4.02
AST > 34 UI/L—n. (%)	68 (27.5%)	52 (29.2%)	64 (33.0%)
ALT > 55 UI/L—n. (%)	30 (12.1%)	30 (16.8%)	41 (21.1%)
NT-proBNP > 260 pg/mL—n. (%)	35 (14.2%)	39 (21.9%)	68 (35.0%) *
ESR—mm	59.96 ± 34	55.53 ± 31.72	70.97 ± 115.94
hs-CRP > 0.5 mg/dL—n. (%)	212 (85.8%)	151 (84.8%)	161 (83.0%)
Procalcitonin > 0.5 µg/L—n. (%)	35 (14.2%)	44 (24.7%) *	51 (26.3%) *
HB—g/dL	11.14 ± 3.25	10.94 ± 2.06	10.62 ± 2.29
INR	1.2 ± 0.33	1.3 ± 0.5 *	1.27 ± 0.4

Data are presented as percentage or mean ± SD. eGFR: estimated glomerular filtration rate; AST: aspartate aminotransferase; ALT: alanine aminotransferase; NT-proBNP: N-terminal pro-brain natriuretic peptide; ESR: erythrocyte sedimentation rate; hs-CRP: high-sensitivity C-reactive protein; HB: hemoglobin; INR: international normalized ratio. * p < 0.05 vs. 2019; † p < 0.05 vs. 2020.

In 2020, in-hospital mortality was significantly higher (17.4% vs. 5.3%, $p = 0.009$). In particular, the major cause of death in 2020 was sepsis (47%). Moreover, the LOS was higher in 2020 than in 2019 (respectively, 12.7 ± 6.8 vs. 11.0 ± 6.2, $p = 0.04$), as well as the number of patients who underwent blood transfusion (respectively, 24.7% vs. 16.6%, $p = 0.04$) and the number of sepsis diagnoses (respectively, 27.5% vs. 19.4%, $p = 0.04$). On the contrary, no differences regarding multidrug-resistant germ isolations were found (Table 3).

Table 3. In-hospital outcomes.

	Pre-COVID-19 Era (2019) (n = 247)	COVID-19 Outbreak Era (2020) (n = 178)	COVID-19 Ongoing Era (2021) (n = 194)
TYPE OF DISCHARGE—n. (%)			
Home discharge	196 (79.3%)	109 (61.2%) *	142 (73.2%) †
Nursing home discharge	16 (6.5%)	16 (9.0%)	16 (8.2%)
Death	13 (5.3%)	31 (17.4%) *	14 (7.2%) * †
Transfer to another department	22 (8.9%)	21 (11.8%)	20 (10.3%)
Voluntary discharge	0 (0%)	1 (0.6%)	2 (1.0%)
Length of in-hospital stay (days)	11 ± 6.2	12.7 ± 6.8 *	11.10 ± 6.64
Blood transfusions—n. (%)	41 (16.6%)	44 (24.7%) *	31 (16.0%) †
Diagnosis of sepsis—n. (%)	48 (19.4%)	49 (27.5%) *	54 (27.8%) *
MDR germs isolation—n. (%)	33 (13.4%)	33 (18.5%)	45 (23.2%) *
Respiratory failure—n. (%)	43 (17.4%)	44 (24.7%)	35 (18.0%)

Data are presented as percentage or mean ± SD. MDR: multidrug resistant. * $p < 0.05$ vs. 2019; † $p < 0.05$ vs. 2020.

In the comparison between the COVID 19 ongoing era (2021) and the COVID-19 outbreak (2020) and pre-COVID 19 eras (2019), we did not find differences regarding age, bedridden patients, or the number of home-therapy drugs. As regards sex and VTE risk data, 2021 was closer to 2020 (42.3% of female patients and a Padua score of 3.53 ± 1.63), but SBP was significantly higher in the post-COVID-19 era than in the pre-COVID-19 era (128.3 ± 20.1 vs. 122.9 ± 17.1 mmHg, $p = 0.03$) as well as MBP (92.5 ± 12.6 vs. 87.1 ± 13.4 mmHg, $p = 0.002$). The percentage of patients transferred from the ED SSU was significantly higher in 2021 than in 2019 (73.7% vs. 29.1%, $p < 0.001$) and the number of elective admissions was lower (0% vs. 9.3%, $p < 0.001$) (Table 1).

In 2021, eGFR and INR showed values closer to the pre-COVID-19 era (eGFR 75.7 ± 33.5 vs. 82.7 ± 31.2, INR 1.27 ± 0.4 vs. 1.2 ± 0.33). Furthermore, in 2021, the number of patients with NT-proBNP > 260 pg/mL was significantly higher than in 2019 (35.0% vs. 14.2%, $p < 0.001$) (Table 2).

Moreover, in 2021, we observed a significant reduction in in-hospital mortality and blood transfusions in comparison to the COVID-19 outbreak era (respectively, 7.2% vs. 17.4%, $p = 0.003$ and 16.0% vs. 24.7%, $p = 0.04$), as well as a significant increase in home discharges (73.2% vs. 61.2%, $p = 0.01$). However, sepsis was the first cause of death in 2021 (85.7%), with an increase in multidrug-resistant germ isolation (23.2% 2021 vs. 13.4% 2019, $p = 0.007$). As regards LOS, there was a decrease in comparison to the COVID-19 outbreak era; however, values did not reach statistical significance and values were closer to those in 2019 (Table 3).

3.2. Analysis of Major Determinants of In-Hospital Mortality in the Study Groups

Subsequently, we performed a logistic regression analysis, which highlighted an association between in-hospital mortality, solid tumors ($\beta = 4.5$, $p = 0.002$) and eGFR ($\beta = -0.094$, $p = 0.003$) in 2019. In 2020, in-hospital mortality was associated with solid tumors ($\beta = 2.98$, $p = 0.005$) and respiratory failure ($\beta = 3.23$, $p = 0.001$). In 2021, we highlighted an association between in-hospital mortality, respiratory failure ($\beta = 3.1$, $p = 0.01$) and serum albumin ($\beta = -2.8$, $p = 0.01$) (Table 4).

Table 4. Logistic regression analysis evaluating major determinants of in-hospital mortality in the three different eras.

	Coefficient β	p
Pre-COVID-19 era (2019)		
Solid tumors	4.5	0.002
eGFR	−0.094	0.003
COVID-19 outbreak era (2020)		
Solid tumors	2.98	0.005
Respiratory failure	3.23	0.001
COVID-19 ongoing era (2021)		
Respiratory failure	3.1	0.01
Serum albumin	−2.8	0.01

eGFR: estimated glomerular filtration rate.

Finally, when evaluating the entire study population (Table 5), we found an association between in-hospital death, being bedridden (β = 1.4, p = 0.004), respiratory failure (β = 1.5, p = 0.001), eGFR (β = −0.16, p = 0.03) and hospitalization in the COVID-19 outbreak era (β = 1.6, p = 0.005).

Table 5. Logistic regression analysis evaluating major determinants of in-hospital mortality considering the entire population.

	Coefficient β	p
Being bedridden	1.4	0.004
Respiratory failure	1.5	0.001
eGFR	−0.16	0.03
Hospitalization in COVID-19 outbreak era (2020)	1.6	0.005

eGFR: estimated glomerular filtration rate.

4. Discussion

In this study, we aimed to investigate the effects of the COVID-19 pandemic on internal medicine departments not directly involved in the management of patients suffering from SARS-CoV-2 infection. The principal findings were: (1) mortality and morbidity increased among patients hospitalized in the COVID-19 era (2020), with a reverse trend the year after the pandemic outbreak; (2) an increased number of diagnoses of sepsis and increased MDR germ isolation in 2020 and 2021; (3) the length of in-hospital stay was significantly longer during 2020. All these results are in line with other studies showing an increase in mortality in patients admitted to the ED and other specialty units during the pandemic [17–23]. These findings could be explained by a large decrease in hospitalizations during the pandemic due to patients' fear of hospital-acquired infection of COVID-19, especially among the elderly, and the reduced capacity of healthcare services to provide timely diagnoses and treatment. Indeed, during this period, the percentage of patients with a diagnosis of acute coronary syndrome decreased by 40% compared to the same period in 2019 [24], and hospitalizations for acute stroke decreased by 80% to 50% in some countries [25]. Furthermore, the number of newly diagnosed cancer patients decreased by 46.5% [26]. As regards hospitalizations, the outpatient volume for all diseases decreased by approximately 60% across the United States [27]. The number of outpatient visits for bronchitis decreased by 76.79%, pneumonia by 71.03%, and acute upper respiratory infection by 56.87% in 2020, compared to the same data observed in 2019 [28]. In addition, Piccolo et al. found that in Campania, Italy, the COVID-19 outbreak was linked to a reduction in percutaneous coronary intervention, and the authors speculate that a possible explanation could be the underestimation of chest pain by patients due to a fear of contracting SARS-CoV-2 infection if they had been to hospital [29]. Furthermore, access to telemedicine was difficult for elderly patients, who often have lower IT skills [30]. Consequently, a delay in seeking medical care led to more critically ill patients being admitted during the pandemic and worse in-hospital outcomes. For instance, our study showed that patients hospitalized during the pandemic had worse kidney function, which is an independent predictor of all-cause mortality [31–33]. In addition, patients hospitalized in 2020 more frequently had an altered coagulation state, with an increase in INR and higher Padua score, which are both associated with higher in-hospital morbidity and mortality, as previously reported [34–37]. Moreover, among our patients, a significantly higher incidence of sepsis and chronic renal failure emerged, and sepsis was associated with an increase in multidrug-resistant germ infections [38,39]. In agreement with the literature, our study confirms a strong association between in-hospital mortality, eGFR, being bedridden and the presence of respiratory failure in the logistic regression analysis. Given the strong association between mortality and respiratory failure, an increase in mortality due to unrecognized SARS-CoV-2 infections could be hypothesized; however, all patients examined had a double negative SARS-CoV-2 nasopharyngeal molecular swab at the time of admission to the internal medicine departments and in patients still suspected of having COVID-19 for radiological and clinical reasons, research using a PCR for SARS-CoV-2 on a sample from bronchus alveolar lavage was performed, according to hospital protocols (see Materials and Methods section). Thus, this hypothesis appears unlikely. Analyzing the causes of death, it is interesting to note that the main cause of in-hospital mortality in the COVID-19 outbreak era was sepsis (47% of the causes of death).

Our study demonstrated an increase in LOS in internal medicine departments in the COVID-19 outbreak era. These data are in disagreement with the findings of studies conducted in ultra-specialized departments such as cardiology [20], neurology, and oncology [22]. In these studies, a shorter LOS was found, assuming a more effective management of patients thanks to a reduction in non-urgent services. However, internal medicine departments mainly manage 'urgent hospitalizations' and not 'elective hospitalizations', thus they hardly benefit from a reduction in outpatient activities. On the contrary, internal medicine patients are complex, suffering from multiple comorbidities and often malnourished [40]. The management of these patients failed due to a reduction in chronic disease assistance during the COVID-19 outbreak era. This fact has a negative impact on internal medicine specialists who often have to deal with both acute and chronic diseases with their home therapies, which, whether properly managed or not, lead to early hospital readmission. Indeed, our study found a higher prevalence of congestive heart failure and higher blood pressure values among hospitalized patients during 2021 than in previous years.

In light of the differences reported between the three years considered in terms of hospital outcomes, we do believe that some strategies could be embraced in order to reduce healthcare-associated infections and avoid worse outcomes. We suggest using web-based tools and learning from the scientific literature so that member hospitals can compare their performance to the best performers and identify strategies for improvement. Moreover, we recommend having multidisciplinary teams in order to ensure better medical management. We should consider telemedicine to enhance the quality of medical services and to coordinate emergency systems. Remote patient monitoring with the transmission of physiological data from a home setting, could be particularly useful for chronic conditions such as diabetes or hypertension [41]. Telehealth has a lot of advantages, especially during an infectious disease outbreak. However, it requires a change in medical training across all specialties [42]. Eventually, given that the leading cause of death in internal medicine departments is sepsis, we could create our own sepsis protocol for identifying patients at risk. This could allow clinicians to identify and treat patients early. This study has some strengths. To the best of our knowledge, this is the first study to evaluate the impact of the COVID-19 pandemic on clinical outcomes in a specific clinical setting such as internal medicine departments not directly involved in the pandemic emergency. Our findings provide a new perspective for targeting vulnerable patients and helping to make healthcare decisions after the epidemic subsides or before the next wave hits. Lastly, this study is one of the few that has evaluated the change in LOS over the pandemic period in patients with different medical conditions. However, there are some limitations. Firstly, this is an observational study that might not deduce the causal effects of the COVID-19 pandemic in different waves on in-hospital mortality and LOS. However, because of the small differences in the prevalence of comorbidities among the three years, increased in-hospital mortality and decreased LOS in the year 2020 are likely attributable to the COVID-19 pandemic. Secondly, our data could show some heterogeneity due to dicentric collection.

5. Conclusions

In conclusion, our study highlights how the COVID-19 pandemic caused an increase in mortality, incidence of sepsis and LOS even in patients not directly suffering from SARS-CoV-2 infection. However, it seems reassuring to note that, just over a year after the onset of the pandemic, the data regarding in-hospital mortality, renal function and coagulation state showed a clear reverse trend. On the other hand, the data concerning an increased prevalence and worse control of chronic diseases at a territorial level such as congestive heart failure and hypertension should be considered as a warning sign. Thus, it could be advisable to have a multidisciplinary approach integrated with telemedicine to ensure better medical management of chronic diseases and avoid worse in-hospital outcomes.

Author Contributions: Conceptualization, M.D.M., N.M. and A.D.P.; methodology, M.D.M., N.M. and A.D.P.; software, G.C., G.L. and S.S.; validation, A.D.P., R.S., S.P., A.G. and L.Z.; formal analysis, M.D.M., N.M., S.M. and A.D.P.; investigation, G.C., G.L., C.S. and S.T.; resources, A.D.P., P.C. and F.P.; data curation, M.D.M., N.M. and A.D.P.; writing—original draft preparation, M.D.M., N.M. and S.M.; writing—review and editing, S.S., A.D.P., L.Z., R.S. and S.P.; visualization, A.G., S.P., P.C. and F.P.; supervision, P.C. and F.P.; project administration, A.D.P. All authors have read and agreed to the published version of the manuscript.

Funding: This research received no external funding.

Institutional Review Board Statement: The study was conducted in accordance with the Declaration of Helsinki and approved by Ethical Board Catania 2 (N° prot. 370/2021).

Informed Consent Statement: The requirement for informed consent was waived because of the retrospective design of the data collection.

Data Availability Statement: Data for this study are available under request addressed to A.D.P.

Acknowledgments: We wish to thank the Scientific Bureau of the University of Catania for language support.

Conflicts of Interest: The authors declare no conflict of interest.

References

1. WHO. Coronavirus (COVID-19) Dashboard. Available online: https://covid19.who.int (accessed on 7 June 2022).
2. Reed, C.; Lim, T.; Montgomery, J.M.; Klena, J.D.; Hall, A.J.; Fry, A.M.; Cannon, D.L.; Chiang, C.-F.; Gibbons, A.; Krapiunaya, I.; et al. Seroprevalence of Antibodies to SARS-CoV-2 in 10 Sites in the United States, 23 March–12 May 2020. *JAMA Intern. Med.* **2020**, *180*, 1576–1586. [CrossRef]
3. Metzger, C.; Leroy, T.; Bochnakian, A.; Jeulin, H.; Gegout-Petit, A.; Legrand, K.; Schvoerer, E.; Guillemin, F. Seroprevalence and SARS-CoV-2 Invasion in General Populations: A Scoping Review over the First Year of the Pandemic. *PLoS ONE* **2023**, *18*, e0269104. [CrossRef] [PubMed]
4. Rosenbaum, L. The Untold Toll—The Pandemic's Effects on Patients without COVID-19. *N. Engl. J. Med.* **2020**, *382*, 2368–2371. [CrossRef] [PubMed]
5. COVID-19 Excess Mortality Collaborators Estimating Excess Mortality Due to the COVID-19 Pandemic: A Systematic Analysis of COVID-19-Related Mortality, 2020–2021. *Lancet* **2022**, *399*, 1513–1536. [CrossRef]
6. Zubiri, L.; Rosovsky, R.P.; Mooradian, M.J.; Piper-Vallillo, A.J.; Gainor, J.F.; Sullivan, R.J.; Marte, D.; Boland, G.M.; Gao, X.; Hochberg, E.P.; et al. Temporal Trends in Inpatient Oncology Census Before and During the COVID-19 Pandemic and Rates of Nosocomial COVID-19 Among Patients with Cancer at a Large Academic Center. *Oncologist* **2021**, *26*, e1427–e1433. [CrossRef] [PubMed]
7. Folino, A.F.; Zorzi, A.; Cernetti, C.; Marchese, D.; Pasquetto, G.; Roncon, L.; Saccà, S.; Themistoclakis, S.; Turiano, G.; Verlato, R.; et al. Impact of COVID-19 Epidemic on Coronary Care Unit Accesses for Acute Coronary Syndrome in Veneto Region, Italy. *Am. Heart J.* **2020**, *226*, 26–28. [CrossRef] [PubMed]

8. Schwarz, V.; Mahfoud, F.; Lauder, L.; Reith, W.; Behnke, S.; Smola, S.; Rissland, J.; Pfuhl, T.; Scheller, B.; Böhm, M.; et al. Decline of Emergency Admissions for Cardiovascular and Cerebrovascular Events after the Outbreak of COVID-19. *Clin. Res. Cardiol.* **2020**, *109*, 1500–1506. [CrossRef]
9. Scicali, R.; Piro, S.; Ferrara, V.; Di Mauro, S.; Filippello, A.; Scamporrino, A.; Romano, M.; Purrello, F.; Di Pino, A. Direct and Indirect Effects of SARS-CoV-2 Pandemic in Subjects with Familial Hypercholesterolemia: A Single Lipid-Center Real-World Evaluation. *J. Clin. Med.* **2021**, *10*, 4363. [CrossRef] [PubMed]
10. Bottle, A.; Liddle, A. Hip Fracture in the COVID-19 Era: What Can We Say about Care and Patient Outcomes? *BMJ Qual. Saf.* **2023**, *32*, 244–246. [CrossRef]
11. Lee, W.-E.; Woo Park, S.; Weinberger, D.M.; Olson, D.; Simonsen, L.; Grenfell, B.T.; Viboud, C. Direct and Indirect Mortality Impacts of the COVID-19 Pandemic in the United States, March 1, 2020 to January 1, 2022. *eLife* **2023**, *12*, e77562. [CrossRef]
12. Pizano-Escalante, M.G.; Anaya-Esparza, L.M.; Nuño, K.; de Rodríguez-Romero, J.J.; Gonzalez-Torres, S.; López-de la Mora, D.A.; Villagrán, Z. Direct and Indirect Effects of COVID-19 in Frail Elderly: Interventions and Recommendations. *J. Pers. Med.* **2021**, *11*, 999. [CrossRef] [PubMed]
13. Redberg, R.F.; Katz, M.; Steinbrook, R. Internal Medicine and COVID-19. *JAMA* **2020**, *324*, 1135–1136. [CrossRef] [PubMed]
14. Pietrantonio, F.; Rosiello, F.; Alessi, E.; Pascucci, M.; Rainone, M.; Cipriano, E.; Di Berardino, A.; Vinci, A.; Ruggeri, M.; Ricci, S. Burden of COVID-19 on Italian Internal Medicine Wards: Delphi, SWOT, and Performance Analysis after Two Pandemic Waves in the Local Health Authority "Roma 6" Hospital Structures. *Int. J. Environ. Res. Public Health* **2021**, *18*, 5999. [CrossRef] [PubMed]
15. Inker, L.A.; Eneanya, N.D.; Coresh, J.; Tighiouart, H.; Wang, D.; Sang, Y.; Crews, D.C.; Doria, A.; Estrella, M.M.; Froissart, M.; et al. New Creatinine- and Cystatin C–Based Equations to Estimate GFR without Race. *N. Engl. J. Med.* **2021**, *385*, 1737–1749. [CrossRef] [PubMed]
16. Barbar, S.; Noventa, F.; Rossetto, V.; Ferrari, A.; Brandolin, B.; Perlati, M.; De Bon, E.; Tormene, D.; Pagnan, A.; Prandoni, P. A Risk Assessment Model for the Identification of Hospitalized Medical Patients at Risk for Venous Thromboembolism: The Padua Prediction Score. *J. Thromb. Haemost.* **2010**, *8*, 2450–2457. [CrossRef] [PubMed]
17. Bodilsen, J.; Nielsen, P.B.; Søgaard, M.; Dalager-Pedersen, M.; Speiser, L.O.Z.; Yndigegn, T.; Nielsen, H.; Larsen, T.B.; Skjøth, F. Hospital Admission and Mortality Rates for Non-COVID Diseases in Denmark during COVID-19 Pandemic: Nationwide Population Based Cohort Study. *BMJ* **2021**, *373*, n1135. [CrossRef] [PubMed]
18. Sokolski, M.; Gajewski, P.; Zymliński, R.; Biegus, J.; Berg, J.M.T.; Bor, W.; Braunschweig, F.; Caldeira, D.; Cuculi, F.; D'Elia, E.; et al. Impact of Coronavirus Disease 2019 (COVID-19) Outbreak on Acute Admissions at the Emergency and Cardiology Departments Across Europe. *Am. J. Med.* **2021**, *134*, 482–489. [CrossRef] [PubMed]
19. Lai, A.G.; Pasea, L.; Banerjee, A.; Hall, G.; Denaxas, S.; Chang, W.H.; Katsoulis, M.; Williams, B.; Pillay, D.; Noursadeghi, M.; et al. Estimated Impact of the COVID-19 Pandemic on Cancer Services and Excess 1-Year Mortality in People with Cancer and Multimorbidity: Near Real-Time Data on Cancer Care, Cancer Deaths and a Population-Based Cohort Study. *BMJ Open* **2020**, *10*, e043828. [CrossRef]
20. Bollmann, A.; Hohenstein, S.; König, S.; Meier-Hellmann, A.; Kuhlen, R.; Hindricks, G. In-Hospital Mortality in Heart Failure in Germany during the COVID-19 Pandemic. *ESC Heart Fail.* **2020**, *7*, 4416–4419. [CrossRef]
21. De Rosa, S.; Spaccarotella, C.; Basso, C.; Calabrò, M.P.; Curcio, A.; Filardi, P.P.; Mancone, M.; Mercuro, G.; Muscoli, S.; Nodari, S.; et al. Reduction of Hospitalizations for Myocardial Infarction in Italy in the COVID-19 Era. *Eur. Heart J.* **2020**, *41*, 2083–2088. [CrossRef]
22. Xiong, J.; Wai, A.K.C.; Wong, J.Y.H.; Tang, E.H.M.; Chu, O.C.K.; Wong, C.K.H.; Rainer, T.H. Impact of Varying Wave Periods of COVID-19 on in-Hospital Mortality and Length of Stay for Admission through Emergency Department: A Territory-Wide Observational Cohort Study. *Influenza Other Respir. Viruses* **2022**, *16*, 193–203. [CrossRef] [PubMed]
23. Liu, J.; Zhang, L.; Yan, Y.; Zhou, Y.; Yin, P.; Qi, J.; Wang, L.; Pan, J.; You, J.; Yang, J.; et al. Excess Mortality in Wuhan City and Other Parts of China during the Three Months of the COVID-19 Outbreak: Findings from Nationwide Mortality Registries. *BMJ* **2021**, *372*, n415. [CrossRef]
24. Mafham, M.M.; Spata, E.; Goldacre, R.; Gair, D.; Curnow, P.; Bray, M.; Hollings, S.; Roebuck, C.; Gale, C.P.; Mamas, M.A.; et al. COVID-19 Pandemic and Admission Rates for and Management of Acute Coronary Syndromes in England. *Lancet* **2020**, *396*, 381–389. [CrossRef]
25. Markus, H.S.; Brainin, M. COVID-19 and Stroke-A Global World Stroke Organization Perspective. *Int. J. Stroke* **2020**, *15*, 361–364. [CrossRef] [PubMed]
26. Kaufman, H.W.; Chen, Z.; Niles, J.; Fesko, Y. Changes in the Number of US Patients With Newly Identified Cancer Before and During the Coronavirus Disease 2019 (COVID-19) Pandemic. *JAMA Netw. Open* **2020**, *3*, e2017267. [CrossRef] [PubMed]
27. The Impact of COVID-19 on Outpatient Visits in 2020: Visits Remained Stable, Despite a Late Surge in Cases. Available online: https://www.commonwealthfund.org/publications/2021/feb/impact-covid-19-outpatient-visits-2020-visits-stable-despite-late-surge (accessed on 7 June 2022).
28. Wang, W.; Zheng, Y.; Jiang, L. Impact of the COVID-19 Epidemic on Outpatient Visits of Common Respiratory Diseases. *Res. Sq.* **2020**. [CrossRef]
29. Piccolo, R.; Bruzzese, D.; Mauro, C.; Aloia, A.; Baldi, C.; Boccalatte, M.; Bottiglieri, G.; Briguori, C.; Caiazzo, G.; Calabrò, P.; et al. Population Trends in Rates of Percutaneous Coronary Revascularization for Acute Coronary Syndromes Associated with the COVID-19 Outbreak. *Circulation* **2020**, *141*, 2035–2037. [CrossRef]

30. Bonora, B.M.; Morieri, M.L.; Avogaro, A.; Fadini, G.P. The Toll of Lockdown Against COVID-19 on Diabetes Outpatient Care: Analysis from an Outbreak Area in Northeast Italy. *Diabetes Care* **2021**, *44*, e18–e21. [CrossRef]
31. Chronic Kidney Disease Prognosis Consortium; Matsushita, K.; van der Velde, M.; Astor, B.C.; Woodward, M.; Levey, A.S.; de Jong, P.E.; Coresh, J.; Gansevoort, R.T. Association of Estimated Glomerular Filtration Rate and Albuminuria with All-Cause and Cardiovascular Mortality in General Population Cohorts: A Collaborative Meta-Analysis. *Lancet* **2010**, *375*, 2073–2081. [CrossRef]
32. Fox, C.S.; Matsushita, K.; Woodward, M.; Bilo, H.J.G.; Chalmers, J.; Heerspink, H.J.L.; Lee, B.J.; Perkins, R.M.; Rossing, P.; Sairenchi, T.; et al. Associations of Kidney Disease Measures with Mortality and End-Stage Renal Disease in Individuals with and without Diabetes: A Meta-Analysis. *Lancet* **2012**, *380*, 1662–1673. [CrossRef]
33. Fried, L.F.; Katz, R.; Sarnak, M.J.; Shlipak, M.G.; Chaves, P.H.M.; Jenny, N.S.; Stehman-Breen, C.; Gillen, D.; Bleyer, A.J.; Hirsch, C.; et al. Kidney Function as a Predictor of Noncardiovascular Mortality. *J. Am. Soc. Nephrol.* **2005**, *16*, 3728–3735. [CrossRef]
34. Arpaia, G.G.; Caleffi, A.; Marano, G.; Laregina, M.; Erba, G.; Orlandini, F.; Cimminiello, C.; Boracchi, P. Padua Prediction Score and IMPROVE Score Do Predict In-Hospital Mortality in Internal Medicine Patients. *Intern. Emerg. Med.* **2020**, *15*, 997–1003. [CrossRef]
35. Benediktsson, S.; Hansen, C.; Frigyesi, A.; Kander, T. Coagulation Tests on Admission Correlate with Mortality and Morbidity in General ICU Patients: An Observational Study. *Acta Anaesthesiol. Scand.* **2020**, *64*, 628–634. [CrossRef] [PubMed]
36. Fischer, C.M.; Yano, K.; Aird, W.C.; Shapiro, N.I. Abnormal Coagulation Tests Obtained in the Emergency Department Are Associated with Mortality in Patients with Suspected Infection. *J. Emerg. Med.* **2012**, *42*, 127–132. [CrossRef] [PubMed]
37. Marcucci, M.; Iorio, A.; Nobili, A.; Tettamanti, M.; Pasina, L.; Djade, C.D.; Marengoni, A.; Salerno, F.; Corrao, S.; Mannucci, P.M.; et al. Prophylaxis of Venous Thromboembolism in Elderly Patients with Multimorbidity. *Intern. Emerg. Med.* **2013**, *8*, 509–520. [CrossRef]
38. Zaccone, V.; Tosoni, A.; Passaro, G.; Vallone, C.V.; Impagnatiello, M.; Li Puma, D.D.; De Cosmo, S.; Landolfi, R.; Mirijello, A.; Internal Medicine Sepsis Study Group. Sepsis in Internal Medicine Wards: Current Knowledge, Uncertainties and New Approaches for Management Optimization. *Ann. Med.* **2017**, *49*, 582–592. [CrossRef] [PubMed]
39. Rossio, R.; Franchi, C.; Ardoino, I.; Djade, C.D.; Tettamanti, M.; Pasina, L.; Salerno, F.; Marengoni, A.; Corrao, S.; Marcucci, M.; et al. Adherence to Antibiotic Treatment Guidelines and Outcomes in the Hospitalized Elderly with Different Types of Pneumonia. *Eur. J. Intern. Med.* **2015**, *26*, 330–337. [CrossRef]
40. Miano, N.; Di Marco, M.; Alaimo, S.; Coppolino, G.; L'Episcopo, G.; Leggio, S.; Scicali, R.; Piro, S.; Purrello, F.; Di Pino, A. Controlling Nutritional Status (CONUT) Score as a Potential Prognostic Indicator of In-Hospital Mortality, Sepsis and Length of Stay in an Internal Medicine Department. *Nutrients* **2023**, *15*, 1554. [CrossRef]
41. Logan, A.G.; McIsaac, W.J.; Tisler, A.; Irvine, M.J.; Saunders, A.; Dunai, A.; Rizo, C.A.; Feig, D.S.; Hamill, M.; Trudel, M.; et al. Mobile Phone-Based Remote Patient Monitoring System for Management of Hypertension in Diabetic Patients. *Am. J. Hypertens.* **2007**, *20*, 942–948. [CrossRef]
42. Witkowska-Zimny, M.; Nieradko-Iwanicka, B. Telemedicine in Emergency Medicine in the COVID-19 Pandemic-Experiences and Prospects-A Narrative Review. *Int. J. Environ. Res. Public Health* **2022**, *19*, 8216. [CrossRef]

Disclaimer/Publisher's Note: The statements, opinions and data contained in all publications are solely those of the individual author(s) and contributor(s) and not of MDPI and/or the editor(s). MDPI and/or the editor(s) disclaim responsibility for any injury to people or property resulting from any ideas, methods, instructions or products referred to in the content.

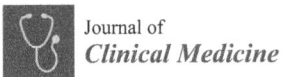

Article

Early Hospital Discharge Using Remote Monitoring for Patients Hospitalized for COVID-19, Regardless of Need for Home Oxygen Therapy: A Descriptive Study

Samy Talha [1,2,*], Sid Lamrous [3], Loic Kassegne [4], Nicolas Lefebvre [5], Abrar-Ahmad Zulfiqar [6], Pierre Tran Ba Loc [7], Marie Geny [8], Nicolas Meyer [7], Mohamed Hajjam [9], Emmanuel Andrès [2,6] and Bernard Geny [1,2]

[1] Physiology and Functional Exploration Service, University Hospital of Strasbourg, 67000 Strasbourg, France; bernard.geny@chru-strasbourg.fr
[2] Research Team 3072 "Mitochondria, Oxidative Stress and Muscle", University of Strasbourg, 90032 Strasbourg, France; emmanuel.andres@chru-strasbourg.fr
[3] UTBM, CNRS, FEMTO-ST Institute, 90000 Belfort, France; sid.lamrous@utbm.fr
[4] Pneumology Department, University Hospital of Strasbourg, 67000 Strasbourg, France; loic.kassegne@chru-strasbourg.fr
[5] Infectious Disease Department, University Hospital Strasbourg, 67000 Strasbourg, France; nicolas.lefebvre@chru-strasbourg.fr
[6] Internal Medicine Department, University Hospital Strasbourg, 67000 Strasbourg, France; abzulfiqar@gmail.com
[7] Public Health Department, University Hospital Strasbourg, 67000 Strasbourg, France; pierre.tranbaloc@chru-strasbourg.fr (P.T.B.L.); nicolas.meyer@chru-strasbourg.fr (N.M.)
[8] Association for Assistance to Victims, Place Alfred de Musset, BP 3314, CEDEX, 27033 Evreux, France; mariegeny.mg@gmail.com
[9] Predimed Technology, 67300 Schiltigheim, France; mohamed.hajjam@predimed-technology.com
* Correspondence: samy.talha@chru-strasbourg.fr

Abstract: Aim: Since beds are unavailable, we prospectively investigated whether early hospital discharge will be safe and useful in patients hospitalized for COVID-19, regardless of their need for home oxygen therapy. Population and Methods: Extending the initial inclusion criteria, 62 patients were included and 51 benefited from home telemonitoring, mainly assessing clinical parameters (blood pressure, heart rate, respiratory rate, dyspnea, temperature) and peripheral saturation (SpO_2) at follow-up. Results: 47% of the patients were older than 65 years; 63% needed home oxygen therapy and/or presented with more than one comorbidity. At home, the mean time to dyspnea and tachypnea resolutions ranged from 21 to 24 days. The mean oxygen-weaning duration was 13.3 ± 10.4 days, and the mean SpO_2 was 95.7 ± 1.6%. The nurses and/or doctors managed 1238 alerts. Two re-hospitalizations were required, related to transient chest pain or pulmonary embolism, but no death occurred. Patient satisfaction was good, and 743 potential days of hospitalization were saved for other patients. Conclusion: The remote monitoring of vital parameters and symptoms is safe, allowing for early hospital discharge in patients hospitalized for COVID-19, whether or not home oxygen therapy was required. Oxygen tapering outside the hospital allowed for a greater reduction in hospital stay. Randomized controlled trials are necessary to confirm this beneficial effect.

Keywords: COVID-19; sanitary crisis; home-telemonitoring; artificial intelligence; remote monitoring; early hospital discharge

1. Introduction

The COVID-19 pandemic affected many patients worldwide, leading to millions of deaths and even more patients suffering greatly from long-COVID or post-COVID conditions. Globally, at the beginning of May 2023, there were 765,222,932 confirmed cases of COVID-19, including 6,921,614 deaths, reported to the WHO [1]. However, nearly

20 million persons might have died worldwide due to COVID-19, 5–15% of whom needed hospitalization. Further, approximately 10% of COVID-19 patients might demonstrate long-lasting symptoms, some of them until two years after the initial viral infection, which significantly limits both quality of life and ability to return to work [2–5]. This viral infection is not yet totally under control and rebounds, likely related to other variants, might result in care facilities becoming congested again, causing further harm to the population. Thus, even if Omicrons variants are generally less severe than the first variant, healthcare systems may be overwhelmed, particularly in countries with low population immunity [6]. Recently, in France, we still observed 422,226 contaminations by COVID-19 in March and April 2023 [1].

In October 2020, we observed, for the second time in France, an accelerated deterioration in COVID epidemic indicators, with many patients hospitalized for COVID-19 every day. The national 7-day incidence rate was above 430 per 100,000 inhabitants (Public Health France). To limit viral transmission in all territories, and thus reduce the impact on the hospital capacity as quickly as possible, the French government decided to take drastic measures, including a population lock-down. Nevertheless, it was necessary to adapt our healthcare system to avoid overflows in critical care hospitalization capacity and preserve conventional hospitalization capacity. Indeed, this is a major issue in the case of severe forms requiring hospitalization [7].

Spare hospital bed vacancies might be obtained by strengthening the link between conventional hospitalization and community medicine, aiming to allow for selected patients to be discharged from hospital earlier. Retrospectives studies have supported the potential usefulness of telemonitoring and telemedicine in COVID-19 patients, allowing for an early return home [8–10].

To this end, a national strategy for facilitated and adapted post-hospital care was implemented within the framework of a coordinated care pathway. We regionally developed TELECOVID-RAD, which is an innovative telemonitoring system set up to favor an early return home for patients hospitalized in the Strasbourg University Hospital for SARS-CoV-2, whether or not oxygen therapy was required. This solution, part of the healthcare pathway, re-enforced the city–hospital link to facilitate the hospitalization/discharge process. This offered healthcare providers the opportunity to closely monitor symptoms and vital parameters of COVID-19 patients in their own homes.

The aim of this prospective and descriptive study was to evaluate a newly created telemonitoring coordinated-care pathway in the setting of the COVID-19 pandemic's resurgence. We investigated whether patients requiring home oxygen therapy might also safely benefit from an early hospital discharge, as presumed in patients not requiring oxygen [11], and whether this can reduce the duration of hospitalization without readmission, facilitating a faster turn-over of beds and thus providing the possibility of other patients being hospitalized.

2. Population and Methods

2.1. Population and Study Design

2.1.1. Patients' Inclusion and Exclusion Criteria

Patients presenting with COVID-19 RT-PCR-confirmed infection and oxygen saturation below 93% on ambient air, whether or not this was associated with major dyspnea, who were hospitalized in the University Strasbourg Hospital, France, from November 2020 to August 2021, were proposed for participation in this prospective study. All patients gave their informed consent, and the study was approved by the ethics committee of the University of Strasbourg (CE-2022-61, 2 October 2022).

For all patients, inclusion criteria related either to their environment or to their clinical characteristics. Thus, a fixed and sanitary home less than 30 min from the referral health care institution with a nearby emergency structure and the possibility to isolate in a single room, together with the presence of a third party 24 h a day/7 days a week with reliable telephone access, were mandatory. For patients still requiring oxygen at home, specific inclusion criteria were autonomy (Katz ADL > 3/6) and oxygen requirement < 4 L/min (nasal cannula or mask) to maintain pulsed oxygen saturation (SpO_2) > 92% at rest.

The French High Heath authority (HAS) initially stated that patients needing home oxygen therapy and presenting with one major or more than one minor exclusion criteria should not be included in home telemonitoring. The major exclusion criteria were refusal of the patient, his entourage or his attending physician, absence of inclusion criteria, destabilized chronic pathologies, cancer under chemotherapy, congenital or acquired immunedepression, solid organ malignancy, hematopoietic stem cell transplantation related to a hematological malignancy under treatment, decompensated cirrhosis, neurological or neurovascular disease that may impair respiratory function, morbid obesity (body mass index-BMI ≥ 40 kg/m^2), suspicion of pulmonary embolism or pulmonary embolism not excluded (positive clinical and D-dimer arguments), or confirmed pregnancy regardless of term.

Minor exclusion criteria were numerous: >70 years old, severe cardiovascular pathologies (arterial hypertension with polytherapy, history of stroke or coronary artery disease, heart surgery, heart failure), balanced diabetes, chronic respiratory pathology, cancer controlled under treatment including radiotherapy < 6 months, no decompensated cirrhosis, moderate to severe obesity (body mass index (BMI) ≥ 30 and <40 kg/m^2). These criteria were designed to encourage patients with the highest risk of severe forms to stay in hospital rather than return home early. Nevertheless, as part of a doctor–patient shared decision, home oxygen therapy was considered regardless of age (HAS 9 November 2020). Further, in view of the numerous comorbidities present in severe forms of COVID-19, we also proposed home telemonitoring to stabilized patients with more than one minor exclusion criteria, considering their specific health status and environmental context.

The medical team decided on early discharge based on significant clinical improvements in patients, and the stability of this amelioration over time.

2.1.2. Telemonitoring Establishment

At least 24 h before the patient's hospital discharge, after obtaining informed consent, the attending hospital physician notified the family doctor and the regional care-coordination platform (regional support platform (PRAG)). The platform was then responsible for coordinating care at home with the patient's healthcare professionals (general practitioner (GP), nurses, physiotherapists, and pharmacists if oxygen therapy was required), as well as the provider of the remote monitoring equipment.

A technician from the remote monitoring solution came to the patient's home on the day of discharge from hospital to install remote monitoring devices (connected devices such as an oximeter, blood pressure monitor and tablet, approved for medical use in Europe). The patient, a caregiver, and the nurse were trained in their use and if there was no WIFI at home, a substitute solution using a 4G key was provided (Figure 1).

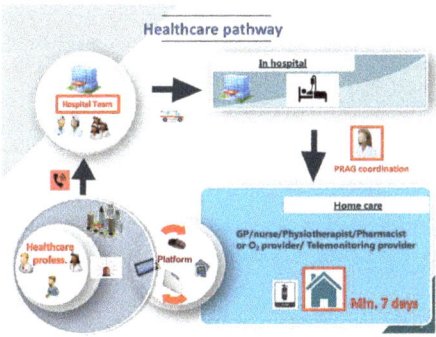

Figure 1. Telemonitoring organization. GP: general practitioner; Healthcare profess.: healthcare professional; PRAG: healthcare regional support platform.

Home care of patients started in the immediate aftermath of hospitalization for 7 days (extendable according to the advice of the attending physician). The nurse received alerts at the patient's bedside via the tablet present in the home, or remotely on his/her smartphone when a relative took measurements. The nurse called the attending physician (GP) in case of an alert.

The telemonitoring care pathway ended when patients no longer needed home monitoring because symptoms sufficiently improved or oxygen weaned, or if patients needed admission to the hospital.

2.1.3. Parameters Determined and Alerts Settings

Patients on oxygen therapy measured the following parameters three times a day: respiratory rate, heart rate, temperature, systolic and diastolic blood pressures, and SpO_2. Patients without oxygen therapy performed these measurements once a day. Connected sensors allowed for the telemonitoring of blood pressure and oxygen saturation, and questionnaires on symptoms (dyspnea using NYHA scale, presence or absence of chest pain, shivers) were filled in daily on the tablet by the patient or his caregiver.

The artificial intelligence platform considered all the parameters to allow for an analysis and trigger eventual alerts. Alerts were color-coded as green (low risk), orange (intermediate risk) or red (high risk), and then automatically sent to the smartphone of the patient's doctor and nurse each day (Figure 2).

Temperature	T < 37.8°	37.8° ≤ T < 38.2°	T ≥ 38.2°
Dyspnea	1	2	3
Chest pain	Yes	No	
Shivers	Yes	No	

Oxygen therapy (O_2 volume ≤ 4 l/min)		
SpO_2 ≥ 96%		no alert
92% ≤ SpO_2 < 96%		orange alert
SpO_2 < 92%		red alert
Without oxygen therapy		
94% ≤ SpO_2 < 96%		orange alert
SpO_2 < 94%		red alert

No alert	No alert		No alert
No alert	Orange alert		Orange alert
Orange alert	Orange alert		Red alert
Orange alert	Red alert		Red alert
Red alert	Red alert		Red alert

Figure 2. Clinical signs and SpO_2 rating for the generation of alerts. One green alert combined with one orange alert generates an orange global alert; two orange alerts generate a red global alert; one red alert combined with one orange alert generates a red global alert; two red alerts generate a red global alert.

2.1.4. Patient's Satisfaction Evaluation

To further determine the usefulness of the remote monitoring of COVID-19 patients, we evaluated patient satisfaction using a questionnaire with three simple key questions. Patients quantified whether they found the device simple to use, whether they felt safe, and whether the care coordination was satisfying on a scale ranging from 1 to 5, with 1 being the lowest and 5 being the highest satisfaction. Data are presented as the mean value.

2.2. Statistical Analysis

Qualitative data were described with frequency (%) and quantitative data, with the mean (SD) or median [Q1–Q3]. Kaplan–Meier estimators were used to evaluate time to resolution of dyspnea and tachypnea. Categorical data were compared with the chi^2 test with no continuity correction. Quantitative data were compared with *t*-test. The level of significance was set at 0.05. All computations were carried out with R 4.2.2.

3. Results

3.1. Flow Chart of the Study

Of the 1834 patients hospitalized in our institution for COVID-19 from November 2020 to August 2021, 62 were included by the regional support platform (PRAG) and 51 were home telemonitored after hospital discharge with My Predi® (Predimed Technology, 667300 Schiltigheim, France) solution. Eleven patients discontinued treatment, mainly due to refusal to continue upon arriving home, or because caregivers were not sufficiently available. Among these 51 patients, 32 (63%) were still receiving nasal oxygen at hospital discharge (Figure 3).

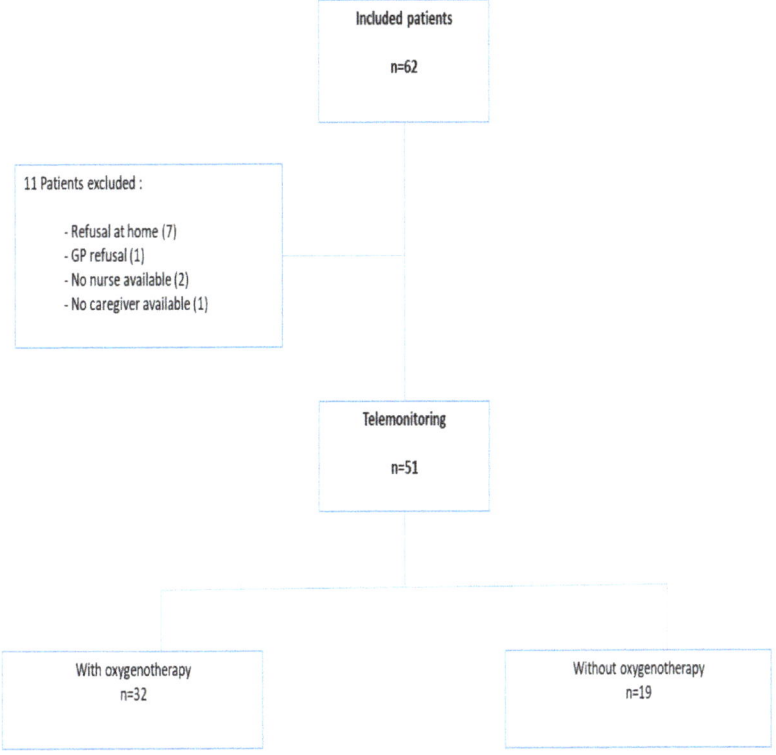

Figure 3. Flow chart of the study.

3.2. Patients' Clinical Characteristics, Main Risk Factors, Comorbidities and Symtoms

The mean age of the patients was 65 years, and 2 (4%), 25 (49%) and 24 (47%) of them were below 45, between 45 and 65 and older than 65 years old, respectively. There were slightly more men than women (55% versus 45%), and mean BMI was 28.6 kg/m^2, ranging from 16.9 to 41.7. Fourteen (27.5%) patients were obese with a BMI > 30 kg/m^2.

The main risk factors and co-morbidities were hypertension (55%), diabetes mellitus (29%), and obesity (27%). Ninety-eight percent of the patients presented with comorbidities, and 63% of them presented with more than one minor comorbidity (Table 1). Charlson's indice of comorbidities was 4.2 (±2.7), despite the absence of active neoplasia in our population (exclusion criteria). Thirty-three percent of the patients were transiently hospitalized in a critical care unit upon their arrival at hospital.

Table 1. COVID-19 patients' clinical characteristics, risk factors, comorbidities and symptoms.

		Total Population (n = 51)	Patients with Oxygen (n = 32)	Patients without Oxygen (n = 19)	p-Value
Clinical characteristics	Age, years Mean (±SD)	64.9 (±14)	65.5 (±15)	63.9 (±12)	0.677
	Male, n (%)	28 (55%)	16 (50%)	12 (63%)	0.361
	Female, n (%)	23 (45%)	16 (50%)	7 (37%)	
	BMI, kg/m^2 Mean (±SD)	28.6 (±5)	27.2 (±5)	30.9 (±5)	0.009
Main risk factors and comorbidities	Hypertension, n (%)	28 (55%)	17 (53%)	11 (58%)	0.741
	Diabetes, n (%)	15 (29%)	7 (22%)	8 (42%)	0.125
	Obesity, n (%)	14 (27%)	7 (22%)	7 (58%)	0.247
	Coronaropathy, n (%)	9 (18%)	6 (19%)	3 (16%)	0.789 *
	Active smoking, n (%)	8 (16%)	5 (16%)	3 (16%)	0.988 *
	Asthma, n (%)	4 (8%)	1 (3%)	3 (16%)	0.190 *
	Chronic obstructive pulmonary disease, n (%)	1 (2%)	0 (0%)	1 (5%)	0.104 *
Symptoms	Dyspnea, n (%)	43 (84)	28 (88)	15 (79)	0.417
	Weakness, n (%)	40 (78)	25 (78)	15 (79)	0.945
	Cough n (%)	38 (75)	27 (84)	11 (58)	0.036
	Digestive troubles, n (%)	20 (39)	14 (44)	6 (32)	0.389
	Anorexia, n (%)	15 (29)	10 (31)	5 (26)	0.708
	Myalgias, n (%)	12 (24)	8 (25)	4 (21)	0.748
	Headache, n (%)	9 (18)	7 (22)	2 (11)	0.304
	Anosmia/dysgeusia, n (%)	6 (12)	3 (9)	3 (16)	0.492
	Thoracic pain, n (%)	4 (8)	2 (6)	2 (11)	0.583

All tests: chi^2 test with no continuity correction. *: Fisher exact test gave the same conclusion as to significance.

3.3. Patients' Evolution at Home

3.3.1. Need for Re-Hospitalization

In our cohort, two patients (4%) were re-admitted to the hospital on day 15 after discharge. One, related to chest pain occurrence, resumed spontaneously, and no cause was found. This patient was discharged from hospital on the same day as readmission. The second patient presented with a pulmonary embolism detected by the platform during home telemonitoring and was re-hospitalized with a favorable clinical evolution. No other significant deleterious situations occurred and no death occurred within 30 days of hospital discharge.

3.3.2. Evolution of Clinical Parameters during Home Telemonitoring

As presented in Table 2, temperature and systemic blood pressure, collected in 51 patients, were in the normal range and stable during home telemonitoring. Very few chests pain or shivering episodes occurred.

Table 2. Telemonitored clinical and functional signs and alerts.

Temperature and Systemic Blood Pressure	First Day	Last Day
Temperatures (°C), mean (±SD)	36.6 (±0.4)	36.6 (±0.5)
BP (mmHg), mean (±SD) Systolic	122 (±15)	125.2 (±17)
Diastolic	76.1 (±13)	79.8 (±14)
Mean	83.5 (±15)	80.9 (±16)
Functional Signs (n = 41)		
Chest pain: no/increasing/decreasing, n (%)	36 (88)/2 (5)/2 (5)	
Shivers: no/yes, n (%)	40 (98)/1 (2)	
Alerts, n (%)		
Cumulative: Total/Red/Orange	1238 (100)/722 (58)/505 (41)	
Mean per patient: Total/Red/Orange	24.1/14.2/9.9	

Cpm: cycle per minute; °C: Celsius, mmHg: millimeters of mercury, BP: blood pressure.

The platform raised a total of 1238 alerts, including 722 (58%) red and 505 (41%) orange alerts. No at-home life-threatening emergencies occurred.

The longest symptoms were dyspnea and tachypnea. The mean time to dyspnea resolution was 21 ± 1 days and 24 ± 1 days in the entire population and in the patients discharged with oxygen, respectively (Figure 4A). The mean time to tachypnea resolution was 23 ± 1 and 24 ± 1 days in the entire population and in the patients discharged with oxygen, respectively (Figure 4B). Among the 19 patients discharged without oxygen therapy, no patients needed new oxygen during the home telemonitoring period.

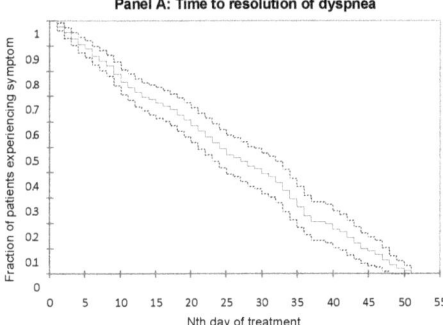 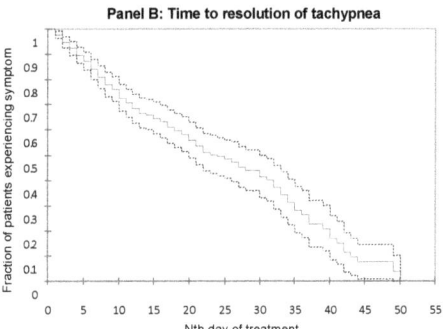

Figure 4. Kaplan–Meier curves showing the time-course of dyspnea (**Panel A**) and tachypnea (**Panel B**) resolutions in patients requiring home oxygen therapy. Blue lines show the fraction of patients still presenting dyspnea (A) and/or tachypnea (B) over time and the black lines indicates the 95% confidence interval of time to symptom resolution.

3.3.3. Oxygen Therapy Evolution during Home Telemonitoring

The data concerning oxygen therapy are presented in Table 3.

Mean oxygen output at hospital discharge and during home telemonitoring was below 2 L/min. Mean SpO_2 during home telemonitoring was 95.7 ± 1.6%.

For all patients weaned from oxygen at home, mean and median oxygen weaning durations were 13.3 ± 10.4 days and 9.5 (1–41) respectively. The cumulative total of days required for oxygen weaning (duration +1 day) was 430 days.

Table 3. Oxygen therapy evolution during home telemonitoring.

	Patients with Oxygen n = 32
Oxygen output (L/min) at hospital discharge mean (±SD)	1.9 (±0.7)
Mean oxygen output (L/min) during home telemonitoring mean (±SD)	1.6 (±0.7)
Oxygen weaning achievement n (%)	32 (100%)
Oxygen weaning duration, in days mean (±SD)	13.3 (±10.4)
Oxygen weaning cumulative days	430

3.3.4. Patients Satisfaction Evaluation

Thirty-six patients filled out the questionnaire and their assessment of the device's simplicity to use, their feeling of safety and their satisfaction with the care coordination team was 3.7, 3.6, and 3.8/5.

3.3.5. Number of Saved Hospital Days Due to Telemonitoring

The mean duration of telemonitoring was 9.2 ± 3.5 and 17.8 ± 13.7 in patients without and with home oxygen therapy, respectively. This corresponds to 743 hospital days being saved due to telemonitoring; with most of these (568 days) being related to patients needing oxygen therapy.

4. Discussion

The main results of this prospective study demonstrate the safety of an early return home of patients hospitalized for COVID-19. Although patients older than 65 years, those presenting with comorbidities, and/or those requiring oxygen therapy were included, no deaths and only two readmissions occurred within the 30 days following hospital discharge. Further, 743 potential days of hospitalization were saved for other patients, with the majority being related to the early return home of patients still under oxygen.

4.1. Feasibility of Early Return Home in Patients Hospitalized for COVID-19

At the time of the study, doubts were raised concerning the feasibility of an early return home in patients hospitalized for COVID-19. Fears of aggravation were particularly strong when oxygen therapy was mandatory. Accordingly, although the need for beds was high in view of the exploding pandemic, restrictive inclusion criteria were proposed to select patients for whom early hospital discharge might be proposed. The aim was to limit the risk of re-admission to hospital, potentially due to an emergency. Thus, initially, the inclusion criteria set by the high health authority (HAS) were quite strict, and a single major criterion or more than one minor criteria excluded patients from this early return home protocol.

These HAS recommendations define good practices, whose purpose is to guide healthcare professionals in designing and implementing the most appropriate preventive, diagnostic or therapeutic care strategies on the basis of proven medical knowledge at the date of their publication [12]. Accordingly, these recommendations evolve with improvements in knowledge.

Although comorbidities likely aggravate COVID-19 patiens' prognosis [13], in view of our population characteristics, we decided to include patients who presented with more than one minor exclusion criteria in cases of clinical stabilization. Indeed, strictly following these exclusion criteria or simply waiting for their official implementation would have excluded many patients from the potential benefits of an early return home. This shared decision greatly improved the clinical feasibility of the study, without any deleterious effects.

Home localization and the need for a rigorous follow-up for patients at home may also reduce the feasibility of such a protocol. Indeed, not all patients live near a hospital or emergency structure, and these patients could benefit from the daily attentions of a relative or available caregivers.

Nevertheless, despite these potential limitations, previous studies reported that an early return home could be proposed for patients suffering from severe forms of COVID-19. Indeed, an overflow of critical care hospitalization capacity occurred in many countries [7]. Retrospective analyses were, therefore, conducted to investigate the feasibility of telemedicine. TELEA in Galicia, a proactive at-home monitoring of patients considered to be high-risk, was associated with lower rates of hospitalization, shorter hospital stays, a lower mortality rate in the first hospitalization, and no at-home life-threatening emergencies [10]. In a primary healthcare center in Barcelona within the context of the first wave of the pandemic—when no rapid diagnostic tests were available—telephone follow-up by healthcare professionals was effective in detecting progression to severe COVID-19 and pneumonia, diagnosing more than 80% of the cases of pneumonia in non-severe COVID-19 patients [14].

In March 2020 in Wisconsin, Annis et al. reported, in 2255 patients, the quick implementation of a remote patient-monitoring program as an effective approach for managing COVID-19 symptoms at home [15]. In France, Covidom was a large telemonitoring solution that was rapidly deployed in the greater Paris area in 70,914 patients during the first wave of the pandemic to monitor patients with COVID-19 at home [16]. This early large-scale solution combined a free web application allowing for patients to fill out short daily questionnaires on their health status with a regional control center that monitored and managed the alerts triggered by questionnaire responses. This solution efficiently alleviated the burden on health care systems' capacities, and cumulatively mobilized more than 2000 volunteers, mostly specialists with decreased activity due to the first lockdown. In contrast, during this wave of the pandemic in France, when hospital activity dramatically increased due due to the preservation of surgery activity while COVID-19 cases progressed, our home system did not require hospital staff and allowed for patients to be efficiently cared for and monitored remotely by their regular GP and nurses at home.

4.2. Safety of Early Return Home in Patients Hospitalized for COVID-19

In the early stages of COVID-19, the safety of this measure has been questioned in view of the gravity of the COVID-19 disease and patients' potential aggravation, particularly when oxygen therapy is needed. In our study, importantly, safety was good in patients, regardless of the requirement for oxygen therapy. Thus, the only two re-admissions at hospital were not directly due to virus-related aggravations. Rather, telemonitoring likely allowed for an earlier diagnosis of pulmonary embolism, detected by the platform during home telemonitoring. Our data are in line with previous studies supporting the safety of an early return home in patients suffering from COVID-19 [10,14–16].

Of particular interest, the need for oxygen therapy, and the increasing length of hospitalization until oxygen weaning, suggests that patients are more vulnerable. However, our results are in line with Covidom in the subgroup of patients requiring nasal oxygen therapy [17] and with Banerjee et al.'s study in the USA, which showed that patients discharged with home oxygen had low rates of mortality and re-hospitalization within 30 days of discharge, preserving safe access to acute care during the COVID-19 pandemic [18]. In the Netherlands, Grutters et al. showed, using retrospective data, that early discharge was possible in severe COVID-19 patients if home telemonitoring included the use of pulse oximetry [19]. Further, van Herwerden et al. showed in 49 patients, that, although 6 patients required readmission, home telemonitoring and oxygen administration can be safely applied in COVID-19 patients [20]. Very interestingly, another study comparing home telemonitoring and oxygen therapy started directly after emergency department (ED) vs. hospital admission, concluded that starting home telemonitoring and oxygen therapy directly after ED assessment was safe [21], with a total home telemonitoring duration of 14 days in both groups.

Thus, early returns home in patients hospitalized for COVID-19, whether or not oxygen is required, appears to be quite safe.

4.3. Usefulness of Early Return Home in Patients Hospitalized for COVID-19

Besides allowing for more personalized care to be delivered to patients, early returns home aimed to avoid hospital overflow, and thus to allow for other patients, whether or not they were suffering from COVID-19, to be hospitalized as needed. Indeed, numerous patients may not have always benefited from an adapted and timely therapy because of the unavailability of the hospital structure during the COVID-19 pandemic. This pitfall will probably also apply in future pandemics, whatever their origin.

Importantly, in our study we observed 17.8 days and 568 days, respectively, of median duration and cumulative days of home telemonitoring in our oxygen sub-group. This is similar to van Herwerden MC's data, showing a potential reduction in hospitalization of 616 days [11]. Similarly, Grutters LA et al. observed that the greatest reduction in hospitalization duration was seen in patients needing home oxygen therapy [10]. Taken together, our clinical protocol appeared efficient; the 743 cumulative days of home monitoring (of which 430 days were needed for oxygen weaning for 32 patients), saved a minimum of 49 hospital beds (based on a COVID-19-related mean hospitalization length of 15.2 days in our hospital). This is consistent with the results of Hanninen (in press) and Suárez-Gil et al., who found shorter hospital stays and lower readmission rates in COVID-19 patients followed at home by telemonitoring [22].

A usefulness assessment including questionnaires on patient's satisfaction and assessments of mental stress and anxiety as an outcome measure would have been interesting. Indeed, patients might experience higher anxiety when managing significant equipment at home without the presence of a doctor, compared to being in the hospital with readily available healthcare professionals. Although not mental stress and anxiety were not specifically investigated, we observed a fair level of satisfaction in our patients. Indeed, a majority found the device simple to use and the organization to be efficient, and accordingly felt safe with at-home monitoring. Our results are consistent with previous data showing high satisfaction levels in telemonitored COVID-19 patients [20].

4.4. Study Limitations and Perspectives

COVID-19 patients' duration of hospitalization was not compared to that of a control group without telemonitoring. A case-control design with a comparison group matching the characteristics of patients still admitted in the hospital would have strengthened the study. While patients on oxygen might fare better at home compared to those discharged without oxygen, this cannot be guaranteed by our design, supporting the need for complementary studies.

Nevertheless, when the length of stay in our hospital of 1756 patients discharged without telemonitoring during the same period was noted, we inferred an important reduction in days spent in a hospital bed (49 days). With the current decline in the number of hospital healthcare professionals, this study shows that this home telemonitoring system is suitable and applicable in the event of hospital tensions linked to strong epidemic periods, such as seasonal flu, which would necessitate increased hospitalization facilities for patients requiring oxygen therapy.

A prospective study including a dedicated nurse coordination unit receiving alerts directly from the homecare remote monitoring system, who could contact patients and their healthcare professionals in return, could further improve the efficiency and safety of homecare. This future study would also allow for a comprehensive implementation analysis, including interviews with doctors, teleproviders, and caregivers, in order to improve the design of this useful help in patient care.

5. Conclusions

This prospective study demonstrates that the remote monitoring of vital parameters and symptoms allows for early hospital discharge in patients hospitalized for COVID-19, whether or not home oxygen therapy is required. Extending these criteria to include patients presenting with more than one comorbidity did not reduce safety.

Interestingly, patients requiring home oxygen therapy likely benefitted more from TELECOVID-RAD, since it allowed for oxygen tapering to occur outside the hospital, and thus a greater reduction in hospital stay compared to patients who did not require oxygen therapy.

Nevertheless, even if our data support the idea that home monitoring reduces the hospital stay of patients with COVID-19, randomized controlled trials are necessary to confirm these beneficial effect [23] and demonstrate that more beds are thus available for other patients. Indeed, this important parameter during sanitary crises also depends on the medical and paramedical team's capacity to take care of more patients.

Author Contributions: Conceptualization, S.T., S.L., M.H., E.A. and B.G.; Methodology, S.T., S.L., A.-A.Z., P.T.B.L., M.H. and B.G.; Validation, S.T., S.L., L.K., N.L., A.-A.Z., P.T.B.L., M.G., N.M., M.H., E.A. and B.G.; Formal analysis, S.T., S.L., N.M. and M.H.; Investigation, S.T., L.K. and N.L.; Writing—original draft, S.T., N.L., P.T.B.L., M.G., N.M., M.H., E.A. and B.G.; Writing—review & editing, S.T. and B.G.; Supervision, S.T. and B.G.; Project administration, S.T. and B.G. All authors have read and agreed to the published version of the manuscript.

Funding: This research received no external funding.

Institutional Review Board Statement: The study was conducted in accordance with the Declaration of Helsinki, and approved by the ethics committee of the University of Strasbourg (CE-2022-61, 2 October 2022).

Informed Consent Statement: Informed consent was obtained from all subjects involved in the study.

Data Availability Statement: Data are available by asking to the corresponding author.

Acknowledgments: We greatly thank B. Boutteau (ARS), M. Rolland (CPAM), M. Rouchon (CPAM), M. Glady (HUS), J. Chartier (HUS), E. Van Wambeke (HUS) and AM. Kasprowicz for their help in performing the study. We greatly thank URPS and PRAG groups.

Conflicts of Interest: Mr. Mohamed Hajjam is the CEO of Predimed Technology, which solution developed by Predimed Technology has been used in this study as part of an institutional project.

References

1. WHO Health Emergency Dashboard WHO (COVID-19) Homepage. Available online: https://covid19.who.int (accessed on 9 May 2023).
2. Wu, Z.; McGoogan, J.M. Characteristics of and Important Lessons from the Coronavirus Disease 2019 (COVID-19) Outbreak in China: Summary of a Report of 72314 Cases from the Chinese Center for Disease Control and Prevention. *JAMA* **2020**, *323*, 1239–1242. [CrossRef]
3. Whitaker, M.; Elliott, J.; Chadeau-Hyam, M.; Riley, S.; Darzi, A.; Cooke, G.; Ward, H.; Elliott, P. Persistent COVID-19 symptoms in a community study of 606,434 people in England. *Nat. Commun.* **2022**, *13*, 1957. [CrossRef]
4. Van Wambeke, E.; Bezler, C.; Kasprowicz, A.-M.; Charles, A.-L.; Andres, E.; Geny, B. Two-Years Follow-Up of Symptoms and Return to Work in Complex Post-COVID-19 Patients. *J. Clin. Med.* **2023**, *12*, 741. [CrossRef]
5. Levy, D.; Giannini, M.; Oulehri, W.; Riou, M.; Marcot, C.; Pizzimenti, M.; Debrut, L.; Charloux, A.; Geny, B.; Meyer, A. Long Term Follow-Up of Sarcopenia and Malnutrition after Hospitalization for COVID-19 in Conventional or Intensive Care Units. *Nutrients* **2022**, *14*, 912. [CrossRef]
6. Pather, S.; Madhi, S.A.; Cowling, B.J.; Moss, P.; Kamil, J.P.; Ciesek, S.; Muik, A.; Türeci, Ö. SARS-CoV-2 Omicron variants: Burden of disease, impact on vaccine effectiveness and need for variant-adapted vaccines. *Front. Immunol.* **2023**, *14*, 1130539. [CrossRef] [PubMed]
7. Mannucci, E.; Silverii, G.A.; Monami, M. Saturation of critical care capacity and mortality in patients with the novel coronavirus (COVID-19) in Italy. *Trends Anaesth. Crit. Care* **2020**, *33*, 33–34. [CrossRef]

8. Martínez-García, M.; Bal-Alvarado, M.; Santos Guerra, F.; Ares-Rico, R.; Suárez-Gil, R.; Rodríguez-Álvarez, A.; Pérez-López, A.; Casariego-Vales, E.; en nombre del Equipo de Seguimiento Compartido TELEA-COVID Lugo; Equipo TELEA COVID-19 (Lugo). Monitoring of COVID-19 patients by telemedicine with telemonitoring. *Rev. Clin. Esp.* **2020**, *220*, 472–479. [CrossRef] [PubMed]
9. O'Keefe, J.B.; Tong, E.J.; O'Keefe, G.D.; Tong, D.C. Description of Symptom Course in a Telemedicine Monitoring Clinic for Acute Symptomatic COVID-19: A Retrospective Cohort Study. *BMJ Open* **2021**, *11*, e044154. [CrossRef] [PubMed]
10. Casariego-Vales, E.; Blanco-López, R.; Rosón-Calvo, B.; Suárez-Gil, R.; Santos-Guerra, F.; Dobao-Feijoo, M.J.; Ares-Rico, R.; Bal-Alvaredo, M.; On Behalf of the Telea-Covid Lugo Comanagement Team. Efficacy of Telemedicine and Telemonitoring in At-Home Monitoring of Patients with COVID-19. *J. Clin. Med.* **2021**, *10*, 2893. [CrossRef]
11. Mattioli, M.; Benfaremo, D.; Fulgenzi, F.; Gennarini, S.; Mucci, L.; Giorgino, F.; Frausini, G.; Moroncini, G.; Gnudi, U. Discharge from the Emergency Department and Early Hospital Revaluation in Patients with COVID-19 Pneumonia: A Prospective Study. *Clin. Exp. Emerg. Med.* **2022**, *9*, 10–17. [CrossRef]
12. Law of April 22, 2005 Relating to the Rights of Patients and the End of Life, LO 2005, Art 10 [V]. Public Health Code. 2005.Gilbert X [2005] Conseil d'Etat 256001, Rec. Lebon, p20. Available online: https://www.legifrance.gouv.fr/ceta/id/CETATEXT000008226250/ (accessed on 9 May 2023).
13. Camacho Moll, M.E.; Mata Tijerina, V.L.; Silva Ramírez, B.; Peñuelas Urquides, K.; González Escalante, L.A.; Escobedo Guajardo, B.L.; Cruz Luna, J.E.; Corrales Pérez, R.; Gómez García, S.; Bermúdez de León, M. Sex, Age, and Comorbidities Are Associated with SARS-CoV-2 Infection, COVID-19 Severity, and Fatal Outcome in a Mexican Population: A Retrospective Multi-Hospital Study. *J. Clin. Med.* **2023**, *12*, 2676. [CrossRef] [PubMed]
14. Baena-Díez, J.M.; Gonzalez-Casafont, I.; Cordeiro-Coelho, S.; Fernández-González, S.; Rodríguez-Jorge, M.; Pérez-Torres, C.U.F.; Larrañaga-Cabrera, A.; García-Lareo, M.; de la Arada-Acebes, A.; Martín-Jiménez, E.; et al. Effectiveness of Telephone Monitoring in Primary Care to Detect Pneumonia and Associated Risk Factors in Patients with SARS-CoV-2. *Healthcare* **2021**, *9*, 1548. [CrossRef] [PubMed]
15. Annis, T.; Pleasants, S.; Hultman, G.; Lindemann, E.; Thompson, J.A.; Billecke, S.; Badlani, S.; Melton, G.B. Rapid Implementation of a COVID-19 Remote Patient Monitoring Program. *J. Am. Med. Inform. Assoc.* **2020**, *27*, 1326–1330. [CrossRef]
16. Yordanov, Y.; Dechartres, A.; Lescure, X.; Apra, C.; Villie, P.; Marchand-Arvier, J.; Debuc, E.; Dinh, A.; Jourdain, P. AP-HP/Universities/Inserm COVID-19 Research Collaboration Covidom, a Telesurveillance Solution for Home Monitoring Patients With COVID-19. *J. Med. Internet. Res.* **2020**, *22*, e20748. [CrossRef]
17. Dinh, A.; Mercier, J.-C.; Jaulmes, L.; Artigou, J.-Y.; Juillière, Y.; Yordanov, Y.; Jourdain, P. AP-HP/Universities/INSERM COVID-19 Research Collaboration Safe Discharge Home with Telemedicine of Patients Requiring Nasal Oxygen Therapy after COVID-19. *Front. Med.* **2021**, *8*, 703017. [CrossRef]
18. Banerjee, J.; Canamar, C.P.; Voyageur, C.; Tangpraphaphorn, S.; Lemus, A.; Coffey, C.; Wald-Dickler, N.; Holtom, P.; Shoenberger, J.; Bowdish, M.; et al. Mortality and Readmission Rates among Patients with COVID-19 after Discharge from Acute Care Setting with Supplemental Oxygen. *JAMA Netw. Open* **2021**, *4*, e213990. [CrossRef]
19. Grutters, L.A.; Majoor, K.I.; Mattern, E.S.K.; Hardeman, J.A.; van Swol, C.F.P.; Vorselaars, A.D.M. Home Telemonitoring Makes Early Hospital Discharge of COVID-19 Patients Possible. *J. Am. Med. Inform. Assoc.* **2020**, *27*, 1825–1827. [CrossRef]
20. Van Herwerden, M.C.; van Steenkiste, J.; El Moussaoui, R.; den Hollander, J.G.; Helfrich, G.; Verberk, I.J.A.M. Home telemonitoring and oxygen therapy in COVID-19 patients: Safety, patient satisfaction, and cost-effectiveness. *Ned. Tijdschr. Geneeskd.* **2021**, *165*, D5740. [PubMed]
21. Van den Berg, R.; Meccanici, C.; de Graaf, N.; van Thiel, E.; Schol-Gelok, S. Starting Home Telemonitoring and Oxygen Therapy Directly after Emergency Department Assessment Appears to Be Safe in COVID-19 Patients. *J. Clin. Med.* **2022**, *11*, 7236. [CrossRef]
22. Suárez-Gil, R.; Casariego-Vales, E.; Blanco-López, R.; Santos-Guerra, F.; Pedrosa-Fraga, C.; Fernández-Rial, Á.; Íñiguez-Vázquez, I.; Abad-García, M.M.; Bal-Alvaredo, M.; On Behalf of the Members of the Lugo Telea-Covid Team. Efficacy of Telemedicine and At-Home Telemonitoring Following Hospital Discharge in Patients with COVID-19. *J. Pers. Med.* **2022**, *12*, 609. [CrossRef]
23. Gruwez, H.; Bakelants, E.; Dreesen, P.; Broekmans, J.; Criel, M.; Thomeer, M.; Vandervoort, P.; Ruttens, D. Remote Patient Monitoring in COVID-19: A Critical Appraisal. *Eur. Respir. J.* **2022**, *59*, 2102697. [CrossRef] [PubMed]

Disclaimer/Publisher's Note: The statements, opinions and data contained in all publications are solely those of the individual author(s) and contributor(s) and not of MDPI and/or the editor(s). MDPI and/or the editor(s) disclaim responsibility for any injury to people or property resulting from any ideas, methods, instructions or products referred to in the content.

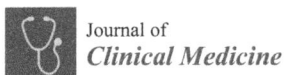

Article

Post-Traumatic Stress Disorder among Polish Healthcare Staff in the Era of the COVID-19 Pandemic

Grzegorz Kobelski [1], Katarzyna Naylor [2], Robert Ślusarz [3] and Mariusz Wysokiński [4,*]

1. Institute of Medical Sciences, University College of Applied Sciences in Chełm, Pocztowa 54, 22-100 Chełm, Poland; gkobelski@panschelm.edu.pl
2. Chair and Department of Didactics and Medical Simulation, Faculty of Medical Sciences, Medical University of Lublin Poland, Chodźki 7, 20-093 Lublin, Poland; katarzyna.naylor@umlub.pl
3. Neurological and Neurosurgical Nursing Department, Faculty of Health Science, Collegium Medicum in Bydgoszcz, Nicolaus Copernicus University in Toruń, 85-821 Bydgoszcz, Poland; robert.slusarz@cm.umk.pl
4. Department of Fundamentals of Nursing, Chair of Nursing Development, Faculty of Health Sciences, Medical University of Lublin Poland, 20-093 Lublin, Poland
* Correspondence: mariusz.wysokinski@umlub.pl

Abstract: Introduction: The COVID-19 pandemic has brought many adverse phenomena, particularly in the area of health for both individuals and society as a whole. Healthcare staff also suffered dire consequences. Aim: The aim of this study was to assess whether the COVID-19 pandemic increased the risk of post-traumatic stress disorder among healthcare professionals in Poland. Material and method: The survey was conducted between 4 April 2022 and 4 May 2022. The study applied the Computer Assisted Web Interview (CAWI) technique using the standardised Peritraumatic Distress Inventory (PDI) questionnaire. Results: The average score obtained by the respondents on the PDI was 21.24 ± 8.97. There was a statistically significant difference between the average PDI score obtained based on the gender of the subject ($Z = 3.873$, $p = 0.0001$.) The score obtained amongst nurses was statistically significantly higher compared to the paramedic group ($H = 6.998$, $p = 0.030$). There was no statistically significant difference between the average PDI score obtained based on the age of the participants ($F = 1.282$, $p = 0.281$), nor with their length of service ($F = 0.934$, $p = 0.424$). A total of 82.44% of the respondents received 14 PDI points, the cut-off point indicating the risk of PTSD that was adopted in the study. It was concluded that 6.12% of respondents did not require intervention (<7 PDI score); 74.28% of respondents needed further follow-up for PTSD and a reassessment of the PDI approximately 6 weeks after the initial testing; and 19.59% required coverage for PTSD prevention and mitigation (>28 PDI score). Conclusions: The study has shown a high risk of post-traumatic stress disorder among healthcare professionals in Poland. This risk is related to the gender of the respondents, with an indication of a higher risk of PTSD among women. The results have also shown a correlation between increased risk of post-traumatic stress disorder and occupation, with nurses being the most affected group. In contrast, no association has been found in terms of age and length of service for an increase in the risk of PTSD, following exposure to trauma in relation to healthcare services during the COVID-19 pandemic.

Keywords: post-traumatic stress disorder; COVID-19 pandemic; healthcare system

Citation: Kobelski, G.; Naylor, K.; Ślusarz, R.; Wysokiński, M. Post-Traumatic Stress Disorder among Polish Healthcare Staff in the Era of the COVID-19 Pandemic. *J. Clin. Med.* **2023**, *12*, 4072. https://doi.org/10.3390/jcm12124072

Academic Editors: Daniel L. Herr and Giovanni Giordano

Received: 28 April 2023
Revised: 4 June 2023
Accepted: 13 June 2023
Published: 15 June 2023

Copyright: © 2023 by the authors. Licensee MDPI, Basel, Switzerland. This article is an open access article distributed under the terms and conditions of the Creative Commons Attribution (CC BY) license (https://creativecommons.org/licenses/by/4.0/).

1. Introduction

Post-traumatic stress disorder, or PTSD, is a psychiatric disorder classified in DSM-5 under the number 309.81, ICD-10 F43.10, characterised by devastating psychological symptoms following the experience of severe trauma [1,2]. Trauma is interpreted as an extremely stressful event that has occurred in a person's life, often described as the 'worst,' such as the experience of war, terror, violence, rape, sexual abuse, kidnapping, disaster, or catastrophe. A traumatic event is also defined as one being directly involved in or witnessing an immediate life-threatening event, such as, but not limited to, a traffic accident, serious illness, suffering or death of a loved one, miscarriage of a child, childbirth under traumatising prolonged exposure to death, suffering and human misfortunes, etc. [3,4].

PTSD can be triggered both by a one-off experience of trauma, as well as by prolonged or repeated exposure to a traumatic event. It can become active a few weeks after exposure to the trauma, as well as remain latent for months or even years [5]. A factor predisposing one to the onset of PTSD is primarily the experience of long-term trauma [6]. Furthermore, according to available analyses, the most frequently mentioned predictor of this phenomenon is the female gender [7,8].

Symptoms manifested by the person affected by PTSD can vary in form and severity, most commonly appearing several weeks after exposure to a severely stressful event and persisting for at least one month, according to the DSM classification, causing significant dysfunction in everyday functioning and widespread psychological suffering. PTSD symptoms in the literature are divided into three categories: intrusion (reliving the trauma in the form of dreams or memories), avoidance (activities related to reliving the event, such as conversations, stimuli and feelings) and arousal (strong emotional reactions, general irritability, difficulty concentrating and falling asleep) [9,10]. The most frequently described symptoms experienced by people affected by post-traumatic stress disorder are an exaggerated avoidance of thoughts and emotions related to the traumatic event experienced, an aversion to adult conversations and discussions, and even a lack of memory about the trauma experience. It is also characteristic that, despite attempts to displace the trauma experienced, it is typical to re-experience it through recurrent, persistent memories, dissociative episodes of re-experiencing the trauma (called "flashbacks"), and numerous nightmares [11,12]. Symptoms of PTSD often include suicidal thoughts, anxiety, panic attacks, outbursts of aggression, and depressive disorders triggered by memories and re-experiencing the trauma. It is also characteristic of people with PTSD to present features of alienation, nihilism, dullness, anhedonia, and avoidance of all activities and situations that might resemble the trauma experienced [13–15].

Determining the magnitude of the prevalence of PTSD in the global and local population is difficult to estimate, despite many diagnostic research tools for post-traumatic stress disorder. This difficulty occurs due to the numerous diagnostic criteria for PTSD requiring the subject to, among other things, identify the exposure of an identifiable traumatic event and the fact that most of the tools refer to an analysis of the subject's entire life and an attempt to identify the most traumatic event in the participant's life. Nevertheless, several studies highlight the fact that PTSD can occur as a result of multiple experiences of challenging trauma, exemplified by those in the medical profession [16]. The WHO Global Mental Health Survey 2014–2020 uncovers that the prevalence of PTSD in the population averages around 4% globally [17–19].

Post-traumatic stress disorder (PTSD) has serious social consequences. Low public awareness of the risk, difficulties in diagnosis, lack of effective methods of preventing PTSD after traumatic experiences, and difficulties in treatment mean that many people who have experienced trauma do not receive help in the early stages of the development of peritraumatic disorders, with serious consequences for mental health. Among these individuals, a large proportion are health system staff, experiencing repeated and chronic exposure to trauma during their working lives. On 11 March 2020, the World Health Organisation declared a SARS-CoV-2 coronavirus-induced COVID-19 pandemic of unprecedented magnitude, involving many countries around the world, claiming more than 6.5 million lives by the end of 2022, which, for health system workers, has become a repeated and chronic exposure to the trauma of experiencing death and human suffering [20–23].

In Poland, the first SARS-CoV-2 infection was detected on 4 March 2020, and by 30 April 2020, there were approximately 12.9 thousand diagnosed cases of COVID-19 [24]. The reality faced by the employees of the Polish healthcare system was unprecedented. The constantly increasing number of patients in serious condition, the lack of places in hospitals, a large number of deaths among patients, including co-workers, working overtime, shortages in personal protective equipment, or the discomfort of long working hours in protective suits caused exhaustion and discouragement. The new realities forced the introduction of novel solutions in the healthcare system, transforming hospitals into the so-called single-name institutions—intended only for patients with COVID-19. Temporary hospitals were created in sports halls, stadiums and multi-surface facilities previously intended for other purposes—such as sales halls. Hospital wards transformed into wards for patients with COVID-19, suspended admissions, procedures and planned operations were limited to emergencies only. Doctors, nurses, and paramedics were delegated by the authorities to forced labour in indicated hospitals providing care for patients with COVID-19. Standard tests for SARS-CoV-2 infection were introduced, where the number of people tested exceeded quantitative capabilities. Numerous infections among healthcare workers (HCWs) resulted in a significant reduction in the availability of employees and medical services. For this reason, many hospital wards, and often hospitals, were temporarily closed due to a lack of staff. There were also situations when, due to staff shortages, patients with COVID-19 were cared for by staff with positive SARS-CoV-2 tests—such as in social care homes. This study aimed to assess whether the COVID-19 pandemic has increased the risk of post-traumatic stress disorder among healthcare staff in Poland.

Leading this research was imperative in displaying the perspective concerning the shifts caused by the new reality of the Polish healthcare system to affect the mental health of HCWs. Furthermore, this study was to show the importance of providing adequate psychological care and support after exposure to trauma that should be ensured to healthcare system employees in Poland to diagnose early and prevent PTSD promptly.

2. Materials and Methods

2.1. Participants and Study Characteristics

The research was conducted between 4 April 2022 and 4 May 2022, among 245 healthcare professionals. The survey used the Computer Assisted Web Interview (CAWI) technique [25–27] using the Microsoft Forms software. The sample selection was based on a search for participants among members of thematic groups of forums and online groups for employees of the Polish healthcare system. The inclusion criteria for the study were:

1. Provides medical services as an employee or collaborator as a healthcare provider in a healthcare facility during the COVID-19 pandemic;
2. The occurrence of a traumatic event related to the provision of medical services during the COVID-19 pandemic.

2.2. Method

The study used a standardised questionnaire, Peritraumatic Distress Inventory (PDI), by A. Brunet et al., 2001 [28] as a screening tool to assess the risk of PTSD. The PDI evaluates the level of physiological and emotional suffering experienced by an individual in relation to exposure to trauma [6,29,30].

The study used a Polish adaptation of the PDI by Rybojad and Aftyka, 2018 [31]. The questionnaire in the Polish adaptation consists of 12 items for self-assessment of perceived discomfort in relation to the experience of the traumatic event, both during and/or after the traumatic event, using a 5-point Likert scale (0–4). Due to the low factor value obtained during the validation, the original PDI scale was rejected—the 5-item "I felt guilty" scale [28,32,33]. A respondent in the Polish adaptation of the PDI can score a maximum of 48 points, and the higher the score obtained, the most prominent the exposure to distress [34].

The study analysis adopted the approach proposed by Guardia et al., 2013 [35] at the parallel most commonly recommended cut-off point of 14, which is an interpretation of the PDI score as a prediction of the occurrence of PTSD after exposure to trauma. In addition, the authors suggested that immediate care and follow-up should be implemented for patients with a PDI score >28; for those with 7–28 points, a follow-up a few weeks after the test; for those with <7 points, no further monitoring [35].

2.3. Statistical Analysis

Statistical analyses were performed using Statistica 9.1 software (StatSoft, Kraków, Poland).

The results obtained in terms of the analysis of quantitative variables are presented using the mean, median and standard deviation, and in terms of qualitative variables using the number and percentage.

The qualitative characteristics between the analysed variables were investigated with the Chi2 test. In addition, the normality of the distribution was tested using the Shapiro–Wilk test. Finally, the differences between groups were assessed with the Mann–Whitney test for two groups; an ANOVA analysis of variance for three or more groups (with Tukey's RIR post hoc test), or, if the requirements for ANOVA use were not fulfilled, the Kruskal–Wallis test was employed.

$p < 0.05$ was set as a significance level to determine the presence of statistically significant correlations or differences.

2.4. Ethical Statement

The research was conducted based on the requirements of the Declaration of Helsinki. All participants were informed of the purpose of the study and took part voluntarily and consciously.

3. Results

3.1. Sociodemographic Analysis of the Study Group

The characteristics of the study group are shown in Table 1. A total of 245 healthcare providers participated in the study; the majority were female (77.14%). The average age of participants was 40.2 years (SD = 10.1). The most numerous professional group were nurses (67.76%) and the average length of service of the respondents was 15.4 years (SD = 11.1).

Table 1. Sociodemographic analysis of the study group.

Variable	Category	Number (N)	Percentage (%)
Gender	Woman	189	77.14
	Man	56	22.86
Age	Up to 30 years of age	54	22.04
	31–40 years of age	76	31.02
	41–50 years of age	78	31.84
	over 50 years of age	37	15.10
Occupation	Nurse	166	67.76
	Paramedic	46	18.78
	Healthcare worker	4	1.63
	Medical Registrar	1	0.41
	Administrative Officer	7	2.86
	Physician	7	2.86
	Midwife	10	4.08
	Electroradiology technician	1	0.41
	Psychologist	2	0.82
	Sanitarian	1	0.41
Length of service	up to 5 years	67	27.35
	6–15 years	69	28.16
	16–25 years	54	22.04
	over 25 years	55	22.45

3.2. PDI Questionnaire

The study results showed that the average score obtained on the PDI by the subjects was 21.24 ± 8.97 (presented in Table 2). There was a statistically significant difference between the mean PDI score obtained based on the participants' gender. Female participants ($n = 189$) obtained a statistically significantly ($Z = 3.873$, $p = 0.0001$) higher score

(M = 22.52, SD = 8.18) compared to the male population (*n* = 56, M = 16.91, SD = 10.18). In the analysed PDI result, there were statistically significant differences between occupational groups (H = 6.998, *p* = 0.030). Similarly, nurses obtained a statistically significantly higher score when compared to paramedics. Due to the variety of occupations of the respondents, other, less numerous occupations were grouped into a single category, 'other occupations', creating the following division into three groups: nurses (*n* = 166), paramedics (*n* = 46) and other professions (*n* = 33). An ANOVA analysis of variance resulted in no statistically significant difference between the average PDI score obtained based on the age of the subjects (F = 1.282, *p* = 0.281), as well as in terms of the average PDI score obtained and the length of service (F = 0.934, *p* = 0.424).

Table 2. Differences in PDI score in relation to the sociodemographic characteristics of the subjects.

Variable	Category	M	Me	SD	Statistical Analysis
Gender	Woman	22.52	23.00	8.18	Z = 3.873
	Man	16.91	16.50	10.19	*p* = 0.0001
Age	Up to 30 years of age	21.76	20.50	10.74	
	31–40 years of age	19.57	19.00	8.70	F = 1.282
	41–50 years of age	22.08	22.00	7.59	*p* = 0.281
	over 50 years of age	22.11	25.00	9.30	
Length of service	up to 5 years	21.88	21.00	10.27	
	6–15 years	19.83	20.00	9.09	F = 0.934
	16–25 years	22.30	22.00	7.26	*p* = 0.425
	over 25 years	21.20	21.00	8.64	
Occupation	Nurse (I)	22.30	22.00	8.49	H = 6.998
	Paramedic (II)	18.32	17.00	9.95	*p* = 0.030
	Other occupation (III)	19.97	21.00	9.13	I > II

M—average, Me—median, SD—standard deviation, H—Kruskal–Wallis test, F—ANOVA analysis of variance, Z—Mann–Whitney test, *p*—statistical significance.

A total of 82.44% of participants obtained the cut-off point of 14 PDI scores indicating the risk of PTSD (Table 3). The result of ≥14 PDI scores was analysed in relation to sociodemographic characteristics; there was a statistical relationship between gender and high PTSD risk (Chi^2 = 23.698, *p* = 0.000). Similarly, analysis with Pearson's chi-square test showed a statistical relationship (Chi^2 = 15.453, *p* = 0.001) in terms of the 14 PDI cut-off score achieved and the represented occupation. The analysis of the results shows that the majority of the respondents (>63%) in all the professional groups represented are at high risk of PTSD, with the highest percentage characterized by a score ≥14 points among nurses—87.95%. Additionally, each age group was dominated by individuals (>75%) at increased risk of post-traumatic stress disorder (age up to 30 years—79.63%; 31–40 years—78.95%; 41–50 years—88.46%; over 50 years—81.08%). However, the Pearson chi-square test showed no statistical relationship (Chi^2 = 2.937, *p* = 0.401) between the age of the participants and the PDI cut-off point. Moreover, in terms of work experience and a score of ≥14 points on PDI, the vast majority of respondents (>80%) in each group were at increased risk of PTSD (up to 5 years of service—80.60%; 6–15 years 76.81%; 16–25 years 90.74%; over 25 years of service—83.64%). Analysis with Pearson chi-square test showed no statistical relationship (Chi^2 = 4.293, *p* = 0.231) of work experience in relation to reaching the cut-off point.

Further analyses included any need for therapeutic intervention in relation to the respondents' PDI scores (Table 4), as recommended by Guardia et al., 2013 [35]. A total of 6.12% of participants did not require intervention (<7 PDI score); 74.28% of respondents required further follow-up for PTSD and reassessment of PDI approximately 6 weeks after the previous survey; and 19.59% required steps concerning PTSD prevention and mitigation (>28 PDI score). Pearson's chi-square test analysis showed that there was statistical significance in the relationship between gender and the level of PDI requiring therapeutic action ($Chi2$ = 12.507, *p* = 0.002), Pearson's chi-square test analysis showed that there was statical significance in the relationship between gender and the level of PDI requiring therapeutic action (Chi^2 = 12.507, p = 0.002), in both groups, the highest number of subjects were those who required further monitoring for PTSD (PDI scores of 7–28 were obtained by 76.72% of women and 66.07% of men). Similarly, relevance was shown for the age of respondents (Chi^2 = 13.01, p = 0.043), where the majority (>59%) required follow-up for PTSD (age up to 30 years—66.67%; 31–40 years—80.26%; 41–50 years—80.77%; over 50 years—59.46%). There was also evidence of statistical significance (Chi^2 = 11.110, p = 0.025) in terms of occupation and type of intervention. In all groups (>69%) there was a need for further follow-up for PTSD warnings (nurses—75.30%; paramedics—69.57%; other occupations—75.76%). In all job tenure groups, most people (>70%) achieved a score (7–28 on the PDI) qualifying them for further follow-up (up to 5 years of service—70.15%; 6–15 years—75.36%; 16–25 years—81.48%; over 25 years of service—70.91%). However, there was no statistical significance found in this respect (Chi^2 = 4.649, p = 0.590).

Table 3. Relationship of PDI cut-off score and sociodemographic characteristics of respondents.

Variable	Category	Cut-Off ≥14 Points PDI - PTSD Risk				Chi^2 p
		≤13 pt		≥14 pt		
		N	%	N	%	
Gender	Woman	21	11.11	168	88.89	Chi^2 = 23.698
	Man	22	39.29	34	60.71	p = 0.000
Age	Up to 30 years of age	11	20.37	43	79.63	
	31–40 years of age	16	21.05	60	78.95	Chi^2 = 2.937
	41–50 years of age	9	11.54	69	88.46	p = 0.401
	over 50 years of age	7	18.92	30	81.08	
Length of service	Up to 5 years	13	19.40	54	80.60	
	6–15 years	16	23.19	53	76.81	Chi^2 = 4.293
	16–25 years	5	9.26	49	90.74	p = 0.231
	over 25 years	9	16.36	46	83.64	
Occupation	Nurse	20	12.05	146	87.95	Chi^2 = 15.453
	Paramedic	17	36.96	29	63.04	p = 0.001
	Other occupation	6	18.18	27	81.82	
Total		43	17.55	202	82.44	-

Table 4. Relationship between the need for intervention concerning PTSD and sociodemographic characteristics of respondents.

Variable	Category	PDI Result—Need for Intervention <7 pt. PDI—Lack of Intervention 7–28 PDI—Further Observation for PTSD >28 PDI—Urgent Intervention						Chi^2 p
		<7 pt		7–28 pt		>28 pt		
		n	%	n	%	n	%	
Gender	Woman	6	3.17	145	76.62	38	20.11	Chi^2 = 12.507
	Man	9	16.07	37	66.07	10	17.86	p = 0.002
Age	Up to 30 years of age	5	9.26	36	66.67	13	24.07	
	31–40	6	7.89	61	80.26	9	11.84	Chi^2 = 13.012
	41–50	2	2.56	63	80.77	13	16.67	p = 0.043
	over 50 years of age	2	5.41	22	59.46	13	35.14	
Length of service	Up to 5 years	5	7.46	47	70.15	15	22.39	
	6–15 years	6	8.70	52	75.36	11	15.94	Chi^2 = 4.649
	16–25 years	1	1.85	44	81.48	9	16.67	p = 0.589
	over 25 years	3	5.45	39	70.91	13	23.64	

Table 4. Cont.

Variable	Category	PDI Result—Need for Intervention <7 pt. PDI—Lack of Intervention 7–28 PDI—Further Observation for PTSD >28 PDI—Urgent Intervention						Chi^2 p
		<7 pt		7–28 pt		>28 pt		
		n	%	n	%	n	%	
Occupation	Nurse	5	3.01	125	75.30	36	21.69	Chi^2 = 11.110 p = 0.025
	Paramedic	5	10.87	32	69.57	9	19.57	
	Other occupation	5	15.15	25	75.76	3	9.09	
	Total	15	6.12	182	74.28	48	19.59	-

4. Discussion

The COVID-19 pandemic, despite the fact it does not constitute a typical factor that can be identified as a direct cause of PTSD, has placed a significant traumatic burden on health professionals. There is a growing trend of anxiety and stress triggers that can lead to the development of PTSD among healthcare professionals as a consequence of experiencing the COVID-19 pandemic [30,36,37]. A review of studies confirms that healthcare professionals worldwide experienced psychological strain during the COVID-19 pandemic and, consequently, an increased risk of PTSD (Kang et al., 2020 [38]; Chen et al., 2020 [39]; Chidiebere Okechukwu et al., 2020 [40]; Shahrour and Dardas, 2020 [41]; Greenberg et al., 2020 [42]; Lamb et al., 2020 [43]). A review of the literature presents the high risk of PTSD among medical aid personnel during the COVID-19 pandemic, particularly affecting the North American region (Norman et al., 2020 [44]; Sagherian et al., 2020 [45]; Ayotte et al., 2020 [46]; Rodriguez et al., 2020 [47]; Shechter et al., 2020 [48]; Mehta et al., 2020 [49]; Crowe et al., 2020 [50]). Similarly, the analysis of studies also portrays a high level of exposure to PTSD among healthcare professionals in Europe (Vlah Tomičević and Lang, 2020 [51]; Alonso et al., 2020 [52]; Marco et al., 2020 [53]; Martínez-Caballeroi et al., 2020 [54]; Blanco-Daza et al., 2020 [55]; Luceño-Moreno et al., 2020 [56]; Steudte-Schmiedgen et al., 2020 [57]), with a particular focus on the high risks in the Italian region: (Di Tella et al., 2020 [58]; Bassi et al., 2020 [59]; Marcomini et al., 2020 [60], Lasalvia et al., 2020 [61]). Polish studies also confirm that caring for patients during the COVID-19 pandemic resulted in an increased risk of PTSD (Nowicki et al., 2020 [62]; Kosydar-Bochenek et al., 2021 [63]). In the Asian region, the findings varied widely from an extremely low 2.3% of healthcare professionals at risk of developing PTSD in the study by Chinvararak et al., 2021 [64] to an extremely high 54.6% in the study by Jiang et al., 2020 [65].

The authors' research has demonstrated that the risk level for PTSD among the population surveyed (N = 245) was very high, 82.44%. Similarly, Mirzaei et al., 2020 [66], and Kabunga and Okalo, 2021 [67] also obtained a high risk for PTSD amongst their respondents, 86% and 65.7% respectively. The average score in our study was 21.24 ± 8.97 PDI, similar results were obtained in studies conducted in Korea—Yoon et al., 2021 [30], PDI: 19.75 ± 8.82—and Italy—Carmassi et al., 2020 [32], PDI: 19.11 ± 8.29—which indicates a similar level of exposure to experiencing PTSD among the Polish population of healthcare professionals as in the Italian and Korean populations.

The conducted study uncovered a relationship between the sociodemographic characteristics and the risk of post-traumatic stress disorder. In terms of gender, females were shown to have a higher exposure to PTSD with a rate of 88.89%. Similar conclusions based on the study were shown by Blekas et al., 2020 [68]; Di Tella et al., 2020 [58]; Işik et al., 2020 [69] and Steudte-Schmiedgen et al., 2020 [57]. Similar conclusions were presented in Polish research by Kosydar-Bochenek et al., 2021 [63]; Bidzan et al., 2020 [70] and Rachubińska et al., 2022 [71]. However, Qutishat et al., 2020 [72], in a study conducted among Jordanian nurses, and Alanazi et al., 2020 [73], in a literature review concerning emergency healthcare professionals during the COVID-19 pandemic, showed that men were characterized by a higher incidence of PTSD. In contrast, no association between gender and the occurrence of increased risk of PTSD was found in studies by Zhou et al., 2020 [74] and Blanco-Daza et al., 2020 [55].

The authors' research also presented a correlation between occupation and the risk of post-traumatic stress disorder among healthcare professionals, demonstrating that nurses are an occupational group particularly vulnerable to PTSD after experiencing trauma related to the COVID-19 pandemic. The above relationship was also found by Bulut et al., 2020 [75]; Geng et al., 2020 [76]; Shechter et al., 2020 [48]; and Song et al., 2020 [77], indicating that nurses are the most-burdened occupational group in terms of the occurrence of PTSD. A study by Lasalvia et al., 2020 [61] amongst 2195 Italian healthcare professionals concludes that being a nurse at least doubles the risk of developing posttraumatic stress symptoms. Research conducted in Poland by Szwamel et al., 2022 [78]; Haor et al., 2023 [79]; and Dymecka et al., 2022 [80] indicated that nurses were the group most exposed to stress in the face of the COVID-19 pandemic. This is mainly due to close contact with COVID-19 patients, the risk of infection, and overwork. In contrast, a different conclusion was drawn by Martínez-Caballero et al. on the basis of their study, 2020 [54], indicating a higher trauma burden for paramedics than for nurses. In contrast, Bahadirli and Sagaltici, 2020/2021 [81] conclude that the risk of PTSD is the highest in the group of doctors. Das et al., 2020 [82] presented no association between occupation and the risk of PTSD after experiencing trauma suffered during the COVID-19 pandemic.

Further, young age was enumerated as a risk factor for PTSD (Geng et al., 2020 [76]; Lamb et al., 2020 [43]; Shahrour and Dardas, 2020 [41]; Alonso et al., 2020 [52]; Chatzittofis et al., 2020 [83]). However, that was not confirmed in authors' research. Other studies also showed that older people were at a greater risk of developing PTSD, such as Di Tella et al. 2020 [58].

The results of our study showed a partial correlation between the age of the respondents and the need for intervention in relation to PTSD risk. There is a relationship between the age and the PDI score, demanding further follow-up or immediate therapeutic support.

The current global research trends (Sanghera et al., 2019/2020 [84]; Luceño-Moreno et al., 2020 [56]; Nowicki et al., 2020 [62]) highlighted the tendency for a shorter length of service to influence the increased risk of PTSD after experiencing COVID-19-related trauma; however, the authors' results showed no association with greater exposure to PTSD due to shorter work experience.

The trends shown in our research and global studies clearly show that the COVID-19 pandemic, although it had similar effects on the mental health of healthcare system employees, did not affect the world similarly. It certainly contributed to the risk burden of PTSD, but the strength of this risk varies across continents, regions, and countries. As shown in the US–Poland comparative study by Szaflarski, 2022 [85], US healthcare workers reported a stronger feeling of being overwhelmed by the COVID-19 pandemic. The geopolitical situation, cultural conditions, experiences of previous epidemic threats, or psychological support provided to healthcare system employees significantly affect the feeling of stress due to the COVID-19 pandemic and the risk of PTSD. In many studies, women and nurses are a group particularly vulnerable to PTSD as a result of the COVID-19 pandemic. It is difficult to determine whether these two characteristics are related, and which is dominant in the influence on the increased risk of PTSD. This is because the female gender predominates in the professional population of nurses. The analysis of the authors' original research also does not give a clear answer to which trait is a predictor of PTSD. In the future, it would be required to conduct research on a representative sample of nurses in terms of a balanced gender division. Indeed, being a nurse and the resulting increased risk of PTSD in the COVID-19 pandemic can be explained by the tasks set for this professional group. The time of exposure to traumatic events in the case of nurses is also of great importance, because this professional group provided prolonged health services to patients with COVID-19. In Poland, nurses in many hospitals were on duty with patients, equipped with personal protective equipment, in a rotational system for several hours, and doctors carried out tasks depending on the needs of patients. The tasks of Polish nurses were based on nursing, continuous health monitoring, support, and the implementation of medical orders for patients, which resulted in heavy time, physical, and mental burden. Each occupational group carrying out tasks during the COVID-19 pandemic was significantly physically and mentally strained, which increased the risk of PTSD. The experience of trauma and the occurrence of PTSD symptoms for healthcare system employees is hazardous because, during this challenging time of the COVID-19 pandemic, they were expected to be fully dedicated, available, physically and mentally resilient, and fully professional in providing medical services. Awareness of this kind of responsibility further increases the risk of PTSD, preventing them from admitting their mental health weaknesses and actively seeking help.

5. Limitations

The authors' study does not take into account all the possible correlations of the characteristics of the subjects with the occurrence of PTSD, nor does it answer the question of whether the next wave of the COVID-19 pandemic in Poland would cause a strong psychological burden on the healthcare system workers, causing long-term consequences in the form of PTSD. Therefore, it seems justified to continue systematic screening for mental stress among employees of the Polish healthcare system. Action must be taken to support those at risk of developing PTSD after experiencing trauma related to healthcare services. The issue of the incidence of PTSD as a result of trauma related to the COVID-19 pandemic is a rather recent topic, and requires further knowledge in this area, and the study presented in this thesis should be repeated in the near future.

In designing the study, it was assumed that the best research tool to assess the risk of PTSD in the long term after the trauma was the Peritraumatic Stress Scale, as opposed to the IES-R Event Impact Scale tool. The PDI has the advantage of being accessible in terms of understanding the questions posed to respondents, and the possibility of deepening the analysis of the results obtained in terms of taking action in response to the result obtained, increasing its sensitivity and reliability. However, the study is not without its limitations, inter alia, because of the risk of respondents referring to a distant past event unrelated to the COVID-19 pandemic, while distorting the overall average PDI scores. A limitation of this study is the way we reached study participants. The selection criterion may inadvertently overestimate the results obtained in the context of high exposure to PTSD by self-selecting for participation in the study. The form of data collection is also an important issue; Internet research has its challenges. The researchers are still determining whether a person participating in the study meets the assumed selection criteria. It is also not possible to observe the response of the examined person to the questions asked, which means that the answers given may not be valid. Another issue is the limited search range of target groups, due to the limited availability in Internet groups and forums. Due to numerous cyberattacks aimed at stealing data, trust in online research is severely limited. People are afraid to open unknown links from unknown addresses, due to the possibility of phishing, malware, ransomware, etc. In addition, the researcher can never be sure whether the person participating in the study is not trying to falsify the results by filling out the questionnaires many times by giving random answers.

6. Conclusions

The conducted study confirmed a high risk of post-traumatic stress disorder among healthcare professionals in Poland who experienced trauma related to the provision of healthcare during the COVID-19 pandemic. This risk is related to the gender of the subjects, with an indication of a higher risk of PTSD among women. The results have further shown a correlation between the increased risk of post-traumatic stress disorder and occupation, with nurses being the most affected group. The findings have demonstrated a partial relationship in relation to the age of the respondents, and the need for intervention in relation to the presence of PTSD hazards.

Author Contributions: G.K.: Conceptualization, data curation, data statistical analysis, methodology, writing—original draft, writing—review and editing. K.N.: Conceptualization, investigation, writing—original draft. M.W.: Conceptualization, preparation, formal analysis, supervision, methodology, writing—original draft, writing—review and editing. R.Ś.: writing—review and editing. All authors have read and agreed to the published version of the manuscript.

Funding: This research received no specific grant from any funding agency in the public, commercial, or not-for-profit sectors.

Institutional Review Board Statement: Bioethics Committe of Lublin Medical University, Approval Code: KE - 0254/290/2018 Approval Date: 29 November 2018.

Informed Consent Statement: Informed consent was obtained from all subjects involved in the study.

Data Availability Statement: Data is available on request from the authors.

Conflicts of Interest: The authors have no conflict to declare.

References

1. American Psychiatric Association (Ed.) *Diagnostic and Statistical Manual of Mental Disorders: DSM-5*, 5th ed.; American Psychiatric Association: Washington, DC, USA, 2013; ISBN 978-0-89042-554-1.
2. Möller, H.-J. Possibilities and Limitations of DSM-5 in Improving the Classification and Diagnosis of Mental Disorders. *Psychiatr. Pol.* **2018**, *52*, 611–628. [CrossRef] [PubMed]
3. Kessler, R.C.; Aguilar-Gaxiola, S.; Alonso, J.; Benjet, C.; Bromet, E.J.; Cardoso, G.; Degenhardt, L.; de Girolamo, G.; Dinolova, R.V.; Ferry, F.; et al. Trauma and PTSD in the WHO World Mental Health Surveys. *Eur. J. Psychotraumatology* **2017**, *8*, 1353383. [CrossRef] [PubMed]
4. Zhou, Y.-G.; Shang, Z.-L.; Zhang, F.; Wu, L.-L.; Sun, L.-N.; Jia, Y.-P.; Yu, H.-B.; Liu, W.-Z. PTSD: Past, Present and Future Implications for China. *Chin. J. Traumatol. Zhonghua Chuang Shang Za Zhi* **2021**, *24*, 187–208. [CrossRef] [PubMed]
5. Charnsil, C.; Narkpongphun, A.; Chailangkarn, K. Posttraumatic Stress Disorder and Related Factors in Students Whose School Burned down: Cohort Study. *Asian J. Psychiatry* **2020**, *51*, 102004. [CrossRef] [PubMed]
6. Bunnell, B.E.; Davidson, T.M.; Ruggiero, K.J. The Peritraumatic Distress Inventory: Factor Structure and Predictive Validity in Traumatically Injured Patients Admitted through a Level I Trauma Center. *J. Anxiety Disord.* **2018**, *55*, 8–13. [CrossRef]
7. Atwoli, L.; Stein, D.J.; Koenen, K.C.; McLaughlin, K.A. Epidemiology of Posttraumatic Stress Disorder: Prevalence, Correlates and Consequences. *Curr. Opin. Psychiatry* **2015**, *28*, 307–311. [CrossRef]
8. Kawakami, N.; Tsuchiya, M.; Umeda, M.; Koenen, K.C.; Kessler, R.C. World Mental Health Survey Japan Trauma and Posttraumatic Stress Disorder in Japan: Results from the World Mental Health Japan Survey. *J. Psychiatr. Res.* **2014**, *53*, 157–165. [CrossRef]
9. Ogińska-Bulik, N. Objawy stresu pourazowego a potraumatyczny wzrost u młodzieży—Ofiar wypadków drogowych. *Psychiatria* **2014**, *11*, 49–58.
10. Ogińska-Bulik, N. Objawy stresu pourazowego u nastoletnich ofiar wypadków drogowych—Rola wsparcia i postaw rodzicielskich. *Psychiatr. Psychoter.* **2015**, *11*, 3–20.
11. Ogińska-Bulik, N.; Juczyński, Z. Rozwój Potraumatyczny—Charakterystyka i Pomiar. *Psychiatria* **2010**, *7*, 129–142.
12. Waltman, S.H.; Shearer, D.; Moore, B.A. Management of Posttraumatic Nightmares: A Review of Pharmacologic and Nonpharmacologic Treatments Since 2013. *Curr. Psychiatry Rep.* **2018**, *20*, 108. [CrossRef]
13. Bossini, L.; Ilaria, C.; Koukouna, D.; Caterini, C.; Olivola, M.; Fagiolini, A. PTSD in victims of terroristic attacks—A comparison with the impact of other traumatic events on patients' lives. *Psychiatr. Pol.* **2016**, *50*, 907–921. [CrossRef]
14. Ogińska-Bulik, N.; Juczyński, Z. Konsekwencje Doświadczanych Negatywnych Wydarzeń Życiowych-Objawy Stresu Pourazowego i Potraumatyczny Wzrost. *Psychiatria* **2012**, *9*, 1–10.
15. Ogłodek, E. Symptoms intensification of posttraumatic stress in individuals performing the job of a medical rescue worker. *Med. Sr.* **2011**, *14*, 54–58.
16. DeLucia, J.A.; Bitter, C.; Fitzgerald, J.; Greenberg, M.; Dalwari, P.; Buchanan, P. Prevalence of Post-Traumatic Stress Disorder in Emergency Physicians in the United States. *West. J. Emerg. Med.* **2019**, *20*, 740–746. [CrossRef]
17. Karam, E.G.; Friedman, M.J.; Hill, E.D.; Kessler, R.C.; McLaughlin, K.A.; Petukhova, M.; Sampson, L.; Shahly, V.; Angermeyer, M.C.; Bromet, E.J.; et al. Cumulative Traumas and Risk Thresholds: 12-Month PTSD in the World Mental Health (WMH) Surveys. *Depress. Anxiety* **2014**, *31*, 130–142. [CrossRef]
18. Koenen, K.C.; Ratanatharathorn, A.; Ng, L.; McLaughlin, K.A.; Bromet, E.J.; Stein, D.J.; Karam, E.G.; Meron Ruscio, A.; Benjet, C.; Scott, K.; et al. Posttraumatic Stress Disorder in the World Mental Health Surveys. *Psychol. Med.* **2017**, *47*, 2260–2274. [CrossRef]
19. Stein, D.J.; Harris, M.G.; Vigo, D.V.; Tat Chiu, W.; Sampson, N.; Alonso, J.; Altwaijri, Y.; Bunting, B.; Caldas-de-Almeida, J.M.; Cía, A.; et al. Perceived Helpfulness of Treatment for Posttraumatic Stress Disorder: Findings from the World Mental Health Surveys. *Depress. Anxiety* **2020**, *37*, 972–994. [CrossRef]

20. Adil, M.T.; Rahman, R.; Whitelaw, D.; Jain, V.; Al-Taan, O.; Rashid, F.; Munasinghe, A.; Jambulingam, P. SARS-CoV-2 and the Pandemic of COVID-19. *Postgrad. Med. J.* **2021**, *97*, 110–116. [CrossRef]
21. Osuchowski, M.F.; Aletti, F.; Cavaillon, J.-M.; Flohé, S.B.; Giamarellos-Bourboulis, E.J.; Huber-Lang, M.; Relja, B.; Skirecki, T.; Szabó, A.; Maegele, M. SARS-CoV-2/COVID-19: Evolving Reality, Global Response, Knowledge Gaps, and Opportunities. *Shock* **2020**, *54*, 416–437. [CrossRef]
22. Ochani, R.; Asad, A.; Yasmin, F.; Shaikh, S.; Khalid, H.; Batra, S.; Sohail, M.R.; Mahmood, S.F.; Ochani, R.; Hussham Arshad, M.; et al. COVID-19 Pandemic: From Origins to Outcomes. A Comprehensive Review of Viral Pathogenesis, Clinical Manifestations, Diagnostic Evaluation, and Management. *Infez. Med.* **2021**, *29*, 20–36. [PubMed]
23. WHO. Coronavirus (COVID-19) Dashboard. Available online: https://covid19.who.int (accessed on 1 January 2023).
24. Śleszyński, P. Prawidłowości przebiegu dyfuzji przestrzennej rejestrowanych zakażeń koronawirusem SARS-CoV-2 w Polsce w pierwszych 100 dniach epidemii. The regularity of spatial diffusion of recorded SARS-CoV-2 coronavirus infections of the epidemic in Poland in the first 100 days. *Czas. Geogr.* **2020**, *91*, 5–18.
25. Mider, D. Dylematy Metodologiczne Badań Kultury Politycznej w Internecie. *Przegląd Politol.* **2018**, *2*, 23–34. [CrossRef]
26. Sowa, P.; Pędziński, B.; Krzyżak, M.; Maślach, D.; Wójcik, S.; Szpak, A. The Computer-Assisted Web Interview Method as Used in the National Study of ICT Use in Primary Healthcare in Poland—Reflections on a Case Study. *Stud. Log. Gramm. Rhetor.* **2015**, *43*, 137–146. [CrossRef]
27. Fowler, F.J.; Mangione, T.W. *Standardized Survey Interviewing; Minimizing Interviewer-Related Error*; Applied Social Research Methods Series; Sage Publications: Newbury Park, CA, USA, 1990; ISBN 978-0-8039-3092-6.
28. Brunet, A.; Weiss, D.S.; Metzler, T.J.; Best, S.R.; Neylan, T.C.; Rogers, C.; Fagan, J.; Marmar, C.R. The Peritraumatic Distress Inventory: A Proposed Measure of PTSD Criterion A2. *Am. J. Psychiatry* **2001**, *158*, 1480–1485. [CrossRef]
29. Antičević, V.; Bubić, A.; Britvić, D. Peritraumatic Distress and Posttraumatic Stress Symptoms during the COVID-19 Pandemic: The Contributions of Psychosocial Factors and Pandemic-Related Stressors. *J. Trauma Stress* **2021**, *34*, 691–700. [CrossRef]
30. Yoon, H.; You, M.; Shon, C. Peritraumatic Distress during the COVID-19 Pandemic in Seoul, South Korea. *Int. J. Environ. Res. Public Health* **2021**, *18*, 4689. [CrossRef]
31. Rybojad, B.; Aftyka, A. Trafność, Rzetelność i Analiza Czynnikowa Polskiej Wersji Skali Dystresu Okołotraumatycznego. *Psychiatr. Pol.* **2018**, *52*, 887–901. [CrossRef]
32. Carmassi, C.; Bui, E.; Bertelloni, C.A.; Dell'Oste, V.; Pedrinelli, V.; Corsi, M.; Baldanzi, S.; Cristaudo, A.; Dell'Osso, L.; Buselli, R. Validation of the Italian Version of the Peritraumatic Distress Inventory: Validity, Reliability and Factor Analysis in a Sample of Healthcare Workers. *Eur. J. Psychotraumatology* **2021**, *12*, 1879552. [CrossRef]
33. Vance, M.C.; Kovachy, B.; Dong, M.; Bui, E. Peritraumatic Distress: A Review and Synthesis of 15 Years of Research. *J. Clin. Psychol.* **2018**, *74*, 1457–1484. [CrossRef]
34. Rybojad, B.; Aftyka, A.; Milanowska, J. Peritraumatic Distress among Emergency Medical System Employees: A Proposed Cut-off for the Peritraumatic Distress Inventory. *Ann. Agric. Environ. Med.* **2019**, *26*, 579–584. [CrossRef]
35. Guardia, D.; Brunet, A.; Duhamel, A.; Ducrocq, F.; Demarty, A.-L.; Vaiva, G. Prediction of Trauma-Related Disorders: A Proposed Cut-off score for the Peritraumatic Distress Inventory. *Prim. Care Companion CNS Disord.* **2013**, *15*, PCC.12l01406. [CrossRef]
36. Bridgland, V.M.E.; Moeck, E.K.; Green, D.M.; Swain, T.L.; Nayda, D.M.; Matson, L.A.; Hutchison, N.P.; Takarangi, M.K.T. Why the COVID-19 Pandemic Is a Traumatic Stressor. *PLoS ONE* **2021**, *16*, e0240146. [CrossRef]
37. Cooke, J.E.; Eirich, R.; Racine, N.; Madigan, S. Prevalence of Posttraumatic and General Psychological Stress during COVID-19: A Rapid Review and Meta-Analysis. *Psychiatry Res.* **2020**, *292*, 113347. [CrossRef]
38. Kang, L.; Ma, S.; Chen, M.; Yang, J.; Wang, Y.; Li, R.; Yao, L.; Bai, H.; Cai, Z.; Xiang Yang, B.; et al. Impact on Mental Health and Perceptions of Psychological Care among Medical and Nursing Staff in Wuhan during the 2019 Novel Coronavirus Disease Outbreak: A Cross-Sectional Study. *Brain. Behav. Immun.* **2020**, *87*, 11–17. [CrossRef]
39. Chen, R.; Sun, C.; Chen, J.; Jen, H.; Kang, X.L.; Kao, C.; Chou, K. A Large-Scale Survey on Trauma, Burnout, and Posttraumatic Growth among Nurses during the COVID-19 Pandemic. *Int. J. Ment. Health Nurs.* **2021**, *30*, 102–116. [CrossRef]
40. Chidiebere Okechukwu, E.; Tibaldi, L.; La Torre, G. The Impact of COVID-19 Pandemic on Mental Health of Nurses. *Clin. Ter.* **2020**, *171*, e399–e400. [CrossRef]
41. Shahrour, G.; Dardas, L.A. Acute Stress Disorder, Coping Self-efficacy and Subsequent Psychological Distress among Nurses amid COVID-19. *J. Nurs. Manag.* **2020**, *28*, 1686–1695. [CrossRef]
42. Greenberg, N.; Weston, D.; Hall, C.; Caulfield, T.; Williamson, V.; Fong, K. Mental Health of Staff Working in Intensive Care during COVID-19. *Occup. Med. Oxf. Engl.* **2021**, *71*, 62–67. [CrossRef]
43. Lamb, D.; Gnanapragasam, S.; Greenberg, N.; Bhundia, R.; Carr, E.; Hotopf, M.; Razavi, R.; Raine, R.; Cross, S.; Dewar, A.; et al. Psychosocial Impact of the COVID-19 Pandemic on 4378 UK Healthcare Workers and Ancillary Staff: Initial Baseline Data from a Cohort Study Collected during the First Wave of the Pandemic. *Occup. Environ. Med.* **2021**, *78*, 801–808. [CrossRef]
44. Norman, S.B.; Feingold, J.H.; Kaye-Kauderer, H.; Kaplan, C.A.; Hurtado, A.; Kachadourian, L.; Feder, A.; Murrough, J.W.; Charney, D.; Southwick, S.M.; et al. Moral Distress in Frontline Healthcare Workers in the Initial Epicenter of the COVID-19 Pandemic in the United States: Relationship to PTSD Symptoms, Burnout, and Psychosocial Functioning. *Depress. Anxiety* **2021**, *38*, 1007–1017. [CrossRef] [PubMed]
45. Sagherian, K.; Steege, L.M.; Cobb, S.J.; Cho, H. Insomnia, Fatigue and Psychosocial Well-being during COVID-19 Pandemic: A Cross-sectional Survey of Hospital Nursing Staff in the United States. *J. Clin. Nurs.* **2020**, *00*, 1–14. [CrossRef] [PubMed]

46. Ayotte, B.J.; Schierberl Scherr, A.E.; Kellogg, M.B. PTSD Symptoms and Functional Impairment among Nurses Treating COVID-19 Patients. *SAGE Open Nurs.* **2022**, *8*, 23779608221074652. [CrossRef] [PubMed]
47. Rodriguez, R.M.; Montoy, J.C.C.; Hoth, K.F.; Talan, D.A.; Harland, K.K.; Eyck, P.T.; Mower, W.; Krishnadasan, A.; Santibanez, S.; Mohr, N.; et al. Symptoms of Anxiety, Burnout, and PTSD and the Mitigation Effect of Serologic Testing in Emergency Department Personnel During the COVID-19 Pandemic. *Ann. Emerg. Med.* **2021**, *78*, 35–43.e2. [CrossRef] [PubMed]
48. Shechter, A.; Chiuzan, C.; Shang, Y.; Ko, G.; Diaz, F.; Venner, H.K.; Shaw, K.; Cannone, D.E.; McMurry, C.L.; Sullivan, A.M.; et al. Prevalence, Incidence, and Factors Associated with Posttraumatic Stress at Three-Month Follow-up among New York City Healthcare Workers after the First Wave of the COVID-19 Pandemic. *Int. J. Environ. Res. Public Health* **2021**, *19*, 262. [CrossRef]
49. Mehta, S.; Yarnell, C.; Shah, S.; Dodek, P.; Parsons-Leigh, J.; Maunder, R.; Kayitesi, J.; Eta-Ndu, C.; Priestap, F.; LeBlanc, D.; et al. The Impact of the COVID-19 Pandemic on Intensive Care Unit Workers: A Nationwide Survey. *Can. J. Anaesth.* **2022**, *69*, 472–484. [CrossRef]
50. Crowe, S.; Howard, A.F.; Vanderspank-Wright, B.; Gillis, P.; McLeod, F.; Penner, C.; Haljan, G. The Effect of COVID-19 Pandemic on the Mental Health of Canadian Critical Care Nurses Providing Patient Care during the Early Phase Pandemic: A Mixed Method Study. *Intensive Crit. Care Nurs.* **2021**, *63*, 102999. [CrossRef]
51. Vlah Tomičević, S.; Lang, V.B. Psychological Outcomes amongst Family Medicine Healthcare Professionals during COVID-19 Outbreak: A Cross-Sectional Study in Croatia. *Eur. J. Gen. Pract.* **2021**, *27*, 184–190. [CrossRef]
52. Alonso, J.; Vilagut, G.; Mortier, P.; Ferrer, M.; Alayo, I.; Aragón-Peña, A.; Aragonès, E.; Campos, M.; Cura-González, I.D.; Emparanza, J.I.; et al. Mental Health Impact of the First Wave of COVID-19 Pandemic on Spanish Healthcare Workers: A Large Cross-Sectional Survey. *Rev. Psiquiatr. Salud Ment.* **2021**, *14*, 90–105. [CrossRef]
53. Marco, C.A.; Larkin, G.L.; Feeser, V.R.; Monti, J.E.; Vearrier, L. Posttraumatic Stress and Stress Disorders during the COVID-19 Pandemic: Survey of Emergency Physicians. *J. Am. Coll. Emerg. Physicians Open* **2020**, *1*, 1594–1601. [CrossRef]
54. Martínez-Caballero, C.M.; Cárdaba-García, R.M.; Varas-Manovel, R.; García-Sanz, L.M.; Martínez-Piedra, J.; Fernández-Carbajo, J.J.; Pérez-Pérez, L.; Madrigal-Fernández, M.A.; Barba-Pérez, M.Á.; Olea, E.; et al. Analyzing the Impact of COVID-19 Trauma on Developing Post-Traumatic Stress Disorder among Emergency Medical Workers in Spain. *Int. J. Environ. Res. Public. Health* **2021**, *18*, 9132. [CrossRef]
55. Blanco-Daza, M.; de la Vieja-Soriano, M.; Macip-Belmonte, S.; Tercero-Cano, M. del C. Posttraumatic Stress Disorder in Nursing Staff during the COVID-19 Pandemic. *Enferm. Clin. Engl. Ed.* **2022**, *32*, 92–102. [CrossRef]
56. Luceño-Moreno, L.; Talavera-Velasco, B.; García-Albuerne, Y.; Martín-García, J. Symptoms of Posttraumatic Stress, Anxiety, Depression, Levels of Resilience and Burnout in Spanish Health Personnel during the COVID-19 Pandemic. *Int. J. Environ. Res. Public Health* **2020**, *17*, 5514. [CrossRef]
57. Steudte-Schmiedgen, S.; Stieler, L.; Erim, Y.; Morawa, E.; Geiser, F.; Beschoner, P.; Jerg-Bretzke, L.; Albus, C.; Hiebel, N.; Weidner, K. Correlates and Predictors of PTSD Symptoms among Healthcare Workers during the COVID-19 Pandemic: Results of the EgePan-VOICE Study. *Front. Psychiatry* **2021**, *12*, 686667. [CrossRef]
58. Di Tella, M.; Romeo, A.; Benfante, A.; Castelli, L. Mental Health of Healthcare Workers during the COVID-19 Pandemic in Italy. *J. Eval. Clin. Pract.* **2020**, *26*, 1583–1587. [CrossRef]
59. Bassi, M.; Negri, L.; Delle Fave, A.; Accardi, R. The Relationship between Posttraumatic Stress and Positive Mental Health Symptoms among Health Workers during COVID-19 Pandemic in Lombardy, Italy. *J. Affect. Disord.* **2021**, *280*, 1–6. [CrossRef]
60. Marcomini, I.; Agus, C.; Milani, L.; Sfogliarini, R.; Bona, A.; Castagna, M. COVID-19 and Posttraumatic Stress Disorder among Nurses: A Descriptive Cross-Sectional Study in a COVID Hospital. *Med. Lav.* **2021**, *112*, 241–249. [CrossRef]
61. Lasalvia, A.; Bonetto, C.; Porru, S.; Carta, A.; Tardivo, S.; Bovo, C.; Ruggeri, M.; Amaddeo, F. Psychological Impact of COVID-19 Pandemic on Healthcare Workers in a Highly Burdened Area of North-East Italy. *Epidemiol. Psychiatr. Sci.* **2020**, *30*, e1. [CrossRef]
62. Nowicki, G.J.; Ślusarska, B.; Tucholska, K.; Naylor, K.; Chrzan-Rodak, A.; Niedorys, B. The Severity of Traumatic Stress Associated with COVID-19 Pandemic, Perception of Support, Sense of Security, and Sense of Meaning in Life among Nurses: Research Protocol and Preliminary Results from Poland. *Int. J. Environ. Res. Public. Health* **2020**, *17*, 6491. [CrossRef]
63. Kosydar-Bochenek, J.; Krupa, S.; Favieri, F.; Forte, G.; Medrzycka-Dabrowska, W. Polish Version of the Post-Traumatic Stress Disorder Related to COVID-19 Questionnaire COVID-19-PTSD. *Front. Psychiatry* **2022**, *13*, 868191. [CrossRef]
64. Chinvararak, C.; Kerdcharoen, N.; Pruttithavorn, W.; Polruamngern, N.; Asawaroekwisoot, T.; Munsukpol, W.; Kirdchok, P. Mental Health among Healthcare Workers during COVID-19 Pandemic in Thailand. *PLoS ONE* **2022**, *17*, e0268704. [CrossRef] [PubMed]
65. Jiang, H.; Huang, N.; Tian, W.; Shi, S.; Yang, G.; Pu, H. Factors Associated with Posttraumatic Stress Disorder among Nurses during COVID-19. *Front. Psychol.* **2022**, *13*, 745158. [CrossRef] [PubMed]
66. Mirzaei, A.; Molaei, B.; Habibi-Soola, A. Post-Traumatic Stress Disorder and Its Related Factors in Nurses Caring for COVID-19 Patients. *Iran. J. Nurs. Midwifery Res.* **2022**, *27*, 106–111. [PubMed]
67. Kabunga, A.; Okalo, P. Frontline Nurses' Posttraumatic Stress Disorder and Associated Predictive Factors during the Second Wave of COVID-19 in Central, Uganda. *Neuropsychiatr. Dis. Treat.* **2021**, *17*, 3627–3633. [CrossRef]
68. Blekas, A.; Voitsidis, P.; Athanasiadou, M.; Parlapani, E.; Chatzigeorgiou, A.F.; Skoupra, M.; Syngelakis, M.; Holeva, V.; Diakogiannis, I. COVID-19: PTSD Symptoms in Greek Health Care Professionals. *Psychol. Trauma Theory Res. Pract. Policy* **2020**, *12*, 812–819. [CrossRef]

69. Işik, M.; Kirli, U.; Özdemir, P.G. The Mental Health of Healthcare Professionals during the COVID-19 Pandemic. *Turk Psikiyatri Derg. Turk. J. Psychiatry* **2021**, *32*, 225–234. [CrossRef]
70. Bidzan, M.; Bidzan-Bluma, I.; Szulman-Wardal, A.; Stueck, M.; Bidzan, M. Does Self-Efficacy and Emotional Control Protect Hospital Staff from COVID-19 Anxiety and PTSD Symptoms? Psychological Functioning of Hospital Staff after the Announcement of COVID-19 Coronavirus Pandemic. *Front. Psychol.* **2020**, *11*, 552583. [CrossRef]
71. Rachubińska, K.; Cybulska, A.M.; Sołek-Pastuszka, J.; Panczyk, M.; Stanisławska, M.; Ustianowski, P.; Grochans, E. Assessment of Psychosocial Functioning of Polish Nurses during COVID-19 Pandemic. *Int. J. Environ. Res. Public. Health* **2022**, *19*, 1435. [CrossRef]
72. Qutishat, M.; Abu Sharour, L.; Al-Dameery, K.; Al-Harthy, I.; Al-Sabei, S. COVID-19-Related Posttraumatic Stress Disorder among Jordanian Nurses during the Pandemic. *Disaster Med. Public Health Prep.* **2021**, *16*, 2552–2559. [CrossRef]
73. Alanazi, T.N.M.; McKenna, L.; Buck, M.; Alharbi, R.J. Reported Effects of the COVID-19 Pandemic on the Psychological Status of Emergency Healthcare Workers: A Scoping Review. *Australas. Emerg. Care* **2022**, *25*, 197–212. [CrossRef]
74. Zhou, T.; Guan, R.; Sun, L. Perceived Organizational Support and PTSD Symptoms of Frontline Healthcare Workers in the Outbreak of COVID-19 in Wuhan: The Mediating Effects of Self-efficacy and Coping Strategies. *Appl. Psychol. Health Well-Being* **2021**, *13*, 745–760. [CrossRef]
75. Bulut, D.; Sefa Sayar, M.; Koparal, B.; Cem Bulut, E.; Çelik, S. Which of Us Were More Affected by the Pandemic? The Psychiatric Impacts of the COVID-19 Pandemic on Healthcare Professionals in the Province Where the First Quarantine Units Were Established in Turkey. *Int. J. Clin. Pract.* **2021**, *75*, e14235. [CrossRef]
76. Geng, S.; Zhou, Y.; Zhang, W.; Lou, A.; Cai, Y.; Xie, J.; Sun, J.; Zhou, W.; Liu, W.; Li, X. The Influence of Risk Perception for COVID-19 Pandemic on Posttraumatic Stress Disorder in Healthcare Workers: A Survey from Four Designated Hospitals. *Clin. Psychol. Psychother.* **2021**, *28*, 1146–1159. [CrossRef]
77. Song, X.; Fu, W.; Liu, X.; Luo, Z.; Wang, R.; Zhou, N.; Yan, S.; Lv, C. Mental Health Status of Medical Staff in Emergency Departments during the Coronavirus Disease 2019 Epidemic in China. *Brain. Behav. Immun.* **2020**, *88*, 60–65. [CrossRef]
78. Szwamel, K.; Kaczorowska, A.; Lepsy, E.; Mroczek, A.; Golachowska, M.; Mazur, E.; Panczyk, M. Predictors of the Occupational Burnout of Healthcare Workers in Poland during the COVID-19 Pandemic: A Cross-Sectional Study. *Int. J. Environ. Res. Public. Health* **2022**, *19*, 3634. [CrossRef]
79. Haor, B.; Antczak-Komoterska, A.; Kozyra, J.; Grączewska, N.; Głowacka, M.; Biercewicz, M.; Królikowska, A.; Jabłońska, R.; Grzelak, L. System of Work and Stress-Coping Strategies Used by Nurses of a Polish Hospital during the COVID-19 Pandemic. *Int. J. Environ. Res. Public Health* **2023**, *20*, 4871. [CrossRef]
80. Dymecka, J.; Machnik-Czerwik, A.; Filipkowski, J. Fear of COVID-19, Risk Perception and Stress Level in Polish Nurses during COVID-19 Outbreak. *J. Neurol. Neurosurg. Nurs.* **2021**, *10*, 3–9. [CrossRef]
81. Bahadirli, S.; Sagaltici, E. Post-Traumatic Stress Disorder in Healthcare Workers of Emergency Departments during the Pandemic: A Cross-Sectional Study. *Am. J. Emerg. Med.* **2021**, *50*, 251–255. [CrossRef]
82. Das, K.; Ryali, V.S.S.R.; Bhavyasree, R.; Sekhar, C.M. Postexposure Psychological Sequelae in Frontline Health Workers to COVID-19 in Andhra Pradesh, India. *Ind. Psychiatry J.* **2021**, *30*, 123–130. [CrossRef]
83. Chatzittofis, A.; Karanikola, M.; Michailidou, K.; Constantinidou, A. Impact of the COVID-19 Pandemic on the Mental Health of Healthcare Workers. *Int. J. Environ. Res. Public Health* **2021**, *18*, 1435. [CrossRef]
84. Sanghera, J.; Pattani, N.; Hashmi, Y.; Varley, K.F.; Cheruvu, M.S.; Bradley, A.; Burke, J.R. The Impact of SARS-CoV-2 on the Mental Health of Healthcare Workers in a Hospital Setting-A Systematic Review. *J. Occup. Health* **2020**, *62*, e12175. [CrossRef] [PubMed]
85. Szaflarski, M. Health-Care Workers during the COVID-19 Pandemic: A Comparative USA-Poland Analysis. In *COVID-19: Cultural Change and Institutional Adaptations*; Routledge: London, UK, 2022; ISBN 978-1-00-330261-2.

Disclaimer/Publisher's Note: The statements, opinions and data contained in all publications are solely those of the individual author(s) and contributor(s) and not of MDPI and/or the editor(s). MDPI and/or the editor(s) disclaim responsibility for any injury to people or property resulting from any ideas, methods, instructions or products referred to in the content.

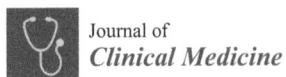

Article

Physical Activity Modifies the Severity of COVID-19 in Hospitalized Patients—Observational Study

Edyta Sutkowska [1,*], Agata Stanek [2], Katarzyna Madziarska [3], Grzegorz K. Jakubiak [2], Janusz Sokołowski [4], Marcin Madziarski [5], Karolina Sutkowska-Stępień [6], Karolina Biernat [1], Justyna Mazurek [1,*], Adrianna Borowkow-Bulek [7], Jakub Czyżewski [8], Gabriela Wilk [8], Arkadiusz Jagasyk [8] and Dominik Marciniak [9]

1. University Rehabilitation Centre, Wroclaw Medical University, 50-556 Wroclaw, Poland
2. Department and Clinic of Internal Medicine, Angiology, and Physical Medicine, Faculty of Medical Sciences in Zabrze, Medical University of Silesia, 41-902 Bytom, Poland; astanek@tlen.pl (A.S.); grzegorz.k.jakubiak@gmail.com (G.K.J.)
3. Clinical Department of Nephrology and Transplantation Medicine, Wroclaw Medical University, 50-556 Wroclaw, Poland; katarzyna.madziarska@umw.edu.pl
4. Clinical Department of Emergency Medicine, Wroclaw Medical University, 50-556 Wroclaw, Poland
5. Clinical Department of Rheumatology and Internal Medicine, University Hospital, 50-556 Wroclaw, Poland; mmadziarski@usk.wroc.pl
6. Department of General, Minimally Invasive and Endocrine Surgery, University Hospital, 50-556 Wroclaw, Poland; ksutkowska@usk.wroc.pl
7. Department of Internal Medicine, Angiology and Physical Medicine, Specialist Hospital No.2, 41-902 Bytom, Poland; adrianna.borowkow@gmail.com
8. Postgraduate–Internship, University Hospital, 50-556 Wrocław, Poland
9. Department of Drugs Form Technology, Wroclaw Medical University, 50-556 Wroclaw, Poland
* Correspondence: edyta.sutkowska@umw.edu.pl (E.S.); justyna.mazurek@umw.edu.pl (J.M.); Tel.: +48-71-734-32-20 (E.S. & J.M.)

Citation: Sutkowska, E.; Stanek, A.; Madziarska, K.; Jakubiak, G.K.; Sokołowski, J.; Madziarski, M.; Sutkowska-Stępień, K.; Biernat, K.; Mazurek, J.; Borowkow-Bulek, A.; et al. Physical Activity Modifies the Severity of COVID-19 in Hospitalized Patients—Observational Study. J. Clin. Med. 2023, 12, 4046. https://doi.org/10.3390/jcm12124046

Academic Editor: Francesco Pugliese

Received: 14 May 2023
Revised: 9 June 2023
Accepted: 11 June 2023
Published: 14 June 2023

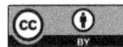

Copyright: © 2023 by the authors. Licensee MDPI, Basel, Switzerland. This article is an open access article distributed under the terms and conditions of the Creative Commons Attribution (CC BY) license (https://creativecommons.org/licenses/by/4.0/).

Abstract: Background and aim: Physical activity (PA) can modulate the immune response, but its impact on infectious disease severity is unknown. We assess if the PA level impacts the severity of COVID-19. Methods: Prospective, cohort study for adults hospitalized due to COVID-19, who filled out the International Physical Activity Questionnaire (IPAQ). Disease severity was expressed as death, transfer to intensive care unit (ICU), oxygen therapy (OxTh), hospitalization length, complications, C-reactive protein, and procalcitonin level. Results: Out of 326 individuals, 131 (57; 43.51% women) were analyzed: age: median—70; range: 20–95; BMI: mean—27.18 kg/m^2; and SD: ±4.77. During hospitalization: 117 (83.31%) individuals recovered, nine (6.87%) were transferred to ICU, five (3.82%) died, and 83 (63.36%) needed OxTh. The median for the hospital stay was 11 (range: 3–49) for discharged patients, and mean hospitalization length was 14 (SD: ±5.8312) for deaths and 14.22 days (SD: ±6.92) for ICU-transferred patients. The median for MET-min/week was 660 (range: 0–19,200). Sufficient or high PA was found in recovered patients but insufficient PA was observed in dead or ICU-transferred patients ($p = 0.03$). The individuals with poor PA had a higher risk of death (HR = 2.63; ±95%CI 0.58–11.93; $p = 0.037$). OxTh was used more often in the less active individuals ($p = 0.03$). The principal component analysis confirmed a relationship between insufficient PA and an unfavorable course of the disease. Conclusion: A higher level of PA is associated with a milder course of COVID-19.

Keywords: COVID-19; IPAQ; disease severity; physical activity level; infection

1. Introduction

The course of coronavirus disease 2019 (COVID-19) was often surprising and sometimes independent of variables previously considered poor prognostic factors [1]. One of the unfavorable prognosis factors was age; however, diabetes and, most of all, obesity were also detected [2–4]. These factors have a common denominator: low physical activity (PA). However, healthy young people also show different levels of PA [5,6]. Thus, also in this group, different disease courses could be observed [7]. This directs our attention to the possible relationship between the course of the disease and PA.

There are a lot of data confirming the impact of physical exercise on human health. Posadzki et al. published in 2020 the systematic Cochrane review [8] which analyzed data from 27,671 participants in the context of the effects of physical activity on health outcomes. One of the most important conclusions was that individuals can significantly modify their physical and mental health by exercising more. The reduction of mortality was also reported, mainly in studies with a longer follow-up, and can reach up to 35% when comparing active people with those characterized by a sedentary lifestyle [9]. Physical activity also improves mental well-being and quality of life (QoL), the very important factors of human life that are involved in the physical status of individuals [10,11].

The balance between the infection and innate as well as adaptive immune response seems to play a crucial role in the course of the infectious disease. The severe acute respiratory syndrome coronavirus-2 (SARS-CoV-2) can effectively evade early innate immune responses, and thus multiply more efficiently before the most effective adaptive immune response is ready. In young, lean, healthy, and active individuals, the first step in the immune response works more effectively and adequately mobilizes T cells from the adaptive immune system to reduce the viral load. In the individuals characterized by a dysfunctional T-cell population (e.g., older, obese people), excessive inflammation with tissue damage is observed as a "response" to diminished adaptive immunity [12–14]. Thus, the impairment in one immune response is compensated by the other. Physical activity can modulate the level of inflammation in pathological states [15–18] so it is also possible that it can modify the cytokine storm, the main cause behind many organ failures and, finally, patient death during severe acute respiratory syndrome coronavirus-2 infection [19,20]. The proposed mechanisms of action of PA in the course of COVID-19 involve irisin production, AMPK pathway activation [21], macrophage activity regulation, and many others [20,22]. The wide aspect of how PA can keep the immune system in a good condition (including immunometabolism) was excellently described in D.C. Nieman and B.D. Pence's review [23]. Regular PA can also provide many "macro" benefits (not only those connected with immune system), such as better cardiovascular and lung health [24,25], which is affected primarily during infection.

Still, their clinical effect on the severity of a disease such as COVID-19 was not part of a prospective study. The main problem which can be detected is the difficulty in assessing the level of PA based on time-consuming questionnaires. The International Physical Activity Questionnaire (IPAQ) is a useful tool for measuring health-related PA in populations [26], and also in its short form (SF). The pandemic provided opportunities to investigate expected relationships between daily PA and disease severity. However, patients hospitalized due to COVID-19 varied in health status, not always having the strength to fill out a questionnaire. In addition, healthcare professionals' PPE clothing (special masks and suits) significantly limited their ability to interview patients. All of these probably made it difficult to assess the above dependencies for healthcare professionals.

Aim

This prospective cohort study aims to investigate whether the level of physical activity measured with the IPAQ-SF modifies the severity of COVID-19. Taking into account the above mention reports, we hypothesized that people who are more physically active have a milder course of the infection.

2. Materials and Methods

All the patients were asked to give their written consent to participate in the study. Patient data and results were analyzed anonymously. The Bioethics Committee of the Wroclaw Medical University approval number is: KB 1081/2021. Trial Registration number: NCT05200767.

2.1. Place

The study was conducted in two hospitals dedicated temporarily to COVID-19 patients: one in Wroclaw, Lower Silesia, and the other in Bytom, Upper Silesia. Initially, the Wroclaw hospital participated in the project, and information from this hospital was collected from 3 January 2022 to March 2022. After obtaining the required approvals, the Bytom hospital joined the project, and data from this hospital covered the period from 31 January to 11 February 2022. After the mentioned periods, both hospitals were no longer COVID-19 treatment centers.

2.2. Participants

Adults (aged 18 at the least) of any sex and race hospitalized for SARS-CoV-2 infection (confirmed by the polymerase chain reaction (PCR) method or equivalent diagnostic technique) at COVID-19 units were asked to give written consent to participate. The exclusion criteria were as follows:

- pregnancy;
- inability to complete the questionnaire during hospitalization or up to a week after discharge;
- history of a significant cardiovascular event in the last 6 months (acute coronary syndrome, stroke, amputation, revascularization of peripheral vessels, and pulmonary or peripheral embolism of any etiology) if the patient did not complete the rehabilitation process;
- symptomatic chronic respiratory disease not responding to therapy before hospitalization for COVID-19 (or no therapy);
- any dyspnea at rest in the last month before COVID-19;
- injury to the locomotor system in the last month before contracting COVID-19;
- hospitalization in the last month before contracting COVID-19.

We proposed these exclusion criteria believing that they could influence the patient's recent PA level and thus not properly reflect its impact on the course of COVID-19. On the contrary, some conditions, such as a cardiovascular incident or stable chronic pulmonary or locomotor system disease, were accepted for evaluation and did not constitute the exclusion criteria. This is because the patient can fully or almost fully recover after rehabilitation or compensate for disability with some form of activity (e.g., wheelchair use after amputation). In addition, because rehabilitation is time-consuming, we tried to account for it with the proposed periods (e.g., 6 months for cardiovascular incidents).

2.3. Methods

The patients were asked to complete the IPAQ during their hospital stay or up to 7 days after discharge. If they were unable to fill out the questionnaire themselves, the patient's next of kin could also do it on their behalf.

IPAQ expresses PA in metabolic equivalent of task (MET)-min/week units. Based on it, the respondents were assigned one of three categories of activity: insufficient (less than 600), sufficient (600–1500 or 600–3000), or high (more than 1500 or 3000 MET-min/week) [27,28]. Example of IPAQ interpretation: two criteria for high activity: a) vigorous-intensity activity on at least 3 days achieving a minimum of at least 1500 MET-min/week OR b) 7 or more days of any combination of walking, moderate-intensity, or vigorous-intensity activities achieving a minimum of at least 3000 MET-min/week.

Due to the expected poor condition of some patients, the short form of the questionnaire was used. It consists of 7 items on all types of PA related to everyday life, work, and leisure. According to the suggestion of adaptation of the IPAQ for the Polish population (IPAQ-PL), the interviewer helped complete the form [27].

The primary outcome measures were death, worsening of the disease (transfer to ICU), or recovery (discharge home). The secondary outcome measure was hospitalization length.

Information on complications, comorbidities, chronic medications, and basic parameters concerning the patient's status and the disease course was obtained from hospital databases. The following parameters determined the severity of the disease (critical data):

death or transfer to ICU, need for oxygen therapy, length of hospitalization, complications other than respiratory failure, and C-reactive protein (CRP) and procalcitonin (PCT) levels on admission.

The funding sources (Wroclaw Medical University-WMU and Medical University of Silesia-MUS, Wroclaw, Poland) had no impact on the study design, data collection, analysis and interpretation; they also had no role in the writing of the manuscript, but agreed to submit the manuscript for publication and gave financial support for proofreading of the translation (WMU) and article processing charge (both universities). The corresponding author had full access to all of the data and the final responsibility to submit for publication.

2.4. Statistical Analysis

Both nominal and ratio variables were analyzed. Basic descriptive statistics were calculated for ratio scale variables: size, mean value—SR, median, 95% confidence interval for the mean value (SR ± 95%CI), and range. Next, size and percentage information was tabulated for nominal variables (including dichotomous ones).

The normality of data distribution was tested with a Shapiro–Wilk test. We used means and standard deviations (SDs) for normally distributed data and medians and ranges for not normally distributed data.

Relationships between variables of nominal scales (including dichotomous ones) were assessed using Pearson's chi-squared test.

Pearson correlation coefficient matrices were calculated to determine correlations between variables of ratio scales. Their statistical significance was determined with a *t*-test.

Principal component analysis (PCA) was used to assess global relationships between the key variables analyzed regardless of scale. The developed PCA model was estimated using the NIPALS algorithm. The convergence criterion was set at 0.00001, and the maximum number of iterations was 100. The number of components was determined by establishing the maximum predictive ability of Q^2 using V-fold cross-validation, adopting $V_{max} = 7$. The resulting optimal PCA model was reduced to 2 principal components (PC 1 and PC 2). The results are presented in a graph, including the contribution of each component to the overall percentage of explained variance and information on their statistical significance.

In addition, survival analysis was performed based on a nonparametric Cox proportional hazards model.

A significance level of $\alpha = 0.05$ was assumed for all statistical analyses carried out.

Statistical analysis was performed using StatSoft's Statistica 13·3 PL.

3. Results

3.1. Basic Information

In the mentioned periods, 326 patients (294 in Wroclaw and 32 in Bytom) were hospitalized due to COVID-19, and 140 gave their written consent to participate in the study (124 from Wroclaw and 16 from Bytom) (Supplements Figure S1). However, the final analysis covered 131 cases (57; 43.51% women) because three patients did not fill out the questionnaire, and hospital data on six participants proved insufficient for analysis. The patient age was: median—70; range: 20–95 (N = 131), mean BMI was 27.18 kg/m^2 (SD: ±4.77; data available for 97 cases); 18 (13.74%) patients were smokers (data available for 125 patients) and 53 (42.06%) were fully vaccinated (data available for 126 individuals) with at least two doses of the vaccine.

A broad characterization of the population is included in the additional documents. They contain information about comorbidities (Supplements Table S1), chronic medications (Supplements Table S2), and laboratory results (Supplements Table S3). Not all of these data were available for the whole group, and the number of analyzed cases is indicated in the tables.

The analysis of the course of hospitalization showed that 117 (83.31%) individuals recovered and were discharged home, nine (6.87%) were transferred to the ICU—their fate is unknown to the researchers, and five (3.82%) died. In 83 (63.36%) individuals, some form of OxTh was necessary. The median for the hospital stay was 11 (range: 3–49) for discharged patients, and mean hospitalization length was 14 days (SD: ±5.8312) for deaths and 14.22 days (SD: ±6.92) for patients transferred to ICU.

3.2. Relationship between IPAQ Score and Severity of the Disease

To analyze the relationship between IPAQ score and survival, the group was divided into two subgroups: recovered patients and patients with unfavorable hospitalization outcomes (death or transfer to ICU; N = 14; 10.69%). None of the patients used the help of a family member to complete the questionnaire, but the interviewers helped them to understand it and marked the correct information for all of them to some extent. The median for energy expenditure was 660 MET-min/week (range: 0–19,200), representing the sufficient level of PA regarding the IPAQ. The results of IPAQ are in Table 1.

Table 1. The IPAQ level and its correlation with recovery or unfavorable hospitalization outcomes (death or transfer to ICU) and need for oxygen therapy.

Variable	IPAQ Level			Chi^2	p-Level
	0	1	2		
Recovery (N = 117)	49 (37.40%)	40 (30.53%)	28 (21.37%)	7.15	0.03
Death or transfer to ICU (N = 5 + 9)	11 (8.40%)	1 (0.76%)	2 (1.53%)		
Does the patient need oxygen therapy?	No (N = 48) 19 (14.50%)	12 (9.16%)	17 (12.98%)	6.78	0.03
	Yes (N = 83) 41 (31.30%)	29 (22.14%)	13 (9.92%)		

Note: IPAQ—International Physical Activity Questionnaire; and ICU—Intensive Care Unit.

Sufficient or high PA was found in patients who recovered, while insufficient activity was more common in patients with unfavorable hospitalization outcomes (death or transfer to ICU) ($p = 0.03$) (Table 1). In addition, the individuals with insufficient PA (IPAQ = 0) had a higher risk of death (HR = 2.63; ±95%CI 0.58–11.93; $p = 0.037$), while patients with sufficient or high PA (IPAQ = 1 or 2) were more likely to recover (HR = 0.39; ±95%CI 0.04–4.39; $p = 0.19$). Survival analysis for the participants is presented in Figure 1.

Oxygen therapy was used more often in the less active individuals (IPAQ = 0 and 1) compared to the more active ones (IPAQ = 2) ($p = 0.03$) (Table 1).

There was no difference in hospitalization length between IPAQ = 0 patients (insufficient activity) (median: 12; range: 5–49) and individuals reporting sufficient or high PA (IPAQ = 1 or 2) (median: 11; range: 3–30) ($p = 0.35$).

In 30 (22.90%) individuals, complications other than respiratory failure were observed: for IPAQ = 0, N= 6 for IPAQ = 1 or 2, N = 26. There was no difference between groups regarding the development of complications ($p = 0.94$) and IPAQ score.

The values for CRP and PCT are in Supplements (Table S3). We observed a negative correlation between PA and CRP level on admission (the higher the PA, the lower the CRP, but with no statistical significance) and a positive correlation for PCT level on admission (the lower the PA, the lower the PCT, but also with no significance).

The PCA (Figure 2) orders the variables according to how close they are together and thus informs about their relationship. The analysis confirmed a relationship between high PA and no need for OxTh. It also corroborated the relationship between insufficient PA and complications, the need for oxygen therapy, a longer hospital stay, unfavorable hospitalization outcome (death or transfer to ICU), and low PCT but higher CRP on admission.

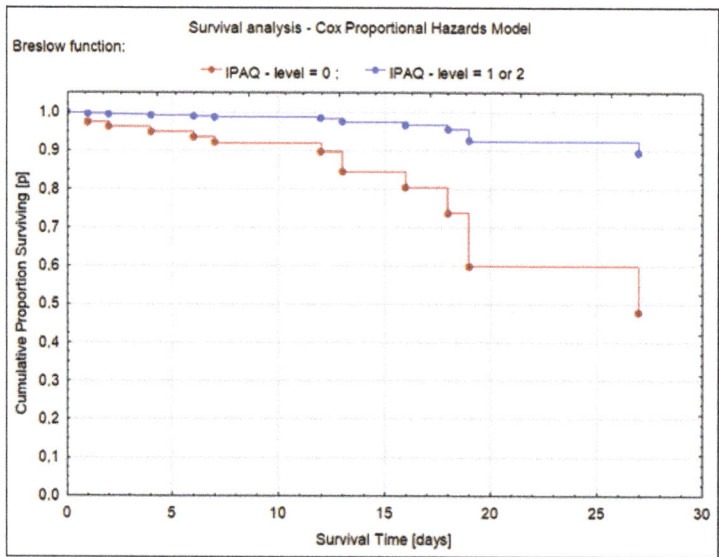

Figure 1. Survival analysis for patients whose physical activity was insufficient (IPAQ = 0) or at least sufficient (IPAQ = 1 or 2).

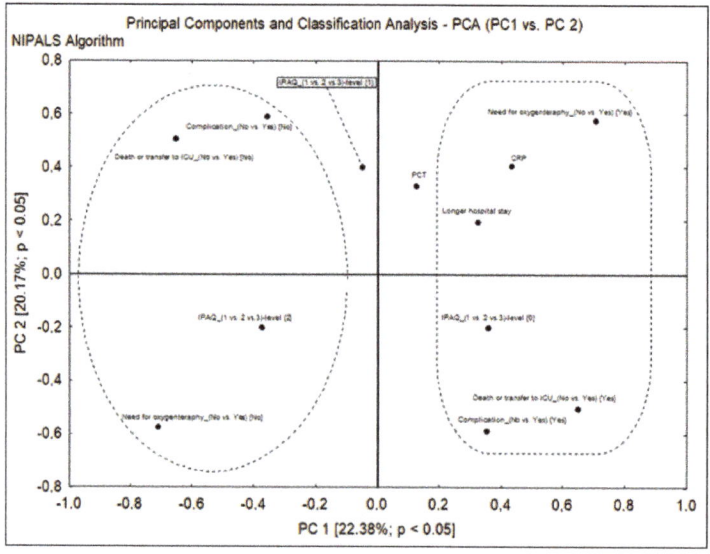

Figure 2. Relationship between physical activity level and selected variables: need for oxygen therapy, complications, duration of hospitalization, and unfavorable hospitalization outcomes (death or transfer to ICU).

4. Discussion

The exercises build muscle mass and produce benefits such as better glucose control or lipid metabolism [29]. Even though the two are connected with a longer life and better life quality, people, especially younger ones, find it difficult to focus on the long-term benefits and take up regular PA. Thus, information on short-term benefits, such as lower incidence of various infections or their milder course, could encourage it in people of all ages. In addition, the much more severe consequences of COVID-19 (compared to other, more trivial respiratory system infectious diseases) and the significantly higher frequency of serious complications (including high death rate) may also reveal potential protective factors. Therefore, the disclosure of factors that help improve the prognosis could more strongly appeal to the public imagination and mobilize people to take action to improve the course of infection or the occurrence of these diseases in general.

Our study confirms with no doubt that people hospitalized due to COVID-19 who had regular PA before getting sick had a better prognosis, with an about 60% higher chance of recovery, for example, due to a reduced hyper-inflammation response [22], as we observed the relationship between PA level and the main marker of inflammation, CRP (higher PA was characterized by lower CRP), but with no statistical significance. In recent decades, a role for muscle as an endocrine organ producing myokines that can contribute to cross-talk between different organs and thus modify the body's response to inflammation has been proposed [30]. Therefore, even minimal PA (referred to as sufficient in IPAQ) protects against death or ICU transfer in our study. This level means one of the following: (a) 3 or more days of vigorous activity for at least 20 min per day, OR (b) 5 or more days of moderate-intensity activity or walking for at least 30 min per day, OR (c) 5 or more days of any combination of walking, moderate-intensity, or vigorous-intensity activities achieving a minimum of at least 600 MET-min/week [31].

It is known that PA improves lung function [32]. We also confirmed that being more active reduces the chances of additional procedures such as oxygen therapy. This gives a smoother disease course and indirectly also proves the efficiency of the patient's respiratory system. Low PA was found by our team to be associated with adverse prognostic factors that appeared during the course of COVID-19, such as the need for oxygen therapy, complications, and, consequently, longer hospital stay, as well as unfavorable hospitalization outcomes (death or transfer to ICU) also in PCA. Thus, our study confirms that, for every person, regardless of fitness and ability, being more active reduces the risk of the adverse, acute consequences of COVID-19 disease. Although we have no information on the long-term complications of COVID-19 up to now, avoiding first-line ones seems to be enough reason to explain to patients the need for minimal but regular PA at least.

In the previous study, we presented patients with type 2 diabetes who declared lower PA levels (mean: 1198•1 MET-min/week) compared to the result of this study, where we focused on the general population [33]. Nonetheless, we are aware that patients with more comorbidities may be less active due to disability [34,35]. The IPAQ analysis combines not only the dynamics of activity but also its regularity and duration as mentioned above. Patients can also pursue a less strenuous PA, such as regular walks, to obtain a higher IPAQ level and reap its benefits. Exercising was found to modulate the AMP-activated protein kinase (AMPK) pathway and decrease cytokine production depending on its intensity, duration, and status [21]. Interestingly, a high-intensity approach is not preferred as it can even be harmful [24,36].

The mean BMI of the studied population was 27 kg/m^2, and less than 20% of the individuals had BMI $\geq$ 30 kg/m^2. As was found in previous studies, obesity was an independent predictor for severity and death in patients suffering from COVID-19 and other infectious diseases [37]. The two hospitals covered in our study were not dedicated to treating the most severe cases; therefore, we cannot exclude that the BMI of the ICU patients was higher [38] as obese individuals are more severely ill and more likely to need mechanical ventilation [39]. Thus, we suggest that the results of our study may be representative of a non-obese population. Due to the independent influence of high BMI mentioned above in the literature on the severity of infection, the analysis of PA's role on the disease course in the obese population should be an element of a separate investigation. Some studies indicate the independent role of muscle mass, volume, and density in the severity of the disease [40,41], so it could be interesting to check if obese but physically active people enjoy the same benefits of regular PA as slim ones.

Just before the COVID-19 pandemic, information on the impact of exercise on the human immune defense was published [42]. Unfortunately, the general impact of PA on infectious disease morbidity and severity was not analyzed as a pure variable but in the context of body composition (reduction of excess body mass) up to now. Our study explored and indicated the connection between PA and the severity of SARS-CoV-2 infection not related to weight loss through exercise. This information seems important not only for individuals but also for health authorities regarding healthcare direction. Although the potential biological mechanism of how PA affects our immunity at the system or cell levels, or how it modulates the release of different substances is explained in a comprehensive review by Jakobsson et al. [43]; our study complements this knowledge with clinical trial results.

5. Limitations

1. IPAQ-PL is dedicated to people aged 15–69. However, for the purpose of the EUPASS (European Physical Activity Surveillance System), residents who had just turned 18 were recruited [28].
2. Respondents were asked to analyze their "usual PA before COVID-19" instead of the recommended "describe your PA during the last 7 days." In our opinion, the disease with mild symptoms/signs probably started a few days before hospitalization, and PA may have been limited. Therefore, "the last 7 days" may not adequately describe the individual's usual status. Although the use of "the last 7 days recall" is recommended, both formulae are available [26].
3. Only patients who were not critically ill during admission were surveyed, which depends on the hospital profile and obvious reasons (patient condition).
4. The analysis of the PA during the COVID period (but not lockdown) cannot be sufficient to properly describe the long-term relationship between analyzed variables in general.
5. The correlation for CRP and PCT and physical activity level was not found as statistically significant.

6. Conclusions

Physical activity importantly modified the course of COVID-19 in a hospitalized population. Regular physical activity before becoming sick gives hospitalized patients about a 60% higher chance of recovery. A higher level of daily PA is associated with a milder course of SARS-CoV-2 infection.

Supplementary Materials: The following supporting information can be downloaded at: https://www.mdpi.com/article/10.3390/jcm12124046/s1, Figure S1: Flow diagram; Table S1: Chronic diseases in patients hospitalized due to COVID-19; Table S2: Chronic medications used by patients hospitalized due to COVID-19; Table S3: Laboratory results on admission to the hospital.

Author Contributions: Conceptualization, E.S., K.M. and J.S.; methodology, E.S., K.M., J.S. and D.M.; software, D.M. and K.B.; validation, E.S., A.S. and K.M.; formal analysis, E.S. and D.M.; investigation, E.S., A.S., K.M., G.K.J., J.S., M.M., K.S.-S., K.B., J.M., A.B.-B., J.C., G.W. and A.J.; resources, E.S., A.S., K.M., J.S., G.K.J., J.M., M.M. and K.S.-S.; data curation, E.S., A.S. and D.M.; writing—original draft preparation, E.S. and D.M.; writing—review and editing, E.S., A.S., K.M., G.K.J., J.S., K.B., J.M., A.J., M.M., K.S.-S., A.B.-B., J.C. and G.W.; visualization, E.S. and D.M.; supervision, E.S., A.S. and K.M.; project administration, E.S.; funding acquisition, E.S. and A.S. All authors have read and agreed to the published version of the manuscript.

Funding: This research received no external funding.

Institutional Review Board Statement: The study was conducted in accordance with the Declaration of Helsinki, and approved by The Bioethics Committee of the Wroclaw Medical University. Approval number: KB 1081/2021. Trial Registration number: NCT05200767.

Informed Consent Statement: Informed consent was obtained from all subjects involved in the study.

Data Availability Statement: Data (individual participant data-row data and statistical analysis, informed consent form, SAP, and study protocol) will be available after publication with no limit to all interested parties on ClinicalTrials and on https://ppm.umw.edu.pl/info/researchdata/UMW9cf7247169fc4d2b8dad0921ad2207fb/.

Acknowledgments: We would like to thank all the patients, their families, students, and young doctors who participated in the study as participants or interviewers.

Conflicts of Interest: The authors declare no conflict of interest.

References

1. Huang, C.; Wang, Y.; Li, X.; Ren, L.; Zhao, J.; Hu, Y.; Zhang, L.; Fan, G.; Xu, J.; Gu, X.; et al. Clinical features of patients infected with 2019 novel coronavirus in Wuhan, China. *Lancet* **2020**, *395*, 497–506. [CrossRef] [PubMed]
2. Rottoli, M.; Bernante, P.; Belvedere, A.; Balsamo, F.; Garelli, S.; Giannella, M.; Cascavilla, A.; Tedeschi, S.; Ianniruberto, S.; Roselli Del Turco, E.; et al. How important is obesity as a risk factor for respiratory failure, intensive care admission and death in hospitalised COVID-19 patients? Results from a single Italian centre. *Eur. J. Endocrinol.* **2020**, *183*, 389–397. [CrossRef] [PubMed]
3. Wu, C.; Chen, X.; Cai, Y.; Xia, J.; Zhou, X.; Xu, S.; Huang, H.; Zhang, L.; Zhou, X.; Du, C.; et al. Risk factors associated with acute respiratory distress syndrome and death in patients with coronavirus disease 2019 pneumonia in Wuhan, China. *JAMA Intern. Med.* **2020**, *180*, 1031. [CrossRef] [PubMed]
4. Romero Starke, K.; Reissig, D.; Petereit-Haack, G.; Schmauder, S.; Nienhaus, A.; Seidler, A. The isolated effect of age on the risk of COVID-19 severe outcomes: A systematic review with meta-analysis. *BMJ Glob. Health* **2021**, *6*, e006434. [CrossRef]
5. Molanorouzi, K.; Khoo, S.; Morris, T. Motives for adult participation in physical activity: Type of activity, age, and gender. *BMC Public Health* **2015**, *15*, 66. [CrossRef]
6. Puciato, D. Sociodemographic associations of physical activity in people of working age. *Int. J. Environ. Res. Public Health* **2019**, *16*, 2134. [CrossRef]
7. De Sanctis, V.; Ruggiero, L.; Soliman, A.T.; Daar, S.; Di Maio, S.; Kattamis, C. Coronavirus Disease 2019 (COVID-19) in adolescents: An update on current clinical and diagnostic characteristics. *Acta Biomed.* **2020**, *91*, 184–194. [CrossRef]
8. Posadzki, P.; Pieper, D.; Bajpai, R.; Makaruk, H.; Könsgen, N.; Neuhaus, A.L.; Semwal, M. Exercise/physical activity and health outcomes: An overview of Cochrane systematic reviews. *BMC Public Health* **2020**, *20*, 1724. [CrossRef]
9. Lan, T.Y.; Chang, H.Y.; Tai, T.Y. Relationship between components of leisure physical activity and mortality in Taiwanese older adults. *Prev. Med.* **2006**, *43*, 36–41. [CrossRef]
10. Fox, K.R. The influence of physical activity on mental well-being. *Public Health Nutr.* **1999**, *2*, 411–418. [CrossRef]
11. Chen, L.J.; Stevinson, C.; Ku, P.W.; Chang, Y.K.; Chu, D.C. Relationships of leisure-time and non-leisure-time physical activity with depressive symptoms: A population-based study of Taiwanese older adults. *Int. J. Behav. Nutr. Phys. Act.* **2012**, *14*, 28. [CrossRef]
12. De Candia, P.; Prattichizzo, F.; Garavelli, S.; Matarese, G. T cells: Warriors of SARS-CoV-2 infection. *Trends Immunol.* **2021**, *42*, 18–30. [CrossRef]
13. Brodin, P. Immune determinants of COVID-19 disease presentation and severity. *Nat. Med.* **2021**, *27*, 28–33. [CrossRef]
14. Sette, A.; Crotty, S. Adaptive immunity to SARS-CoV-2 and COVID-19. *Cell* **2021**, *184*, 861–880. [CrossRef]
15. Dutra, P.M.L.; Da-Silva, S.A.G.; Mineo, J.R.; Turner, J.E. Editorial: The effects of physical activity and exercise on immune responses to infection. *Front. Immunol.* **2022**, *13*, 842568. [CrossRef]
16. Nieman, D.C.; Wentz, L.M. The compelling link between physical activity and the body's defense system. *J. Sport Health Sci.* **2019**, *8*, 201–217. [CrossRef]
17. Denay, K.L.; Breslow, R.G.; Turner, M.N.; Nieman, D.C.; Roberts, W.O.; Best, T.M. ACSM call to action statement: COVID-19 considerations for sports and physical activity. *Curr. Sports Med. Rep.* **2020**, *19*, 326–328. [CrossRef]
18. Nieman, D.C. Coronavirus disease-2019: A tocsin to our aging, unfit, corpulent, and immunodeficient society. *J. Sport Health Sci.* **2020**, *9*, 293–301. [CrossRef]
19. Hu, B.; Huang, S.; Yin, L. The cytokine storm and COVID-19. *J. Med. Virol.* **2021**, *93*, 250–256. [CrossRef]
20. Nieman, D.C. Exercise Is Medicine for Immune Function: Implication for COVID-19. *Curr. Sports Med. Rep.* **2021**, *20*, 395–401. [CrossRef]
21. Rothschild, J.A.; Islam, H.; Bishop, D.J.; Kilding, A.E.; Stewart, T.; Plews, D.J. Factors influencing AMPK activation during cycling exercise: A pooled analysis and meta-regression. *Sports Med.* **2022**, *52*, 1273–1294. [CrossRef] [PubMed]
22. Alves, H.R.; Lomba, G.S.B.; Gonçalves-de-Albuquerque, C.F.; Burth, P. Irisin, exercise, and COVID-19. *Front. Endocrinol.* **2022**, *13*, 879066. [CrossRef] [PubMed]
23. Nieman, D.C.; Pence, B.D. Exercise immunology: Future directions. *J. Sport Health Sci.* **2020**, *9*, 432–445. [CrossRef] [PubMed]
24. Schnohr, P.; O'Keefe, J.H.; Marott, J.L.; Lange, P.; Jensen, G.B. Dose of jogging and long-term mortality: The Copenhagen City Heart Study. *J. Am. Coll. Cardiol.* **2015**, *65*, 411–419. [CrossRef]

25. Myers, J.; Kokkinos, P.; Nyelin, E. Physical activity, cardiorespiratory fitness, and the metabolic syndrome. *Nutrients* **2019**, *11*, 1652. [CrossRef]
26. Craig, C.L.; Marshall, A.L.; Sjöström, M.; Bauman, A.E.; Booth, M.L.; Ainsworth, B.E.; Pratt, M.; Ekelund, U.; Yngve, A.; Sallis, J.F.; et al. International physical activity questionnaire: 12-country reliability and validity. *Med. Sci. Sports Exerc.* **2003**, *35*, 1381–1395. [CrossRef]
27. Biernat, E.; Stupnicki, R.; Gajewski, A.K. International Physical Activity Questionnaire (IPAQ)-Polish version. *Wych Fiz. Spor.* **2007**, *51*, 47–54. (In Polish)
28. Rütten, A.; Vuillemin, A.; Ooijendijk, W.T.M.; Schena, F.; Sjöströmet, M.; Stahl, T.; Auweele, Y.V.; Welshman, J.; Ziemainz, H. Physical activity monitoring in Europe. The European Physical Activity Surveillance System (EUPASS) approach and indicator testing. *Public Health Nutr.* **2003**, *6*, 377–384. [CrossRef]
29. Borghouts, L.B.; Keizer, H.A. Exercise and insulin sensitivity: A review. *Int. J. Sports Med.* **2000**, *21*, 302–307. [CrossRef]
30. Pedersen, B.K.; Febbraio, M.A. Muscle as an endocrine organ: Focus on muscle-derived interleukin-6. *Physiol. Rev.* **2008**, *88*, 1379–1406. [CrossRef]
31. IPAQ International Physical Activity Questionnaire. Available online: https://www.physio-pedia.com/images/c/c7/Quidelines_for_interpreting_the_IPAQ.pdf (accessed on 12 June 2022).
32. Novotová, K.; Pavlů, D.; Dvořáčková, D.; Arnal-Gómez, A.; Espí-López, G.V. Influence of walking as physiological training to improve respiratory parameters in the elderly population. *Int. J. Environ. Res. Public Health* **2022**, *19*, 7995. [CrossRef]
33. Available online: https://virtual.cvot.org/wp-content/uploads/2022/11/CVOT_Summit_2022_Programme_Booklet.pdf (accessed on 10 November 2022).
34. Martinez-Gomez, D.; Guallar-Castillon, P.; Garcia-Esquinas, E.; Bandinelli, S.; Rodríguez-Artalejo, F. Physical activity and the effect of multimorbidity on all-cause mortality in older adults. *Mayo Clin. Proc.* **2017**, *92*, 376–382. [CrossRef]
35. Vancampfort, D.; Koyanagi, A.; Ward, P.B.; Rosenbaum, S.; Schuch, F.B.; Mugisha, J.; Richards, J.; Firth, J.; Stubbs, B. Chronic physical conditions, multimorbidity and physical activity across 46 low-and middle-income countries. *Int. J. Behav. Nutr. Phys. Act.* **2017**, *14*, 6. [CrossRef]
36. Simpson, R.; Kunz, H.; Agha, N.; Graff, R. Exercise and the regulation of immune functions. *Prog. Mol. Biol. Transl. Sci.* **2015**, *135*, 355–380. [CrossRef]
37. Fezeu, L.; Julia, C.; Henegar, A.; Bitu, J.; Hu, F.B.; Grobbee, D.E.; Kengne, A.-P.; Hercberg, S.; Czernichow, S. Obesity is associated with higher risk of intensive care unit admission and death in influenza A (H1N1) patients: A systematic review and meta-analysis. *Obes. Rev.* **2011**, *12*, 653–659. [CrossRef]
38. Biscarini, S.; Colaneri, M.; Ludovisi, S.; Seminari, E.; Pieri, T.C.; Valsecchi, P.; Gallazzi, I.; Giusti, E.; Camma, C.; Zuccaro, V.; et al. The obesity paradox: Analysis from the SMAtteo COvid-19 REgistry (SMACORE) cohort. *Nutr. Metab. Cardiovasc. Dis.* **2020**, *30*, 1920–1925. [CrossRef]
39. Simonnet, A.; Chetboun, M.; Poissy, J.; Raverdy, V.; Noulette, J.; Duhamel, A.; Labreuche, J.; Mathieu, D.; Pattou, F.; Jourdain, M.; et al. High prevalence of obesity in severe acute respiratory syndrome coronavirus-2 (SARS-CoV-2) requiring invasive mechanical ventilation. *Obesity* **2020**, *28*, 1195–1199. [CrossRef]
40. Yang, Y.; Ding, L.; Zou, X.; Shen, Y.; Hu, D.; Hu, X.; Li, Z.; Kamel, I.R. Visceral adiposity and high intramuscular fat deposition independently predict critical illness in patients with SARS-CoV-2. *Obesity* **2020**, *28*, 2040–2048. [CrossRef]
41. Chandarana, H.; Pisuchpen, N.; Krieger, R.; Dane, B.; Mikheev, A.; Feng, Y.; Kambadakone, A.; Rusinek, H. Association of body composition parameters measured on CT with risk of hospitalization in patients with Covid-19. *Eur. J. Radiol.* **2021**, *145*, 110031. [CrossRef]
42. Jakobsson, J.; Cotgreave, I.; Furberg, M.; Arnberg, N.; Svensson, M. Potential physiological and cellular mechanisms of exercise that decrease the risk of severe complications and mortality following SARS-CoV-2 infection. *Sports* **2021**, *9*, 121. [CrossRef]
43. Lim, Y.; Lee, M.H.; Jeong, S.; Han, H.W. Association of Physical Activity with SARS-CoV-2 Infection and Severe Clinical Outcomes Among Patients in South Korea. *JAMA Netw. Open* **2023**, *6*, e239840. [CrossRef] [PubMed]

Disclaimer/Publisher's Note: The statements, opinions and data contained in all publications are solely those of the individual author(s) and contributor(s) and not of MDPI and/or the editor(s). MDPI and/or the editor(s) disclaim responsibility for any injury to people or property resulting from any ideas, methods, instructions or products referred to in the content.

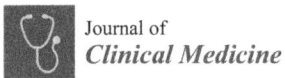

Article

Correlation of ENT Symptoms with Age, Sex, and Anti-SARS-CoV-2 Antibody Titer in Plasma

Aleksandra Kwaśniewska [1,*], Krzysztof Kwaśniewski [2], Andrzej Skorek [3], Dmitry Tretiakow [3,*], Anna Jaźwińska-Curyłło [4] and Paweł Burduk [5]

1. Department of Otolaryngology, Laryngological Oncology and Maxillofacial Surgery, University Hospital No. 2, 85-168 Bydgoszcz, Poland
2. Department of Vascular Surgery and Angiology, University Hospital No. 1, 85-094 Bydgoszcz, Poland
3. Department of Otolaryngology, Medical University of Gdańsk, 80-210 Gdańsk, Poland
4. Regional Center of Blood Donation and Treatment, 80-210 Gdańsk, Poland
5. Department of Otolaryngology, Phoniatrics and Audiology, Collegium Medicum, Nicolaus Copernicus University, 85-168 Bydgoszcz, Poland
* Correspondence: kwasniewska.aleks@gmail.com (A.K.); d.tret@gumed.edu.pl (D.T.)

Abstract: Our objective is to evaluate the correlation between ENT symptom occurrence and antibody titer in convalescent plasma, as well as the influence of age and gender on ENT manifestations of COVID-19. We measured the levels of antibodies in 346 blood donors, who had PCR-confirmed previous infection and met the study inclusion criteria. We recorded otolaryngological symptoms during infection: dry cough, dyspnea, sore throat, smell/taste disturbances, vertigo, dizziness, nausea and vomiting, sudden unilateral loss of hearing, progressive loss of hearing, and tinnitus. In addition, we statistically analyzed the correlation between patients' antibody levels, symptoms, age, and gender using a chi-square test or Fisher exact test. A p-value less than 0.05 determined statistical significance. The mean age of the convalescents was 39.8 ± 9.56 SD and the median of the measured anti-SARS-CoV2 plasma antibodies was 1:368.5. The most common ENT symptoms were smell/taste disturbances (62.43%), dry cough (40.46%), sore throat (24.86%), and dyspnea (23.7%). Smell and taste disturbances were more frequent in younger patients and the marked antibody titer was lower, which was contrary to a higher antibody titer associated with dry cough, dyspnea, and dizziness. Occurrence of sore throat was not correlated with age, sex, or antibody level. There were no significant differences in otological symptoms in female patients. Gender does not affect the occurrence of ENT symptoms. The symptomatic course of SARS-CoV-2 infection is not always associated with higher levels of antibodies in the blood. The age of the infected patients, unlike gender, affects the occurrence of some ENT symptoms.

Keywords: COVID-19; convalescent plasma; SARS-CoV-2; ENT symptoms

1. Introduction

Coronavirus disease 2019 (COVID-19) is an ongoing problem caused by severe acute respiratory syndrome coronavirus 2 (SARS-CoV-2). Initial infection appeared in Wuhan (China) in December 2019 and was declared a pandemic by the World Health Organization (WHO) in March 2020. According to the WHO, COVID-19 has infected over 600 million people and caused over 6.5 million deaths worldwide [1].

Symptoms of the disease are varied; besides general manifestations such as fever or chills, ear, nose, and throat (ENT) symptoms are also prevalent [2]. According to various authors, ENT symptoms associated with COVID-19 could include sore throat, headache, cough, dyspnea, pharyngeal erythema, nasal congestion and obstruction, rhinorrhea, nasal itching, upper respiratory tract infection, tonsil enlargement, sneezing, dysphagia, voice impairment, olfactory and taste dysfunction, dizziness, vertigo, tinnitus, and hearing impairment [2–5].

However, their frequencies differ in patients, as do anti-SARS-CoV-2 antibody levels in their plasma [6]. Treatment with convalescent plasma rich in anti-SARS-CoV-2 antibodies has proven effective in reducing the severe course and mortality of COVID-19 [7]. The correlation of demographic factors and the level of antibodies in relation to their effects on disease symptomatology has been evaluated previously [8–11]. However, only correlation with the severity of the disease was tested, without stratification by each symptom. Furthermore, it was investigated only for the general symptoms of COVID-19 infection, and not with a specific focus on otorhinolaryngological symptoms.

As has been shown by other authors, the severity of the disease affects anti-SARS-CoV2 antibody levels [12–14]. We aimed to analyze if particular otolaryngological symptoms could have a similar predictive value. Investigating the relationship between ENT symptoms and the level of antibodies may facilitate the prediction of the severity, duration and complications of COVID-19 based on the presence or absence of respective symptoms. This research may help otolaryngologists identify patients with COVID-19 infection, and, after further research, predict the course of infection. This could have both scientific and clinical significance.

This study aimed to show the frequency of ENT symptoms among COVID-19 patients, their occurrence depending on sex and age, and the correlation with IgG anti-SARS-CoV-2 antibody titers in convalescent plasma.

2. Materials and Methods

COVID-19 convalescents (n = 346) who donated blood at the Regional Center of Blood Donation and Treatment in Gdańsk (Poland) were enrolled in the study. The objective of blood donation was to acquire plasma rich in anti-SARS-CoV-2 antibodies to be used for the treatment of severe COVID-19 cases. SARS-CoV-2 infection was confirmed by polymerase chain reaction (PCR) testing of nasopharyngeal swabs. The convalescents' blood was donated from 10 to 120 days after a fourteen-day isolation period. None of the donors were vaccinated or hospitalized due to COVID-19. Patients were asked about otolaryngological symptoms of the disease: dry cough, dyspnea, sore throat, smell/taste disturbances, vertigo, dizziness, nausea and vomiting, sudden unilateral loss of hearing, progressive loss of hearing, and tinnitus. The inclusion criteria were confirmed SARS-CoV-2 infection, 18–64 years of age, and normal complete blood count, blood pressure, pulse, and body temperature. The exclusion criteria were autoimmune diseases, anti-HLA antibodies in the blood, active infection (including Treponema pallidum) or oncological illness, history of HIV, Hepatitis B or Hepatitis C infection, and being under the influence of psychoactive substances. The testing methodology of a study by Skorek et al. was replicated [11]. Blood tests were performed using the SARS-CoV-2 S-RBD IgG test of a MAGLUMI 800 device (Snibe Co., Shenzhen, China). Serological tests were performed using the in vitro chemiluminescent kit (Cat. No. SARS-CoV-2 S-RBD IgG122, Mindray, China) for the quantification of S-RBD IgG neutralizing antibodies (nAbs) against SARS-CoV-2. After collecting blood from the examined person, it was placed in test tubes with a separating gel or clot activator. After centrifugation (>10,000 RCF for 10 min), a sample (10 μL volume) containing no fibrin or other solids was collected. Subsequently, the sample, along with the buffer and magnetic particles coated with the recombinant S-RBD antigen, were mixed and incubated, resulting in the formation of immune complexes. After magnetic field precipitation, the supernatant was removed and washed. After the addition of ABEI-labeled anti-human IgG antibodies, the sample was subjected to another incubation and precipitation followed by washing to remove unbound proteins from the sample. Finally, the chemiluminescence reaction was initiated and the light signals were measured with a photomultiplier for 3 s in relative light units (RLUs), which are proportional to the SARS-CoV-2 S-RBD IgG concentration. In the case of a test performed 15 days after the onset of symptoms, the sensitivity of the test (according to the manufacturer) is 100.0% and its specificity is 99.6% (CE REF 30219017 M) [15]. Participation in the study was voluntary and written consent was obtained. The data collected were statistically analyzed using the chi-square test or Fisher exact test when the chi-square test assumption was not fulfilled (theoretical values in each cell of the contingency table equal to at least 5) to derive *p*-values. A post hoc Bonferroni correction was applied. A *p*-value less than 0.05 (typically ≤ 0.05) determined statistical significance. Cohen's h effect size was calculated and classified as small (h = 0.20), medium (h = 0.50) or large (h = 0.80). These calculations were prepared using the Statistica 13.3 StatSoft PL software (Collegium Medicum, Nicolaus Copernicus University, Bydgoszcz, Poland) and the R statistical package version 4.0.2. (Biostat, Warsaw, Poland).

The study was approved by the Regional Independent Bioethics Committee, Gdansk Medical University, Poland (NKBBN 199/2021).

3. Results

The study included 302 males and 44 females, whose mean age was 39.8 ± 9.56 SD (age range 18–64) (Table 1). The median of the measured plasma IgG anti-SASR-CoV2 antibody titers was 1:368.5. Median rather than mean antibody titer levels were calculated to minimize outlier values and for a more accurate predictive value. The FDA recommends 1:160–1:640 as the standard antibody level, which coincides with our work (the mean in the standard range is 1:400). Patients were divided into groups depending on sex and plasma antibody level.

Table 1. Demographic data.

Index	N
Mean age (95% CI)	39.80 (38.79–40.81)
Gender	
Male	302
Female	44
Antibody titer	
<1:368.5 (male:female ratio)	6:1
>1:368.5 (male:female ratio)	9:1
Clinical information	
Hypertension	9 (only males)
Familial hypercholesterolemia	1 (only females)
No comorbidities (male:female ratio)	7:1
Ethnicity	
Polish (%)	346 (100%)

The most common ENT manifestations of COVID-19 infection were smell/taste disturbances (62.43% of patients), dry cough (40.46%), sore throat (24.86%), and dyspnea (23.7%). Others included in the study were vertigo (11.85%), dizziness (8.09%), tinnitus (6.07%), nausea and vomiting (3.76%), sudden unilateral loss of hearing (1.73%), and progressive loss of hearing (0.58%).

We noted a statistically significant correlation between otolaryngological symptoms manifested during COVID-19 infection and measured antibody levels. The occurrence of dry cough, dyspnea, and dizziness was associated with higher antibody titers (Figure 1; Table 2). Additionally, in male patients there was a positive correlation between dry cough, dyspnea, dizziness, vertigo, and higher antibody titers ($p < 0.05$). Interestingly, smell/taste disturbances were correlated with lower antibody titers (Figures 2 and 3; Table 2).

Our study showed no statistically significant differences between sex and occurrence of any ENT symptom of COVID-19 (Table 2). An exception was seen in patients with lower antibody titers, whereby nausea and vomiting were more common in women than in men.

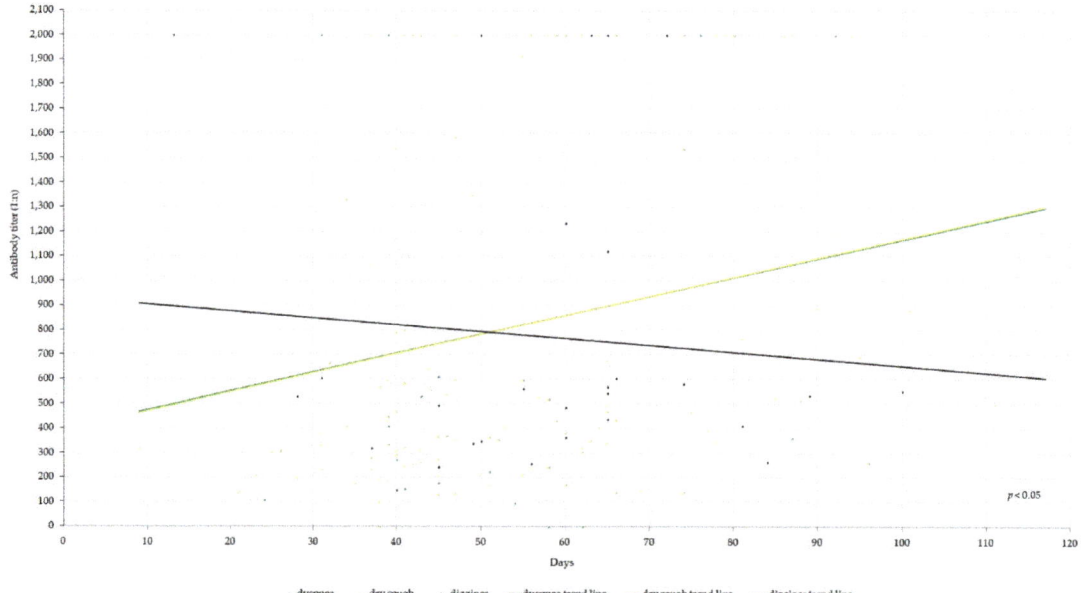

Figure 1. Anti-SARS-CoV-2 antibody titers depending on the symptoms of dizziness, dyspnea, and dry cough. Spots may represent more than one symptom. The chi-square test was used to derive the p-values.

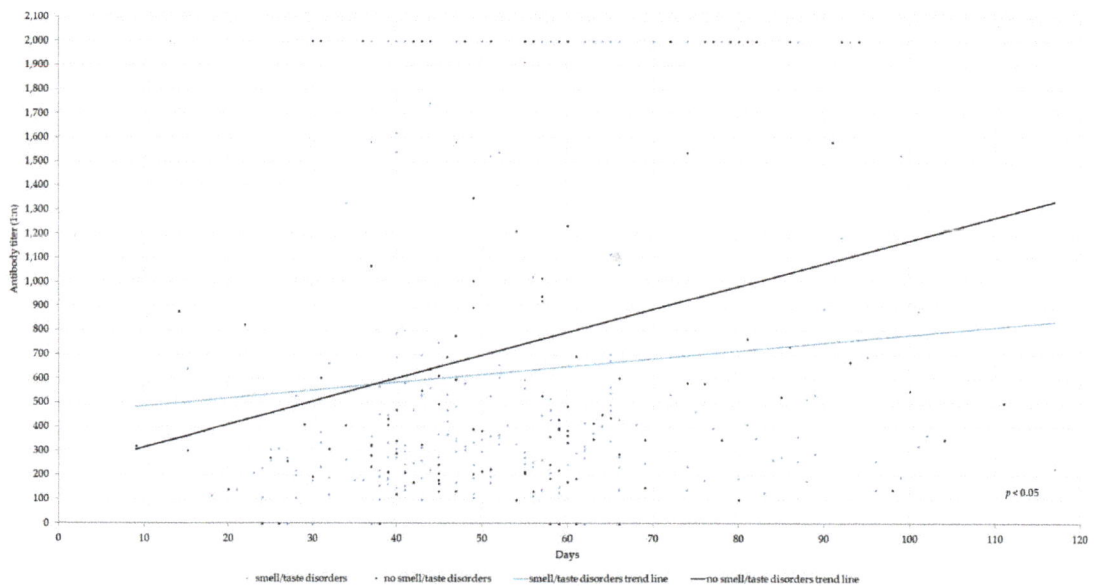

Figure 2. Anti-SARS-CoV-2 antibodies among patients depend on smell/taste disturbances. The chi-square test was used to derive the p-values.

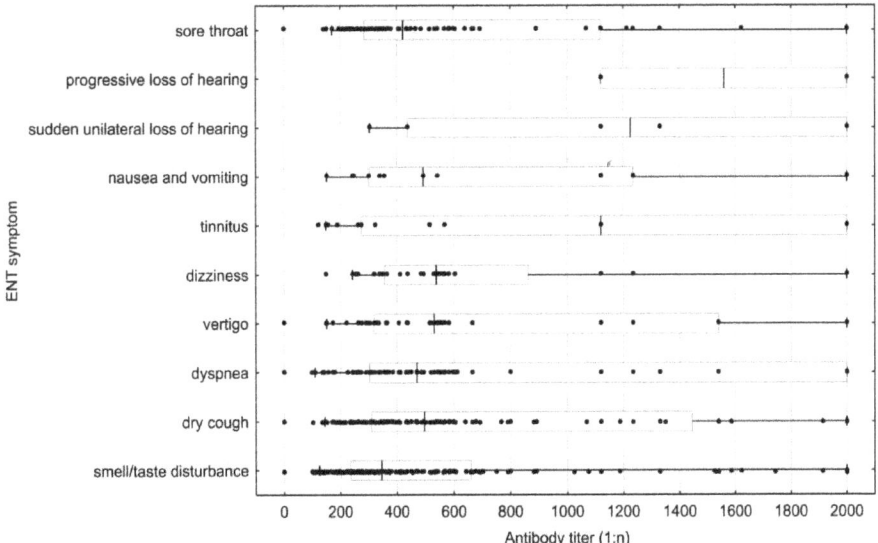

Figure 3. Antibody titer by reported ear, nose, and throat (ENT) symptom. Values for individuals with multiple symptoms are shown for each symptom individually. The center line denotes the median value (50th percentile), the box contains the 25th to 75th percentiles of the dataset, the whiskers mark the 5th and 95th percentiles, and values beyond these upper and lower bounds are considered outliers.

Patients were divided into younger and older groups based on mean age (under and above the age of 38.9). Smell/taste disturbances were more common in younger convalescents (statistically significant difference, $p < 0.05$) (Table 2). Likewise, this difference was maintained both within the male and female patient distributions ($p < 0.05$). There were no statistically significant correlations between sore throat and age, sex, or antibody level. In addition, there was no correlation between antibody titers and ENT symptoms in women ($p > 0.05$). Furthermore, there were no differences ($p > 0.05$) in otological symptoms (tinnitus, sudden unilateral loss of hearing, progressive loss of hearing) in female patients. Unfortunately, the proportion of female patients was too small to facilitate statistically significant results. According to Cohen's classification, the effect sizes observed in the statistically significant comparisons can be considered small effect sizes, which results from large disparity between group sizes.

Table 2. Statistical analysis of ear, nose, and throat (ENT) ENT symptoms by antibody titer; sex, and (age. The chi-square test and the Fisher exact test were used to derive the p-values; $p < 0.05$—outcome statistically significant (marked in bold); Cohen's h effect size was presented; 1:368.5—median antibody titer.

ENT Symptom	<1:368.5 (N = 173)	>1:368.5 (N = 173)	p Value	Cohen's h	Males (N = 302)	Females (N = 44)	p Value	Cohen's h	Age < 39.8 (N = 167)	Age > 39.8 (N = 179)	p Value	Cohen's h
smell/taste disturbance	117	99	**0.046** [a]	0.215	184	32	0.131 [a]	0.252	119	97	**0.001** [a]	0.355
dry cough	51	89	**<0.0001** [a]	0.452	125	15	0.357 [a]	0.151	65	75	0.573 [a]	0.061
sore throat	39	47	0.32 [a]	0.107	72	14	0.253 [a]	0.178	38	48	0.382 [a]	0.094
dyspnea	30	52	**0.005** [a]	0.302	72	10	0.871 [a]	0.026	45	37	0.17 [a]	0.148
vertigo	15	26	0.067 [a]	0.198	37	4	0.544 [a]	0.103	19	22	0.793 [a]	0.028
dizziness	8	20	**0.018** [a]	0.26	26	2	0.554 [b]	0.166	15	13	0.558 [a]	0.063
tinnitus	8	13	0.26 [a]	0.122	19	2	1 [b]	0.077	8	13	0.336 [a]	0.104
nausea and vomiting	6	7	0.786 [a]	0.03	10	3	0.221 [b]	0.162	6	7	0.885 [a]	0.017
sudden unilateral loss of hearing	1	5	0.215 [b]	0.189	6	0	1 [b]	0.283	2	4	0.686 [b]	0.081
progressive loss of hearing	0	2	0.499 [b]	0.215	2	0	1 [b]	0.163	1	1	1 [b]	0.005

[a] p-value calculated with chi-squared test, [b] p-value calculated with Fisher exact test.

4. Discussion

ENT symptoms were frequently observed in COVID-19 infection; however, much variability has been reported in the literature. El-Anwar et al. reported the most common manifestations to be cough (63.3%), dyspnea, (45%) sore throat (30%), nasal congestion (28.3%), nasal obstruction (26.7%), sneezing (26.6%), headache (25%) and smell/taste dysfunction (25%) [3]. However, another study by the same author presented sore throat (11.3%) and headache (10.7%) as the most frequently occurring symptoms [2]. Zięba et al. pointed out olfactory disorders (72%), taste disturbance (68%), and vertigo and dizziness (34%) [4]. Korkmaz et al. mentioned sore throat and smell/taste disturbances as prevailing symptoms [5]. We assume that results differed substantially between studies due to various factors influencing the tested groups. Possible factors might be age, comorbidities, research unit (blood donation center or ENT clinic), and geographical region, which could be associated with non-specific mutations of SARS-CoV-2. Furthermore, the ENT symptoms that the authors considered influenced the study results.

Our study showed no significant differences in ENT symptom manifestation in younger patients as compared with older patients, except for smell/taste disturbance, which occurred more often in patients under 39.8 years of age (Table 2). Elibol et al. report that otolaryngological symptoms are more frequent in the 18–30 age group, which is consistent with our smell/taste disturbance results. The authors noted that ENT manifestations of COVID-19 occurred more often in women [16]. Moreover, Takahashi et al. found gender differences in immune responses to SARS-CoV-2 and in prognostic factors for disease progression [17]. However, in our research, symptoms had different frequencies, e.g., sore throat occurred more often in women (31.82%) than men (23.84%), yet statistical significance was not achieved. As such, we are unable to conclude from our data that gender affects otolaryngological symptoms (Table 2). Furthermore, the female patient group in our study was small, probably caused by the exclusion criteria, as HLA antibodies in the blood appear after pregnancy. Therefore, statistical significance could be underestimated.

This study assessed otolaryngological symptom correlation with the level of anti-SARS-CoV-2 antibody titers; to the authors' knowledge, this is the first study to investigate this. This work may give rise to new considerations if ENT symptom occurrence could become a predictor of immune response; however, this requires further research with larger groups of people.

Plasma substance concentration could have a significant impact on the body's functioning; e.g., potassium disorders can lead to life-threatening conditions [18]. Zheng et al. measured serum albumin levels in patients with sudden sensorineural hearing loss (SSNHL) and proved low albumin levels to be associated with the worse SSNHL functional outcome [19]. We expect that plasma anti-SARS-CoV-2 antibody titer could contribute as a predictive factor for disease severity, duration, and complications.

Convalescent plasma is an accepted method of severe SARS-CoV-2 treatment [20,21]. Song et al. noted that the month after SARS-CoV-2 infection was the time of highest immunoglobulin titer [6]. Another study showed that the persistence of antibodies in plasma after COVID-19 infection was a minimum of 39 weeks [22]. Research has shown that administering convalescent plasma reduced mortality, the need for intubation, and the length of hospitalization [7,23]. However, complications of convalescent plasma immunotherapy, such as transfusion-related acute lung injury (TRALI), were reported [24]. After COVID-19 vaccination was introduced, it became the main method of prevention and thus also of fighting the virus. However, it did not completely eliminate the symptomatic course of the disease. Higher antibody titers post-vaccination were associated with worsening COVID-19 symptoms, which is likely due to an excessive immune response [25]. Every treatment has its side effects and possible complications, thus requiring an individualized approach and patient observation.

5. Conclusions

The most common ENT symptoms of SARS-CoV2 infection are smell/taste disturbances, dry cough, sore throat, and dyspnea. Smell or taste disturbances more often occur in younger patients and are related to lower anti-SARS-CoV-2 antibody titers in convalescent plasma. This study showed a statistically significant correlation between the occurrence of some otolaryngological symptoms and anti-SARS-CoV-2 antibody levels in convalescent plasma. Gender does not affect the occurrence of ENT symptoms during COVID-19 infection.

Author Contributions: Conceptualization, A.K. and K.K.; methodology, A.K.; software, K.K.; validation, A.K., K.K. and A.S.; formal analysis, A.K. and P.B.; investigation, P.B. and A.S.; resources, A.K. and A.J.-C.; data curation, A.K., K.K. and A.S.; writing—original draft preparation, A.K.; writing—review and editing, P.B. and D.T.; visualization, A.K. and K.K.; supervision, A.K.; project administration, A.K. All authors have read and agreed to the published version of the manuscript.

Funding: This research received no external funding.

Institutional Review Board Statement: The study was conducted according to the guidelines of the Declaration of Helsinki and approved by the Regional Independent Bioethics Committee, Gdansk Medical University, Poland (NKBBN 199/2021).

Informed Consent Statement: Informed consent was obtained from all subjects involved in the study.

Data Availability Statement: No public database has been created. All data are available from the authors of the work.

Conflicts of Interest: The authors declare no conflict of interest.

References

1. WHO. Available online: https://covid19.who.int/ (accessed on 28 September 2022).
2. El-Anwar, M.W.; Elzayat, S.; Fouad, Y.A. ENT manifestation in COVID-19 patients. *Auris Nasus Larynx* **2020**, *47*, 559–564. [CrossRef]
3. El-Anwar, M.W.; Eesa, M.; Mansour, W.; Zake, L.G.; Hendawy, E. Analysis of Ear, Nose and Throat Manifestations in COVID-19 Patients. *Int. Arch. Otorhinolaryngol.* **2021**, *25*, e343–e348. [CrossRef]
4. Zięba, N.; Lisowska, G.; Dadok, A.; Kaczmarek, J.; Stryjewska-Makuch, G.; Misiołek, M. Frequency and Severity of Ear-Nose-Throat (ENT) Symptoms during COVID-19 Infection. *Medicina* **2022**, *58*, 623. [CrossRef]
5. Özçelik Korkmaz, M.; Eğilmez, O.K.; Özçelik, M.A.; Güven, M. Otolaryngological manifestations of hospitalised patients with confirmed COVID-19 infection. *Eur. Arch. Oto-Rhino-Laryngol.* **2021**, *278*, 1675–1685. [CrossRef] [PubMed]
6. Song, K.H.; Kim, D.M.; Lee, H.; Ham, S.Y.; Oh, S.M.; Jeong, H.; Jung, J.; Kang, C.K.; Park, J.Y.; Kang, Y.M.; et al. Dynamics of viral load and anti-SARS-CoV-2 antibodies in patients with positive RT-PCR results after recovery from COVID-19. *Korean J. Intern. Med.* **2021**, *36*, 11–14. [CrossRef] [PubMed]
7. Abolghasemi, H.; Eshghi, P.; Cheraghali, A.M.; Imani Fooladi, A.A.; Bolouki Moghaddam, F.; Imanizadeh, S.; Moeini Maleki, M.; Ranjkesh, M.; Rezapour, M.; Bahramifar, A.; et al. Clinical efficacy of convalescent plasma for treatment of COVID-19 infections: Results of a multicenter clinical study. *Transfus. Apher. Sci. Off. J. World Apher. Assoc. Off. J. Eur. Soc. Haemapheresis* **2020**, *59*, 102875. [CrossRef] [PubMed]
8. Klein, S.L.; Pekosz, A.; Park, H.S.; Ursin, R.L.; Shapiro, J.R.; Benner, S.E.; Littlefield, K.; Kumar, S.; Naik, H.M.; Betenbaugh, M.J.; et al. Sex, age, and hospitalization drive antibody responses in a COVID-19 convalescent plasma donor population. *J. Clin. Investig.* **2020**, *130*, 6141–6150. [CrossRef]
9. Uysal, E.B.; Gümüş, S.; Bektöre, B.; Bozkurt, H.; Gözalan, A. Evaluation of antibody response after COVID-19 vaccination of healthcare workers. *J. Med. Virol.* **2022**, *94*, 1060–1066. [CrossRef]
10. Li, K.; Huang, B.; Wu, M.; Zhong, A.; Li, L.; Cai, Y.; Wang, Z.; Wu, L.; Zhu, M.; Li, J.; et al. Dynamic changes in anti-SARS-CoV-2 antibodies during SARS-CoV-2 infection and recovery from COVID-19. *Nat. Commun.* **2020**, *11*, 6044. [CrossRef]
11. Skorek, A.; Jaźwińska-Curyłło, A.; Romanowicz, A.; Kwaśniewski, K.; Narożny, W.; Tretiakow, D. Assessment of anti-SARS-CoV-2 antibodies level in convalescents plasma. *J. Med. Virol.* **2022**, *94*, 1130–1137. [CrossRef]
12. Weisberg, S.P.; Connors, T.J.; Zhu, Y.; Baldwin, M.R.; Lin, W.H.; Wontakal, S.; Szabo, P.A.; Wells, S.B.; Dogra, P.; Gray, J.; et al. Distinct antibody responses to SARS-CoV-2 in children and adults across the COVID-19 clinical spectrum. *Nat. Immunol.* **2021**, *22*, 25–31. [CrossRef] [PubMed]
13. Kritikos, A.; Gabellon, S.; Pagani, J.L.; Monti, M.; Bochud, P.Y.; Manuel, O.; Coste, A.; Greub, G.; Perreau, M.; Pantaleo, G.; et al. Anti-SARS-CoV-2 Titers Predict the Severity of COVID-19. *Viruses* **2021**, *14*, 1089. [CrossRef] [PubMed]

14. Wang, Y.; Zhang, L.; Sang, L.; Ye, F.; Ruan, S.; Zhong, B.; Song, T.; Alshukairi, A.N.; Chen, R.; Zhang, Z.; et al. Kinetics of viral load and antibody response in relation to COVID-19 severity. *J. Clin. Investig.* **2020**, *130*, 5235–5244. [CrossRef] [PubMed]
15. Flisiak, R.; Horban, A.; Jaroszewicz, J.; Kozielewicz, D.; Mastalerz-Migas, A.; Owczuk, R.; Parczewski, M.; Pawłowska, M.; Piekarska, A.; Simon, K.; et al. Management of SARS-CoV-2 infection: Recommendations of the Polish Association of Epidemiologists and Infectiologists as of April 26, 2021. *Pol. Arch. Intern. Med.* **2021**, *131*, 487–496. [CrossRef]
16. Elibol, E. Otolaryngological symptoms in COVID-19. *Eur. Arch. Oto-Rhino-Laryngol.* **2021**, *278*, 1233–1236. [CrossRef]
17. Takahashi, T.; Ellingson, M.K.; Wong, P.; Israelow, B.; Lucas, C.; Klein, J.; Silva, J.; Mao, T.; Oh, J.E.; Tokuyama, M.; et al. Sex differences in immune responses that underlie COVID-19 disease outcomes. *Nature* **2020**, *588*, 315–320. [CrossRef]
18. Heras, M.; Fernández-Reyes, M.J. Serum potassium concentrations: Importance of normokalaemia. Concentraciones séricas de potasio: Importancia de la normopotasemia. *Med. Clin.* **2017**, *148*, 562–565. [CrossRef]
19. Zheng, Z.; Liu, C.; Shen, Y.; Xia, L.; Xiao, L.; Sun, Y.; Wang, H.; Chen, Z.; Wu, Y.; Shi, H.; et al. Serum Albumin Levels as a Potential Marker for the Predictive and Prognostic Factor in Sudden Sensorineural Hearing Loss: A Prospective Cohort Study. *Front. Neurol.* **2021**, *12*, 747561. [CrossRef]
20. Duan, K.; Liu, B.; Li, C.; Zhang, H.; Yu, T.; Qu, J.; Zhou, M.; Chen, L.; Meng, S.; Hu, Y.; et al. Effectiveness of convalescent plasma therapy in severe COVID-19 patients. *Proc. Natl. Acad. Sci. USA* **2020**, *117*, 9490–9496. [CrossRef]
21. Cunningham, A.C.; Goh, H.P.; Koh, D. Treatment of COVID-19: Old tricks for new challenges. *Crit. Care* **2020**, *24*, 91. [CrossRef]
22. Johannesen, C.K.; St Martin, G.; Lendorf, M.E.; Gerred, P.; Fyfe, A.; Paton, R.S.; Thompson, C.; Molsted, S.; Kann, C.E.; Jensen, C.A.; et al. Prevalence and duration of anti-SARS-CoV-2 antibodies in healthcare workers. *Dan. Med. J.* **2022**, *69*, A11210843. [PubMed]
23. Soo, Y.O.; Cheng, Y.; Wong, R.; Hui, D.S.; Lee, C.K.; Tsang, K.K.; Ng, M.H.; Chan, P.; Cheng, G.; Sung, J.J. Retrospective comparison of convalescent plasma with continuing high-dose methylprednisolone treatment in SARS patients. *Clin. Microbiol. Infect.* **2004**, *10*, 676–678. [CrossRef] [PubMed]
24. Chun, S.; Chung, C.R.; Ha, Y.E.; Han, T.H.; Ki, C.S.; Kang, E.S.; Park, J.K.; Peck, K.R.; Cho, D. Possible Transfusion-Related Acute Lung Injury Following Convalescent Plasma Transfusion in a Patient With Middle East Respiratory Syndrome. *Ann. Lab. Med.* **2016**, *36*, 393–395. [CrossRef]
25. Tsuchida, T.; Hirose, M.; Inoue, Y.; Kunishima, H.; Otsubo, T.; Matsuda, T. Relationship between changes in symptoms and antibody titers after a single vaccination in patients with Long COVID. *J. Med. Virol.* **2022**, *94*, 3416–3420. [CrossRef] [PubMed]

Disclaimer/Publisher's Note: The statements, opinions and data contained in all publications are solely those of the individual author(s) and contributor(s) and not of MDPI and/or the editor(s). MDPI and/or the editor(s) disclaim responsibility for any injury to people or property resulting from any ideas, methods, instructions or products referred to in the content.

Article

Post-COVID-19 Status and Its Physical, Nutritional, Psychological, and Social Effects in Working-Age Adults—A Prospective Questionnaire Study

Tamara Nikolic Turnic [1,2,*], Ivana Vasiljevic [1], Magdalena Stanic [1], Biljana Jakovljevic [3], Maria Mikerova [2], Natalia Ekkert [2], Vladimir Reshetnikov [2] and Vladimir Jakovljevic [4,5]

1. Department of Pharmacy, Faculty of Medical Sciences, University of Kragujevac, 34000 Kragujevac, Serbia
2. N.A. Semashko Public Health and Healthcare Department, F.F. Erisman Institute of Public Health, I.M. Sechenov First Moscow State Medical University, 119435 Moscow, Russia
3. Academy for Applied Studies, The College of Health Studies, 11070 Belgrade, Serbia
4. Department of Physiology, Faculty of Medical Sciences, University of Kragujevac, 34000 Kragujevac, Serbia
5. Department of Human Pathology, 1st Moscow State Medical, University IM Sechenov, Trubetskaya Street 8, Str. 2, 119991 Moscow, Russia
* Correspondence: tnikolict@gmail.com or tamara.nikolic@medf.kg.ac.rs; Tel.: +381-656856185

Abstract: Background: The main objective of this study was to evaluate the evolution of physical and daily routine, dietary habits, and mental and social health in individuals with recent COVID-19 infection. Methods: A qualitative prospective cross-sectional study was conducted from 01 October 2021 to 01 March 2022, which included 80 working-age adults from the territory of Central Serbia who had PCR-confirmed SARS-CoV-2 infection in the previous six months. Two structured pre-coded closed-ended questionnaires were submitted to the participants: a questionnaire about post-COVID-19 status (pCOVq) and a shortened version of the World Health Organization's Quality of Life Scale (WHOQOL-BREF). Results: The presence of the COVID-19 disease in the previous period of 6 months among the working-age participants significantly affected the duration of aerobic, anaerobic, and high-intensity physical activities, but also the possibility of performing certain activities such as walking, which represents basic aerobic activity and a measure of general health among middle-aged participants. In the majority of cases (78%), in the post-COVID-19 period, participants indicated a decline in educational and productive activities. Conclusion: Post-COVID status in working-aged participants consists of reduced physical activity, lower quality of life, and similar nutritional habits. Health policies should be more focused on these findings.

Keywords: post-COVID-19 status; physical activities; nutritional habits; social activity; working-age adults

1. Introduction

After the December outbreak of COVID-19 in Wuhan, China, the infection spread rapidly to other parts of the world, and the increasing number of cases suggests that the disease continues to spread steadily [1]. Initially, it was thought that people who had been to the seafood market or consumed food prepared with infected animals had been infected with COVID-19. However, it was later found that a number of people who had not traveled to the seafood market were also infected, i.e., tested positive for COVID-19 [2,3]. This showed that human-to-human transmission of the virus was possible, which was later confirmed in many countries around the world [1–4]. Thanks to the interventions and control measures taken by governments around the world, the number of newly confirmed cases is decreasing worldwide [5]. Although all important measures are being implemented, the risk of transmission has not yet been eliminated, and the epidemic remains a major challenge for clinicians. A large proportion of patients have a mild or moderate course of disease, but a number of patients have a severe and even life-threatening course of disease [6,7].

Social distancing and confinement have been very important in the fight against the spread of the virus [8]. However, all these restrictions affect the health and well-being of the general population. In these circumstances, some sudden and stressful situation after a long stay at home can greatly affect the change of lifestyle, i.e.: physical activity, eating habits, alcohol consumption, mental health, quality of sleep, etc. [9,10].

Further, recommended travel restrictions and regulations against participation in outdoor activities, which includes physical activity and exercise, have greatly affected the routine daily activities of a wide variety of people [11].

Post-COVID syndrome was described as a clinical entity for the first time in the spring of 2020 when patients with COVID-19 still had symptoms several weeks after acute infection [12]. Currently, this syndrome is one of the challenges for health systems, which is becoming more common as the pandemic develops. Recent studies suggest that 10 to 20% of patients with SARS-CoV-2 who go through the acute symptomatic phase have disease sequelae in the form of unexplained, persistent signs or symptoms for 12 weeks after SARS-CoV-2 infection, called "post-COVID syndrome". In general, patients with this syndrome had experience fatigue, extreme tiredness, and symptoms that persist beyond the active phase of the disease [13–15].

Although many patients recover without sequelae, many patients may have symptoms for a long time after recovering from the infection, and others may develop new symptoms. The most common persistent symptoms in the post-infection period (more than 4 weeks from onset) are shortness of breath, cognitive impairment, fatigue, anxiety, and depression [13–15].

The cause of this post-viral syndrome remains unknown, although it resembles chronic fatigue syndrome, which is now referred to as post-viral fatigue syndrome. If these symptoms are simply due to critical illness or hypoxia in ventilator-dependent patients, this would not explain the reason why they occur in non-hospitalized patients and why they are not clearly related to the severity of the original infection [14].

Future research is very important to explain the pathogenesis, clinical spectrum, and prognosis of post-COVID syndrome. In addition, markers that allow for the rapid diagnosis of this syndrome and monitoring of its associated morbidity and prognosis are needed.

The main objective of this study was to assess the evolution of physical and daily routine, as well as mental and social health in individuals with a recent COVID-19 infection over a six-month period after infection and to identify factors associated with (unfavorable) evolution. Secondary objectives were to assess general health and vital energy in working-age individuals, social functioning, and dietary behaviors in the period after COVID.

2. Materials and Methods

2.1. Ethics Approval and Consent to Participate

This study protocol was approved by the Institutional Ethics Committee of the Faculty of Medical Sciences of the University of Kragujevac (No. 147/20) and is in accordance with the principles of the Declaration of Helsinki (2013 revision). Participation in this study was voluntary and anonymous.

2.2. Protocol of the Study

A qualitative prospective cross-sectional study was conducted from 1 October 2021 to 1 March 2022, involving 80 working-age adults from the area of central Serbia who had PCR-confirmed SARS-CoV-2 infection in the previous six months.

2.3. Recruitment of Participants

The inclusion criteria were the presence of SARS-CoV-2 infection in the previous 6 months from inclusion in the study (positive PCR test), ambulatory treatment during COVID-19 disease, an absence of other chronical diseases/treatments, place of residence in the cities of central Serbia, and a positive answer to the question from the first part of the questionnaire (voluntary consent to the study). Exclusion criteria were age less than 18 years and more than 50 years old, place of residence in other countries/regions of the world, as well as an incompletely completed survey and previous hospital treatment regarding COVID-19 disease.

2.4. Instruments

Two structured pre-coded closed-ended questionnaires were submitted to the participants: a questionnaire about post-COVID-19 status (pCOVq) and a shortened version of the World Health Organization's Quality of Life Scale (WHOQOL-BREF).

2.5. A Questionnaire about the Post-COVID-19 Status (pCOVq)

The questionnaire on the post-COVID-19 status of adults in the territory of the municipality of Kragujevac is a standardized tool constructed by the author Kang-Hyun Park and associated and validated on the population of adult respondents during 2020 [16]. The pCOVq is an anonymous questionnaire that consists of 26 questions; each question has up to 6 sub-questions related to the period before and after the infection, and the time allotted for filling it is less than 60 min. The questionnaire consisted of domains, each of which separately analyzed one aspect of life related to the patient, i.e., the respondent (1) physical activity, (2) participation in activities, and (3) nutrition. In previous studies, the pCOVq questionnaire showed high internal reliability, with a Cronbach alpha of 0.83. The intraclass correlation coefficient was 0.97 for the total score of the questionnaire in terms of test–retest reliability [16].

2.6. Physical Activity as a Lifestyle Indicator in Post-COVID Period

A total of six physical activity items were assessed using a five-point Likert scale to measure respondents' frequency of participation in six different physical activities and their satisfaction with participating in these physical activities. The six physical activities included aerobic physical activity; anaerobic physical activity; low-intensity physical activity equivalent to 2–2.9 metabolic equivalents of the task (MET), including gardening, house cleaning, etc.; moderate-intensity physical activity equivalent to 3–5.9 METs, including swimming, doubles tennis, etc.; high-intensity physical activity equivalent to 6–9.9 MET, such as running, climbing, etc.; and walking exercises. According to the American College of Sports Medicine (ACSM), physical activity can be divided into three types, based on intensity. To assess the impact of the COVID-19 pandemic on physical activity, questions were asked about the frequency and satisfaction of participating in physical activity weekly before and after the onset of COVID-19. The higher the score, the higher the level of participation and satisfaction with physical activity.

2.7. Daily Activity as a Lifestyle Indicator in POSt-COVID Period

Six items about the daily activity were also assessed using a five-point Likert scale to measure the frequency of and satisfaction with the variety of present daily activities, such as activities of daily living (ADL), leisure, social activities, work, education, and sleep during the week before and after COVID-19. A higher score indicates more frequent participation in various activities as well as greater satisfaction with participation in activities.

2.8. Nutrition as a Lifestyle Indicator in Post-COVID Period

Finally, nine items on diet were assessed using a five-point Likert scale to assess diet in the week before and after COVID-19 and to measure participants' nutritional status. The amounts of carbohydrates, proteins, fats, vitamins, minerals, water, and alcohol that participants consumed, as well as the frequency of drinking and smoking, were measured. For example, participants were asked, "Before the COVID-19 pandemic, how often did you consume carbohydrate-rich foods such as rice, bread, and flour in the last week?" Participants responded to these questions by selecting one of the five-point Likert scale options: (1) never, (2) 1–2 times a week, (3) 3–4 times a week, (4) 5–6 times a week, and (5) every day. A higher score indicates a higher consumption of each type of food.

2.9. A Shortened Version of the World Health Organization's Quality of Life Scale (WHOQOL-BREF)

A shortened version of the World Health Organization's Quality of Life Scale (WHOQOL-BREF) was used to assess quality of life [17,18]. It contains 26 items rated on a five-point Likert scale and measures four domains: physical, psychological, social and environmental. Raw domain scores were converted to a scale ranging from 0 to 100 to facilitate comparison with other instruments, with higher scores indicating higher quality of life. Cronbach's alpha was 0.91 and 0.94 before and after COVID-19, respectively. Each question has 7 possible answers scored on a Likert scale from 0 to 6, with 0 corresponding to the feeling that it "never" happens and 6 indicating that it happens "every day". Quality of life was assessed only six months after COVID-19, since we could not predict who will be infected [17,18].

2.10. Data Management and Statistical Analysis

This cross-sectional prospective study included the participants who satisfied the inclusion criteria mentioned before. According to the results of the previous study, the sample size was arrived at using the margin of error approach as seen in the equation below: $n = Z2P(1-P)/d2$. The sample size was set at 80 participants. In the evaluation of the quality of life and clinical status, 4 (5%) participants were excluded because of an incompletely filled survey, which is permissible exclusion. Statistical analyses were performed in the SPSS program version 26 using descriptive and statistical analytical tests. Results are presented as frequencies in percent (%) or as arithmetic means and standard deviations (X; SD). A Chi-square test was used to estimate the statistical differences in the distributions of categorical variables. The statistical threshold was set at the level of 0.05.

3. Results

3.1. Basic Demographic Characteristics of Study Population

Table 1 shows the basic demographic characteristics of the study population. Most participants were female, with a mean age of 30.64 ± 1.54 years. In addition, most participants were under 30 years of age, single, employed, and living in a medium-sized city (Table 1).

Table 1. Basic socio-economic characteristics of the study population ($n = 80$). Results are presented as distributions [%]/mean ± stand. deviation.

Variables	Categories ($n = 80$)	Distribution [%]/Mean ± SD
Gender [%]	Male	20 [25%]
	Female	60 [75%]
Age category [%]	20–29 years old	54 [68%]
	30–39 years old	9 [12%]
	40–49 years old	17 [20%]
Age [years; X ± SD]		30.64 ± 1.54
Education level [%]	Elementary school	25 [32.9%]
	High school	6 [2.6%]
	Faculty	21 [27.6%]
	Student	28 [36.8%]

Table 1. Cont.

Variables	Categories (n = 80)	Distribution [%]/Mean ± SD
Marital status [%]	Single	33 [43.4%]
	Married	23 [30.3%]
	Bisexual/homosexual relationship	21 [22.4%]
	Divorced	2 [2.6%]
	Widow/er	1 [1.3%]
Place of living [%]	Big city (above 500,000 inhabitants)	10 [7.9%]
	Middle city (100,000–500,000 inhabitants)	70 [82.1%]
Occupation level [%]	Employed	80 [100%]

3.2. Clinical Status of the Working-Age Study Population

In the form of Table 2, the clinical symptoms among the study population during the period after COVID-19 are shown. During COVID-19, most patients had many current symptoms such as sleep problems, bowel and bladder dysfunction, and respiratory problems. Some of the participants had joint movement restrictions, odor disturbances, circulatory problems, and pain. Interestingly, in the period after COVID, many of these complaints were still present, such as limitations in the sense of smell (17.1%) and taste (15.8%) and breathing problems (14.5%), and most participants had persistent increased fatigue (23.7%). Further, there was a not insignificant number of participants with other persistent symptoms six months after COVID-19 (Table 2).

Table 2. Post-COVID-19 clinical status of participants (n = 76). Results are presented as frequency of responses [%]. Statistical significance was obtained using the Chi-square test (X^2). Single or double asterisks represents the statistically significant difference (* $p < 0.05$; ** $p < 0.01$) in distribution of responses among study population.

Health Problems	Severity of Clinical Problem	Frequency [%]	Do the Above Problems Still Exist?		p Values
			Yes (%)	No (%)	
Sleep problems (this includes problems falling asleep, sleeping through the night, and waking up early)	None	52 (68.4%)	11 (14.5%)	65 (85.5%)	0.021 *
	Mild problem	8 (10.5%)			
	Moderate problem	11 (14.5%)			
	Big problem	5 (6.6%)			
	Extreme problem	0 (0%)			
Bowel dysfunction (e.g., diarrhea and constipation)	None	56 (73.7%)	4 (5.3%)	72 (94.7%)	0.688
	Mild problem	13 (17.1%)			
	Moderate problem	6 (7.9%)			
	Big problem	1 (1.3)			
	Extreme problem	0 (0%)			
Bladder dysfunction (e.g., incontinence, kidney or bladder stones, kidney problem, urine leakage, and reflux)	None	68 (89.5%)	3 (3.9%)	71 (96.1%)	0.216
	Mild problem	4 (5.3%)			
	Moderate problem	3 (3.9%)			
	Big problem	0 (0%)			
	Extreme problem	1 (1.3%)			

Table 2. *Cont.*

Health Problems	Severity of Clinical Problem	Frequency [%]	Do the Above Problems Still Exist?		p Values
			Yes (%)	No (%)	
Limitation of movement (restricted range of motion of the joints)	None	45 (59.2%)	6 (7.9%)	70 (92.1%)	0.275
	Mild problem	16 (21.1%)			
	Moderate problem	11 (14.5%)			
	Big problem	2 (2.6%)			
	Extreme problem	2 (2.6%)			
Muscle problems (uncontrolled, spasmodic muscle movements, such as uncontrollable twitching or spasm)	None	48 (63.2%)	8 (10.5%)	68 (89.5%)	0.216
	Mild problem	16 (21.1%)			
	Moderate problem	10 (13.2%)			
	Big problem	1 (1.3%)			
	Extreme problem	1 (1.3%)			
Respiratory problems (difficulty breathing and increased secretion)	None	32 (42.1%)	11 (14.5%)	65 (85.5%)	0.005 **
	Mild problem	21 (27.6%)			
	Moderate problem	13 (17.1%)			
	Big problem	8 (10.5%)			
	Extreme problem	2 (2.6%)			
Limitation of the sense of smell (e.g., reduced or increased perception of smell)	None	33 (43.4%)	13 (17.1%)	63 (82.9%)	0.021 *
	Mild problem	16 (21.1%)			
	Moderate problem	8 (10.5%)			
	Big problem	9 (11.8%)			
	Extreme problem	10 (13.2%)			
Limitations of the sense of taste (e.g., reduced or increased perception of taste)	None	38 (50%)	12 (15.8%)	64 (84.2%)	0.026 *
	Mild problem	14 (18.4%)			
	Moderate problem	8 (10.5%)			
	Big problem	7 (9.2%)			
	Extreme problem	9 (11.8%)			
Circulation problems or circulatory disorders (including swelling of veins, feet, hands, legs)	None	62 (81.6%)	4 (5.3%)	72 (94.7%)	0.125
	Mild problem	10 (13.2%)			
	Moderate problem	3 (3.9%)			
	Big problem	1 (1.3%)			
	Extreme problem	0 (0%)			
Malaise (e.g., increased fatigue)	None	19 (25%)	18 (23.7%)	58 (76.3%)	0.003 **
	Mild problem	16 (21.1%)			
	Moderate problem	16 (21.1%)			
	Big problem	13 (17.1%)			
	Extreme problem	12 (15.8%)			
Fears and anxiety	None	50 (65.8%)	9 (11.8%)	67 (88.2%)	0.043 *
	Mild problem	14 (18.4%)			
	Moderate problem	5 (6.6%)			
	Big problem	5 (6.6%)			
	Extreme problem	2 (2.6%)			
Pain	None	40 (52.6%)	6 (7.9%)	70 (82.1%)	0.162
	Mild problem	18 (23.7%)			
	Moderate problem	10 (13.2%)			
	Big problem	4 (5.3%)			
	Extreme problem	4 (5.3%)			

3.3. Changes in Different Types and Intensities of Physical Activity in the Working-Age Study Population after SARS-CoV-2 Infection

In this study, we examined the effects of SARS-CoV-2 infection on the different types and intensities of physical activity six months after the onset of the disease (Table 3). We asked participants about the frequency of aerobic, anaerobic, daily, light, and high-intensity physical activity. Interestingly, both aerobic and anaerobic activity changed, and a greater number of participants reduced these physical activities in the period after COVID. Similarly, the number of participants who engaged in high-intensity physical activity decreased, whereas the consumption of low- and moderate-intensity physical activity did not decrease (Table 3).

Table 3. Differences in the frequency of aerobic and anaerobic physical activity, as well as in low-, middle-, and high-intensity activity before and six months after COVID-19. Results are presented as frequency in percent from total number of participants [%]. Statistical significance was obtained using Chi-square test (X2) as follows: [a] = statistically significantly higher number of participants compared to activity before and after COVID-19, [b] = statistically significantly lower number of participants compared to activity before and after COVID-19.

Type of Activity		Aerobic Activity	Anaerobic Activity	Low-Intensity Physical Activity	Middle-Intensity Physical Activity	High-Intensity Physical Activity
Period	Frequency	Percent [%]	Percent [%]	Percent [%]	Percent [%]	Percent [%]
Exercise before COVID-19	Neither day	48.8	56.3	20.0	51.2	50.0
	1–2 days per week	32.5	22.5	23.8	28.7	33.8
	3–4 days per week	11.3	15.0	30.0	15.0	10.0
	5–6 days per week	2.5	5.0	6.3	1.3	5.0
	Every day	5.0	1.3	20.0	3.8	1.3
Exercise after COVID-19	Neither day	60.0 [a]	62.5 [a]	16.3	53.8	56.3 [a]
	1–2 days per week	22.5 [b]	22.5	36.3 [a]	32.5	30.0 [b]
	3–4 days per week	12.5	10.0 [b]	25.0	75.0 [a]	6.3
	5–6 days per week	2.5	2.5	8.8	3.8	6.3 [a]
	Every day	2.5 [b]	2.5	13.8 [b]	2.5	1.3
Duration of physical exercise before COVID-19	None	46.3	53.8	12.5	51.2	46.3
	10–20 min	22.5	18.8	16.3	15.0	11.3
	21–40 min	16.3	17.5	25.0	16.3	23.8
	41–60 min	7.5	6.3	18.8	6.3	10.0
	Above 60 min	7.5	3.8	27.5	11.3	8.8
Duration of physical exercise after COVID-19	None	55 [a]	61.3 [a]	16.3 [a]	51.2	57.5 [a]
	10–20 min	23.8	22.5	20.0	25.0	17.5
	21–40 min	11.3 [b]	7.5 [b]	25.0	11.3 [b]	11.3
	41–60 min	2.5 [b]	5.0	17.3	6.3	10.0 [b]
	Above 60 min	7.5	3.8	21.3	6.3	3.8

Table 3. Cont.

Period	Type of Activity / Frequency	Aerobic Activity Percent [%]	Anaerobic Activity Percent [%]	Low-Intensity Physical Activity Percent [%]	Middle-Intensity Physical Activity Percent [%]	High-Intensity Physical Activity Percent [%]
Possibility of doing exercises before infection	Always less than I wanted	51.2	51.2	25.0	45.0	42.5
	Sometimes less than I wanted	12.5	12.5	6.3	10.0	10.0
	As much as I could	31.3	33.8	46.3	37.5	42.5
	Sometimes more than I wanted	2.5	0	13.8	1.3	1.3
	Always more than I wanted	2.5	2.5	8.8	6.3	3.8
Possibility of doing exercises after infection	Always less than I wanted	57.5 [a]	52.5	26.3	46.3	52.5 [a]
	Sometimes less than I wanted	8.8 [b]	12.5	10.0 [b]	15.0 [b]	10.0
	As much as I could	27.5 [b]	30.0 [b]	43.8	35.0 [b]	31.3 [b]
	Sometimes more than I wanted	1.3	1.3	13.8	1.3	2.5
	Always more than I wanted	5.0	3.8	6.3	2.5	3.8

In terms of duration, there was an increase in the number of participants who did not engage in physical activity during the period after COVID. The opportunity to engage in physical activity after SARS-CoV-2 infection was also reduced, especially for aerobic and high-intensity activities (Table 3).

Regarding the other activities, Table 4 shows the statistical differences in the period before and six months after COVID-19 in the study population. Statistically significant reductions were observed in the frequency and duration of daily and social activities and in the duration of productive and educational activities. As expected, social activities were most reduced in our working-age population (Table 4).

Table 4. Participation in different activities in the period before and six months after COVID-19 among the study population. Statistical significance was obtained using the Chi-square test (X^2). Asterisks (*) represent the statistically significant difference in selected characteristic of activity before and six months after COVID-19, and the double asterisk (**) represents high significance (<0.001).

Activity and Its Characteristics ($n = 80$)		p Values
Daily activity	Frequency [days per week]	0.000 **
	Duration of activity [hours]	0.000 **
	Ability to perform [yes/no]	0.345
Other free-daily activity	Frequency [days per week]	0.013 *
	Duration of activity [hours]	0.040 *
	Ability to perform [yes/no]	0.987
Social activities	Frequency [days per week]	0.016 *
	Duration of activity [hours]	0.001 **
	Ability to perform [yes/no]	0.012 *

Table 4. *Cont.*

Activity and Its Characteristics (n = 80)		p Values
Productive activities	Frequency [days per week]	0.081
	Duration of activity [hours]	0.000 **
	Ability to perform [yes/no]	0.670
Educational activities	Frequency [days per week]	0.023 *
	Duration of activity [hours]	0.222
	Ability to perform [yes/no]	0.035 *
Sleeping/Resting	Duration of activity [hours]	0.662
	Ability to perform [yes/no]	1.000

3.4. Nutrition Habits in the Post-COVID Period among Study Population

From Figure 1 and Table 5, we can see that dietary habits changed significantly in the period after COVID, although most of the changes were not statistically significant. Interestingly, the frequency of water consumption changed in the period after COVID, with a large number of participants consuming water five to six times per week or daily (Figure 1; Table 5). In general, the National Academies of Sciences, Engineering, and Medicine suggests that each day, women drink a total of about 2.7 L (L) or 11 cups of fluid and men consume about 3.7 L (16 cups). Every additional cup is recognized as additional water consumption (Figure 1; Table 5).

Table 5. Change in dietary habits in relation to frequency of consumption per week in the study population. Results were obtained using the Chi-square test. Single asterisks represent the statistically significant difference (* $p < 0.05$) in distribution of responses among study population.

Weekly Intake [Times Per Week]	p Values
Carbohydrates	0.827
Proteins	0.564
Lipids	0.251
Vitamins	0.128
Minerals	0.157
Water	0.049 *
Cigarettes	0.987
Alcohol	0.788

3.5. Quality of Life of Working-Age Participants after SARS-CoV-2 Infection

Table 6 shows the frequency of responses related to self-satisfaction and quality of life. Most participants were satisfied in many ways, but there are still a large number of participants who were generally not satisfied. All questions refer to post-infection symptoms (COVID), so we found that a statistically significant number of participants were only dissatisfied to very dissatisfied with life, health status, daily activities, and personal relationships, which can be considered as decreased satisfaction (Table 6).

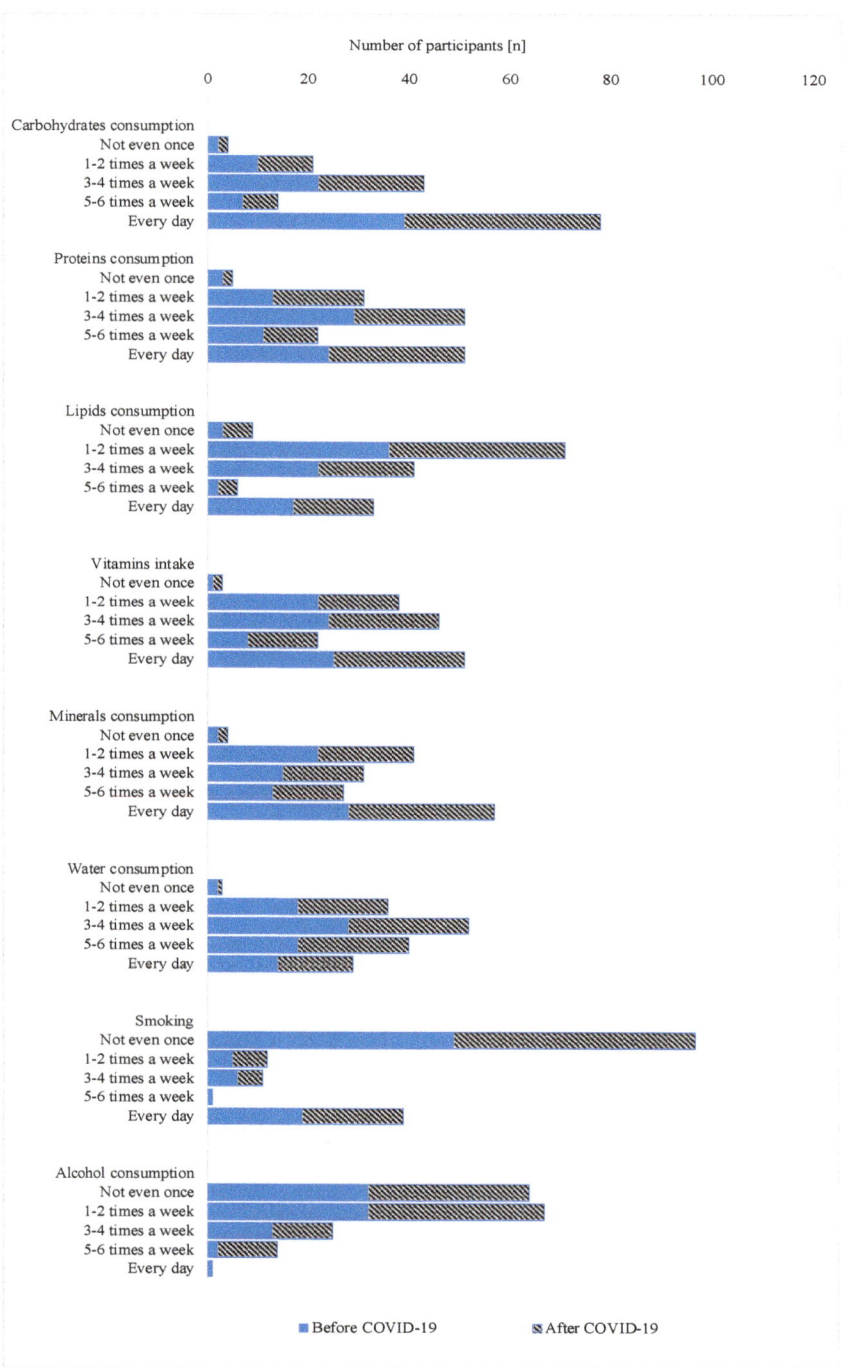

Figure 1. Assessment of weekly food intake and dietary habits of participants before and 6 months after COVID-19. Results are presented as number of patients out of total ($n = 80$).

Table 6. Quality of life of participants six months after COVID-19. Results are presented as frequency of responses [%]. Statistical significance was obtained using the Chi-square test (X2). Asterisks (*) represent the statistically significant difference in distribution of responses among study population ($p < 0.05$).

Item	Graded Responses	Frequency [%]	p Values
How would you rate the quality of your life?	Very satisfied	18 (23,7%)	0.045 *
	Satisfied	52 (68,4%)	
	Neither satisfied nor dissatisfied	6 (7,9%)	
	Dissatisfied	0 (0%)	
	Very dissatisfied	0 (0%)	
How satisfied are you with your health?	Very satisfied	15 (19.7%)	0.035 *
	Satisfied	53 (69.7%)	
	Neither satisfied nor dissatisfied	8 (10.5%)	
	Dissatisfied	0 (0%)	
	Very dissatisfied	0 (0%)	
How satisfied are you with your ability to perform daily life activities?	Very satisfied	26 (34.2%)	0.039 *
	Satisfied	42 (55.3%)	
	Neither satisfied nor dissatisfied	8 (10.5%)	
	Dissatisfied	0 (0%)	
	Very dissatisfied	0 (0%)	
How satisfied are you with yourself?	Very satisfied	29 (38.2%)	0.055
	Satisfied	40 (52.6%)	
	Neither satisfied nor dissatisfied	7 (9.2%)	
	Dissatisfied	0 (0%)	
	Very dissatisfied	0 (0%)	
How satisfied are you with your personal relationships?	Very satisfied	24 (31.6%)	0.028 *
	Satisfied	44 (57.9%)	
	Neither satisfied nor dissatisfied	8 (10.5%)	
	Dissatisfied	0 (0%)	
	Very dissatisfied	0 (0%)	
How satisfied are you with the conditions of your housing?	Very satisfied	34 (44.7%)	0.571
	Satisfied	37 (48.7%)	
	Neither satisfied nor dissatisfied	5 (6.6%)	
	Dissatisfied	0 (0%)	
	Very dissatisfied	0 (0%)	

4. Discussion

The primary objective of this study was to assess the evolution of physical and daily routine, as well as mental and social health in individuals with recent COVID-19 infection over a six-month period after infection and the factors associated with (un)favorable evolution. Secondary objectives were to assess general health and vital energy in working-age individuals, social functioning, and dietary behaviors in the post-COVID period.

For the first time, a study addresses the assessment of the impact of acute infection on the range of other vital activities in young people of working age [19,20]. A variety of questionnaires were used to assess behavior, satisfaction, and objective interference with physical activities. The identification of risk factors for prolonged disease progression is necessary, and early identification and monitoring of patients at increased risk for developing post-syndromal COVID must be a priority.

It has been proven that more than 60% of patients who had COVID-19 have many persistent symptoms and syndromes in the period after COVID [21]. This information could be important not only for healthcare professionals, but also for the economy and people in general, because protracted illness is a global problem, not just an individual disability.

Post-COVID syndrome is a serious condition that includes a variety of new, recurrent, or persistent symptoms that people usually experience at least four weeks after a positive SARS-CoV-2 test [22]. In some cases, symptoms persist for more than 3 months when this syndrome begins as a chronic form of the disease [23].

The results of our study show that there is a statistically significant difference in certain segments before and after infection. Regarding aerobic and anaerobic exercise, the number of subjects who performed these activities decreased significantly after infection. A statistically significant difference was found in the performance of low- and high-intensity physical activities before and after infection.

The duration of low-intensity physical activity decreased sharply, and for high-intensity physical activity, the duration, frequency, and opportunity to engage in it decreased after infection (Tables 2–4). There was also a difference in the duration and opportunity to walk before and after infection, with a decrease in the length of walking and an increase in the number of respondents who reported walking as much as possible. Responses on activities of daily living and leisure showed a statistically significant difference in the performance of these activities before and after infection. The frequency with which daily activities were performed decreased, as did the duration of leisure activities. There was a difference in the frequency with which social and educational activities were performed and in the opportunity to perform them (Table 4). The questions about productive and social activities showed a difference in the duration of these activities, with a significant decrease in the number of respondents who engaged in sports activities for more than one hour. Regarding dietary habits before and after infection in terms of carbohydrates, proteins, vitamins, minerals, and fatty foods, statistical analysis showed that there was no statistically significant difference in the consumption of these nutrients (Figure 1, Table 4).

Regular physical activity is one of the most effective ways to prevent morbidity and early death. The World Health Organization recommends at least 150 min of moderate physical activity per week [24,25]. Individual factors such as gender, age, and health status influence the physical activity that people engage in. During the COVID-19 pandemic, a large proportion of the population remained confined to their homes [24,25]. To prevent physical inactivity, experts recommended getting up, walking around the house, and exercising online. During the pandemic, there were negative effects on physical activity intensity and an increase in the consumption of less healthy foods, as well as an increase in sedentary lifestyle. A decrease in physical activity was also observed in college students, but an increase in anxiety was also observed in individuals aged 18–34 years [26,27].

A study by Bakhsh et al. [24] was conducted with the aim of determining whether the dietary and physical activity patterns of the adult Saudi population changed during the COVID-19 quarantine. The methodology of the study was based on an electronic questionnaire that assessed changes in body weight, eating habits, and physical activity among the adult population of Saudi Arabia (n = 2255) during the COVID-19 quarantine and was disseminated through social networks during the period between June and July 2020. The results of this study showed that over 45% of participants reported consuming larger amounts of food and snacks, which led to weight gain in approximately 28% of subjects. Feeling bored and empty, as well as the availability of time to prepare meals, were the main reasons for changing eating habits. Honey and vitamin C were the most commonly consumed foods to boost immunity. COVID-19 negatively affected physical activity in 52% of respondents, which was associated with a significant increase in body weight ($p < 0.001$) [21]. The aforementioned study examined the changes in dietary habits of the adult population of Saudi Arabia from the aspect of respondents' weight gain, whereas our study examined the difference in micro- and macronutrient intake before and after Corona virus infection. However, our results did not show that there was a statistically significant difference in the intake of macro- and micronutrients analyzed in our questionnaire.

A study by the author Ferreira Rodrigues et al. [25] was conducted with the aim of showing changes in food consumption and food product choices during the pandemic COVID-19 in the Brazilian population. Consumer perceptions of food safety and marketing issues were also studied. An online survey was conducted, and the data were analyzed using descriptive analysis. The results of the study show that the COVID-19 pandemic has affected the consumption and purchase of food. Respondents reported eating and buying larger quantities of food, indicating an increased tendency to eat less healthy food, especially among women. On the other hand, homemade preparations and fresh foods were preferred [25].

Theis et al.'s [26] cross-sectional study was conducted to examine the impact of COVD-19 pandemic-related limitations on physical activity and mental health in children and adolescents. The electronic survey was conducted from June to July 2020. Respondents reported negative effects of isolation, with 61% reporting a decline in physical activity levels and over 90% reporting a negative impact on mental health, including poorer behavior, mood, fitness, and regression in social activities and learning [26].

Since most studies on COVID-19 virus infection have focused on transmission, morbidity, and mortality, a study by Poudel was conducted with the aim of assessing the impact of the virus on health-related quality of life (HRQoL) [27]. The results of this study suggest that a greater impact on HRQoL was achieved in acute infections, women, elderly patients, patients with more severe disease, and patients from low-income countries [27].

COVID-19 can lead to many permanent symptoms such as fatigue, shortness of breath, and decreased ability to perform activities of daily living [28,29]. Clearly, recovery or rehabilitation is necessary to return to a normal state after infection. Pulmonary rehabilitation is an evidence-based intervention that addresses many of the symptoms experienced by long-term infected individuals of COVID-19 (defined as symptoms that persist ≥ 3 months after infection), such as shortness of breath, low energy, impaired ability to perform daily tasks, sleep disturbances, and lower self-confidence. At the molecular level, fatigue and fatigue after COVID-19 could be related to persistent inflammation [28–31]. Pandemic lockdowns have been thought to lead to inactivity and an increase in sedentary behavior, and all necessary measures should be taken to prevent these effects. During isolation, people change their lifestyle habits, increasing the time spent sitting and decreasing the time spent exercising [29–33].

In a study conducted in Spain [34] related to students, it was confirmed that the time spent sitting increased, but surprisingly, the time spent in physical activity also increased, as well as the number of days participants were active. It was found that students who ate a Mediterranean diet exercised more, whereas there was little change in their physical activity behavior. This only goes to show that those who lead a healthy lifestyle also pay attention to their diet and exercise and maintain their habits regardless of the environment. Although the results are positive in terms of physical activity, it should be noted that this population could experience health problems in the future due to the increase in sitting. The most likely reason for the increase in physical activity among young people is that they have realized that their time spent sitting has increased (not going to school, shopping, etc.) and have compensated for this by exercising [34,35]. Another reason could be that students are primarily studying in the health sciences, so they were more inclined to exercise during the pandemic than students in other majors, such as engineering [35].

The limitation of this study is the lack of objective methods of measurement, such as laboratory tests before and after COVID-19, but because infection as well as prolongation of symptoms could not be predicted, this limitation must be justified. Further, the measurement of the costs in case of work loss of these individuals affected by the COVID syndrome could be of importance and interesting to evaluate.

5. Conclusions

The presence of the disease of COVID-19 in the previous 6 months in working-age participants significantly affected the duration of aerobic, anaerobic, and high-intensity physical activities, but also the ability to perform certain activities such as walking, which is a basic aerobic activity and a measure of overall health in middle-aged participants. In the majority of cases (78%), participants reported a decrease in educational and productive activities after COVID-19 compared with the period before COVID-19. Statistical analysis of dietary habits, such as consumption of carbohydrates, proteins, vitamins, minerals, and fatty foods, showed that there was no statistically significant difference in the consumption of these nutrients before and after infection. Health policies should be further guided by these findings.

Author Contributions: Conceptualization, methodology, software, validation: T.N.T. and V.J.; formal analysis, investigation, resources, and data curation: M.S., I.V. and B.J.; writing—original draft preparation, writing—review and editing, visualization, supervision, project administration, funding acquisition: M.M., N.E. and V.R. All authors have read and agreed to the published version of the manuscript.

Funding: This research received no external funding.

Institutional Review Board Statement: Not applicable.

Informed Consent Statement: Informed consent was obtained from all subjects involved in the study.

Data Availability Statement: All data are available on request.

Conflicts of Interest: The authors declare no conflict of interest.

References

1. Khan, M.; Adil, S.F.; Alkhathlan, H.Z.; Tahir, M.N.; Saif, S.; Khan, M.; Khan, S.T. COVID-19: A Global Challenge with Old History, Epidemiology and Progress So Far. *Molecules* **2020**, *26*, 39. [CrossRef]
2. Gavriatopoulou, M.; Ntanasis-Stathopoulos, I.; Korompoki, E.; Fotiou, D.; Migkou, M.; Tzanninis, I.G.; Psaltopoulou, T.; Kastritis, E.; Terpos, E.; Dimopoulos, M.A. Emerging treatment strategies for COVID-19 infection. *Clin. Exp. Med.* **2021**, *21*, 167–179. [CrossRef]
3. Castañeda-Babarro, A.; Arbillaga-Etxarri, A.; Gutiérrez-Santamaría, B.; Coca, A. Physical Activity Change during COVID-19 Confinement. *Int. J. Environ. Res. Public Health* **2020**, *17*, 6878. [CrossRef]
4. Umakanthan, S.; Sahu, P.; Ranade, A.V.; Bukelo, M.M.; Rao, J.S.; Abrahao-Machado, L.F.; Dahal, S.; Kumar, H.; Dhananjaya, K.V. Origin, transmission, diagnosis and management of coronavirus disease 2019 (COVID-19). *Postgrad. Med. J.* **2020**, *96*, 753–758.
5. Chen, P.; Mao, L.; Nassis, G.P.; Harmer, P.; Ainsworth, B.E.; Li, F. Coronavirus disease (COVID-19): The need to maintain regular physical activity while taking precautions. *J. Sport Health Sci.* **2020**, *9*, 103–104. [CrossRef]
6. Jimeno-Almazán, A.; Pallarés, J.G.; Buendía-Romero, Á.; Martínez-Cava, A.; Franco-López, F.; Sánchez-Alcaraz Martínez, B.J.; Bernal-Morel, E.; Courel-Ibáñez, J. Post-COVID-19 Syndrome and the Potential Benefits of Exercise. *Int. J. Environ. Res. Public Health* **2021**, *18*, 5329. [CrossRef]
7. Lechner-Scott, J.; Levy, M.; Hawkes, C.; Yeh, A.; Giovannoni, G. Long COVID or post COVID-19 syndrome. *Mult. Scler. Relat. Disord.* **2021**, *55*, 103268. [CrossRef]
8. Anaya, J.M.; Rojas, M.; Salinas, M.L.; Rodríguez, Y.; Roa, G.; Lozano, M.; Rodríguez-Jiménez, M.; Montoya, N.; Zapata, E.; Monsalve, D.M.; et al. Post-COVID syndrome. A case series and comprehensive review. *Autoimmun. Rev.* **2021**, *20*, 102947. [CrossRef]
9. Yong, S.J. Long COVID or post-COVID-19 syndrome: Putative pathophysiology, risk factors, and treatments. *Infect. Dis.* **2021**, *53*, 737–754. [CrossRef]
10. Pavli, A.; Theodoridou, M.; Maltezou, H.C. Post-COVID Syndrome: Incidence, Clinical Spectrum, and Challenges for Primary Healthcare Professionals. *Arch. Med. Res.* **2021**, *52*, 575–581. [CrossRef]

11. Garrigues, E.; Janvier, P.; Kherabi, Y.; Le Bot, A.; Hamon, A.; Gouze, H.; Doucet, L.; Berkani, S.; Oliosi, E.; Mallart, E.; et al. Post-discharge persistent symptoms and health-related quality of life after hospitalization for COVID-19. *J. Infect.* **2020**, *81*, e4–e6. [CrossRef]
12. Carfi, A.; Bernabei, R.; Landi, F. Gemelli Against COVID-19 Post-Acute Care Study Group. Persistent Symptoms in Patients After Acute COVID-19. *JAMA* **2020**, *324*, 603–605. [CrossRef]
13. Hoyois, A.; Ballarin, A.; Thomas, J.; Lheureux, O.; Preiser, J.C.; Coppens, E.; Perez-Bogerd, S.; Taton, O.; Farine, S.; Van Ouytsel, P.; et al. Nutrition evaluation and management of critically ill patients with COVID-19 during post-intensive care rehabilitation. *J. Parenter. Enteral Nutr.* **2021**, *45*, 1153–1163. [CrossRef]
14. Naureen, Z.; Dautaj, A.; Nodari, S.; Fioretti, F.; Dhuli, K.; Anpilogov, K.; Lorusso, L.; Paolacci, S.; Michelini, S.; Guda, T.; et al. Proposal of a food supplement for the management of post-COVID syndrome. *Eur. Rev. Med. Pharmacol. Sci.* **2021**, *25* (Suppl. 1), 67–73. [CrossRef]
15. Muscogiuri, G.; Barrea, L.; Savastano, S.; Colao, A. Nutritional recommendations for COVID-19 quarantine. *Eur. J. Clin. Nutr.* **2020**, *74*, 850–851. [CrossRef]
16. Park, K.H.; Hong, I.; Park, J.H. Development and Validation of the Yonsei Lifestyle Profile-Satisfaction (YLP-S) Using the Rasch Measurement Model. *Inquiry* **2021**, *58*, 1–8. [CrossRef]
17. Group WHOQOL. Development of the World Health Organization WHOQOL-BREF quality of life assessment. *Psychol. Med.* **1998**, *28*, 551–558. [CrossRef]
18. Skevington, S.M.; Lotfy, M.; O'Connell, K.A. The World Health Organization's WHOQOL-BREF quality of life assessment: Psychometric properties and results of the international field trial. A report from the WHOQOL group. *Qual. Life Res.* **2004**, *13*, 299–310. [CrossRef]
19. Kang, E.; Lee, H.; Sohn, J.H.; Yun, J.; Lee, J.Y.; Hong, Y.C. Impact of the COVID-19 Pandemic on the Health Status and Behaviors of Adults in Korea: National Cross-sectional Web-Based Self-report Survey. *JMIR Public Health Surveill.* **2021**, *7*, e31635. [CrossRef]
20. Suka, M.; Yamauchi, T.; Yanagisawa, H. Changes in health status, workload, and lifestyle after starting the COVID-19 pandemic: A web-based survey of Japanese men and women. *Environ. Health Prev. Med.* **2021**, *26*, 37. [CrossRef]
21. Klok, F.A.; Boon, G.J.A.M.; Barco, S. The post-COVID-19 functional status scale: A tool to measure functional status over time after COVID-19. *Eur. Respir. J.* **2020**, *56*, 2001494. [CrossRef]
22. Lemhöfer, C.; Gutenbrunner, C.; Schiller, J.; Loudovici-Krug, D.; Best, N.; Bökel, A.; Sturm, C. Assessment of rehabilitation needs in patients after COVID-19: Development of the COVID-19-rehabilitation needs survey. *J. Rehabil. Med.* **2021**, *53*, jrm00183. [CrossRef]
23. Poudel, A.N.; Zhu, S.; Cooper, N.; Roderick, P.; Alwan, N.; Tarrant, C.; Ziauddeen, N.; Yao, G.L. Impact of COVID-19 on health-related quality of life of patients: A structured review. *PLoS ONE* **2021**, *16*, e0259164. [CrossRef]
24. Bakhsh, M.A.; Khawandanah, J.; Naaman, R.K.; Alashmali, S. The impact of COVID-19 quarantine on dietary habits and physical activity in Saudi Arabia: A cross-sectional study. *BMC Public Health* **2021**, *21*, 1487. [CrossRef]
25. Rodrigues, J.F.; dos Santos Filho, M.T.C.; de Oliveira, L.E.A.; Siman, I.B.; de Fátima Barcelos, A.; Ramos, G.L.D.P.A.; Esmerino, E.A.; da Cruz, A.G.; Arriel, R.A. Effect of the COVID-19 pandemic on food habits and perceptions: A study with Brazilians. *Trends Food Sci. Technol.* **2021**, *116*, 992–1001. [CrossRef]
26. Theis, N.; Campbell, N.; De Leeuw, J.; Owen, M.; Schenke, K.C. The effects of COVID-19 restrictions on physical activity and mental health of children and young adults with physical and/or intellectual disabilities. *Disabil. Health J.* **2021**, *14*, 101064. [CrossRef]
27. Daynes, E.; Gerlis, C.; Chaplin, E.; Gardiner, N.; Singh, S.J. Early experiences of rehabilitation for individuals post-COVID to improve fatigue, breathlessness exercise capacity and cognition—A cohort study. *Chron. Respir. Dis.* **2021**, *18*, 14799731211015691. [CrossRef]
28. Romero-Blanco, C.; Rodríguez-Almagro, J.; Onieva-Zafra, M.D.; Parra-Fernández, M.L.; Prado-Laguna, M.D.C.; Hernández-Martínez, A. Physical Activity and Sedentary Lifestyle in University Students: Changes during Confinement Due to the COVID-19 Pandemic. *Int. J. Environ. Res. Public Health* **2020**, *17*, 6567. [CrossRef]
29. Mahmud, R.; Rahman, M.M.; Rassel, M.A.; Monayem, F.B.; Sayeed, S.K.J.B.; Islam, M.S.; Islam, M.M. Post-COVID-19 syndrome among symptomatic COVID-19 patients: A prospective cohort study in a tertiary care center of Bangladesh. *PLoS ONE* **2021**, *16*, e0249644. [CrossRef]
30. Munblit, D.; Bobkova, P.; Spiridonova, E.; Shikhaleva, A.; Gamirova, A.; Blyuss, O.; Nekliudov, N.; Bugaeva, P.; Andreeva, M.; DunnGalvin, A.; et al. Incidence and risk factors for persistent symptoms in adults previously hospitalized for COVID-19. *Clin. Exp. Allergy* **2021**, *51*, 1107–1120. [CrossRef]
31. LaVergne, S.M.; Stromberg, S.; Baxter, B.A.; Webb, T.L.; Dutt, T.S.; Berry, K.; Tipton, M.; Haberman, J.; Massey, B.R.; McFann, K.; et al. A longitudinal SARS-CoV-2 biorepository for COVID-19 survivors with and without post-acute sequelae. *BMC Infect. Dis.* **2021**, *21*, 677. [CrossRef]
32. McFann, K.; Baxter, B.A.; LaVergne, S.M.; Stromberg, S.; Berry, K.; Tipton, M.; Haberman, J.; Ladd, J.; Webb, T.L.; Dunn, J.A.; et al. Quality of Life (QoL) Is Reduced in Those with Severe COVID-19 Disease, Post-Acute Sequelae of COVID-19, and Hospitalization in United States Adults from Northern Colorado. *Int. J. Environ. Res. Public Health* **2021**, *18*, 11048. [CrossRef]

33. Sneller, M.C.; Liang, C.J.; Marques, A.R.; Chung, J.Y.; Shanbhag, S.M.; Fontana, J.R.; Raza, H.; Okeke, O.; Dewar, R.L.; Higgins, B.P.; et al. A Longitudinal Study of COVID-19 Sequelae and Immunity: Baseline Findings. *Ann. Intern. Med.* **2022**, *175*, 969–979. [CrossRef]
34. Groff, D.; Sun, A.; Ssentongo, A.E.; Ba, D.M.; Parsons, N.; Poudel, G.R.; Lekoubou, A.; Oh, J.S.; Ericson, J.E.; Ssentongo, P.; et al. Short-term and Long-term Rates of Postacute Sequelae of SARS-CoV-2 Infection: A Systematic Review. *JAMA Netw. Open* **2021**, *4*, e2128568. [CrossRef]
35. Giszas, B.; Trommer, S.; Schüßler, N.; Rodewald, A.; Besteher, B.; Bleidorn, J.; Dickmann, P.; Finke, K.; Katzer, K.; Lehmann-Pohl, K.; et al. Post-COVID-19 condition is not only a question of persistent symptoms: Structured screening including health-related quality of life reveals two separate clusters of post-COVID. *Infection* **2022**, 1–13. [CrossRef]

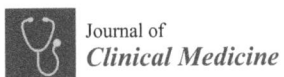

Article

Quality of Life in COVID-19 Outpatients: A Long-Term Follow-Up Study

Vincent Tarazona [1], David Kirouchena [1,*], Pascal Clerc [1,2], Florence Pinsard-Laventure [1] and Bastien Bourrion [1,3]

1. Department of Family Medicine, Faculty of Health Sciences Simone Veil, University Versailles-Saint-Quentin-en-Yvelines (UVSQ), 78180 Montigny le Bretonneux, France
2. Clinical Epidemiology and Ageing Unit, University Paris-Est Creteil (UPEC), 94000 Créteil, France
3. Center for Research in Epidemiology and Population Health, French National Institute of Health and Medical Research (INSERM), University Paris-Saclay, UVSQ, Paul-Brousse Hospital, 94800 Villejuif, France
* Correspondence: kirouchena@protonmail.com

Abstract: Background: The long-term issues faced by COVID-19 survivors remain unclear. Symptoms may persist for several months, even in non-hospitalized patients, probably impacting the quality of life. Objective: To assess the health-related quality of life of outpatients one year after SARS-CoV-2 infection. Design, Settings, and Participants: This prospective multicentre study, conducted in France from February 2020 to February 2022, compared 150 COVID-19 cases (PCR+ and/or CT scan+) and 260 controls (PCR-) selected from a database of four COVID centres. Main outcomes: Health-related quality of life assessed using the EQ-5D-5L scale. Results: COVID-19 outpatients (n = 96) had significantly lower health-related quality of life than controls (n = 81) one year after SARS-CoV-2 infection: the EQ-5D-5L index averaged 0.87 in cases and 0.95 in controls ($p = 0.002$); the EQ-VAS averaged 78 in cases and 86.7 in controls ($p < 0.001$). This alteration in quality of life was more intense in the areas of pain or discomfort and daily activities. Conclusions: This study is the first to show an alteration in the quality of life of COVID-19 outpatients after one year. Appropriate guidance and community rehabilitation programs are required for outpatients with persistent symptoms of COVID-19. Research must continue to confirm these results in larger cohorts.

Keywords: COVID-19; long COVID outpatients; quality of life

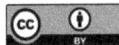

1. Introduction

The coronavirus disease (COVID-19) pandemic has changed humanity's way of life. Since the spring of 2020, there have been more than 30 million confirmed cases in France, causing more than 150,000 deaths [1]. However, death is not the only outcome to measure. Many patients had a slow and painful return to their former state of health [2]. Of specific concern, this finding was not limited to patients recovering from severe COVID-19 (requiring admittance to intensive care unit [ICU]), but also to patients with mild or moderate COVID-19. The sharing of personal experiences of patients and medical professionals [3–5] led to the emergence of the term "long COVID", used to describe the disease in people who report lasting effects of the infection [6].

The persistence of symptoms has been reported in survivors of SARS-CoV-1, with a deficiency in the pulmonary diffusion capacity of carbon monoxide (DLCO) accompanied by significantly lower quality of life and exercise capacities [7]. Recent publications tend to confirm the persistence of symptoms several months after the end of the acute phase of the infection in a considerable number of patients [8,9], and non-hospitalised patients in particular [10]. These patients' feelings of hopelessness are compounded by uncertainty expressed by medical professionals [11]. They feel ignored [12], suggesting that the opinion of the public, the media, and health professionals on COVID is focused only on one of two extremes: mild or severe. These individuals ask their general practionner to validate their symptoms and show empathy [13]. Patients often attempted to "manage" their symptoms independently, without seeking medical advice.

A few studies focusing on hospitalised patients have shown a significant impairment in the quality of life assessed by the EQ-5D-5L scale, up to approximately three months of follow-up [14,15]. However, the impact of persistent COVID-19 symptoms on quality of life in non-hospitalised patients may be underestimated: the consequences of viral infections remain poorly understood. This assessment also helps healthcare professionals to identify risk factors and recognise areas that can be improved to relieve patient symptoms [16].

This study aimed to assess the health-related quality of life of outpatients one year after SARS-CoV-2 infection.

2. Methods

2.1. Design, Settings, and Population

This prospective, multicentre, community-based study, conducted in France from February 2020 to February 2022, used a database created by the Department of General Medicine of Simone Veil University. This database combines the demographic and clinical data of patients who consulted one of the four main COVID outpatient centres in the territory of the Yvelines (78) during the first wave of the epidemic: Les Mureaux, Mantes-La-Jolie, Trappes, and Triel-sur-Seine.

This database included 522 patients who underwent polymerase chain reaction test (PCR), of whom approximately 30% were positive. In addition, out of 116 chest computed tomography (CT) scans performed, approximately 75% were positive for COVID-19.

The inclusion criteria included all the adult patients who consulted in one of these four centres between February and September 2020. COVID patients were included based on positive PCR and/or positive CT scan results. Controls were included based on negative PCR results and without positive CT scan results. All the patients hospitalised during the initial phase were excluded from the outpatient population analysis. Thus, we started this study with 410 outpatients (150 cases and 260 controls).

The patients were contacted by phone after November 2021: the time range between the infection and the follow-up was 14 to 20 months. Initial questions were established on the symptoms presented on the day of call and vaccination status. Quality of life was assessed using the EQ-5D-5L scale with a telephone version validated by the EuroQol group [17]. Data collection by phone was more relevant for this multicentre research during the COVID time because of several lockdowns and travel restrictions.

Secondary exclusion criteria were unreachable patients and those with communication problems. Among the control population, we also asked and excluded patients who presented a positive test for COVID-19 (PCR, antigen, and/or serology) between the initial consultation and telephone call.

2.2. Main Outcomes

We considered the health-related quality of life assessed using the EQ-5D-5L scale as the main outcome. The EQ-5D-5L is a generic questionnaire that is not specific to a particular pathology. This scale is simple and quick to administer and includes five dimensions: mobility, autonomy, daily activities, pain or discomfort, and anxiety or depression. Each dimension was evaluated on a scale of 1 to 5 (1: no problems, 2: slight problems, 3: moderate problems, 4: severe problems, and 5: extreme problems/unable to). This scale is supplemented by a subjective quality of life score (EQ-EVA) from 0 ("the worst possible health") to 100 ("the best possible health").

The EQ-5D-5L is one of the most commonly used instruments for measuring the health-related quality of life in clinical research. This instrument was translated into French and confirmed by the EuroQol group [17].

2.3. Statistical Analysis

Using the EQ-5D-5L scale, we evaluated the health status of the patients from 1 to 5 in five domains and from 0 to 100 with the EQ-EVA. This health state classifier can describe health states that are often reported as vectors ranging from 11111 (full health) to 55555 (worst health). Numerous societal value sets have been derived from population-based valuation studies of a country, when applied to the health state vector, result in a preference-based score that typically ranges from states worse than dead (<0) to 1 (full health), anchoring dead at 0. For example, "11112" meaning slight problems in the anxiety or depression dimension and no problems in any of the other dimensions, is associated with a EQ-5D-5L score of 0.929 in France.

The number of subjects required was calculated assuming a mean score of 0.86 with a variance of 0.2^2 and tolerance of 0.04 to the mean. It was estimated to be 49 individuals per group, or 98 individuals in total. This hypothesis was based on a French study comparing the post-COVID quality of life in two groups [15].

We estimated the proportion of people lost to follow-up to be between 25% and 55%, according to studies evaluating quality of life by phone call [15,18].

Continuous variables are presented as means and standard deviations, and categorical variables are presented as numbers and proportions.

To compare categorical variables between the two groups, a Chi^2 test was used, or a Fisher's exact test was used when the former was not applicable (theoretical numbers less than five). For continuous variables, we performed Student's t-test in the case of a normal distribution or Wilcoxon rank-sum test.

All statistical tests were two-sided, and statistical significance was set at $p < 0.05$. Data were analysed using Statistical Analysis System.

2.4. Regulatory Procedures

This was a non-interventional study involving a human patient (RIPH). Procedures regulated by the "Jarde law" are required to guarantee the protection of people participating in research. The agreement of the French Data Protection Authority (National Commission on Informatics and Liberty) was obtained for reference methodology MR-003. This methodology governs research including health data with a character of public interest, and patients consented to participation after being informed. This study was approved by the French Institutional Review Board.

3. Results

3.1. Sample Characteristics

The study population included 177 patients (96 cases and 81 controls; Figure 1).

We were able to reach 73% of the patients via phone call and obtained 43% complete responses to the questionnaire. Epidemiological and clinical characteristics of the study population are shown in Table 1.

The two groups were comparable in terms of age and sex (no statistically significant difference, $p > 0.05$). There was no significant difference in COVID vaccination between the two groups. Hwever, there was a significant difference in cardiological history ($p = 0.005$) and obesity ($p = 0.013$).

COVID-19 outpatients had significantly higher fatigue (39.6%), dyspnoea (24%), chest pain (8.3%), and ageusia (5.21%) one year after SARS-CoV-2 infection.

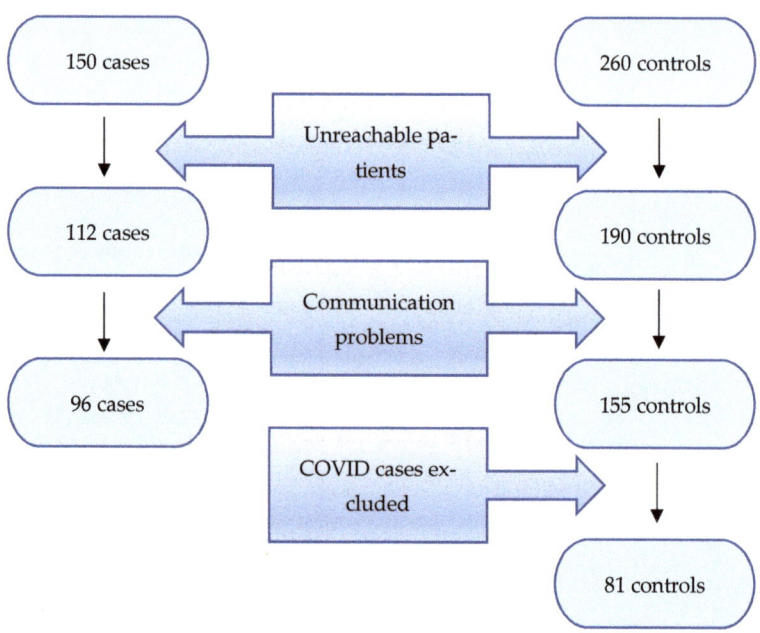

Figure 1. Flowchart.

Table 1. Symptoms and quality of life of 177 patients at 1 year after their visit in a COVID ambulatory center.

	Cases n = 96	Controls n = 81	p Value
Age (years)	45.8 (14.9)	43.2 (14.5)	0.242
Sex (male)	39 (40.6)	30 (37.0)	0.625
Vaccination	87 (90.6)	77 (95.0)	0.260
Comorbidities			
Cardiological	22 (23.1)	5 (6.94)	0.005
Respiratory	9 (9.5)	11 (15.3)	0.253
Diabetes	4 (4.2)	4 (5.6)	0.727
Obesity	11 (11.8)	1 (1.4)	0.013
Tobacco	7 (7.9)	8 (11.2)	0.463
Immune deficiency	8 (8.4)	5 (6.9)	0.724
Symptoms			
Fatigue	38 (39.6)	17 (21)	0.008
Cough	11 (11.5)	8 (9.9)	0.734
Dyspnea	23 (24)	3 (3.7)	<0.001
Chest pain	8 (8.3)	1 (1.2)	0.032
Anosmia	9 (9.4)	2 (2.5)	0.058
Ageusia	5 (5.21)	0 (0)	0.037
Throat sore	4 (4.2)	2 (2.5)	0.534
Headaches	12 (12.5)	4 (4.9)	0.081
Quality of life			
EQ-5D-5L index	0.87 (0.19)	0.95 (0.11)	0.002
EQ-EVA	78 (17.6)	86.7 (9.7)	<0.001

Results are expressed as count (%) for categorical variables and as mean (standard derivation) for continuous variables.

3.2. Quality of Life

Regarding our main outcome, the EQ-5D-5L index mean (SD), which evaluates quality of life in five domains, was at 0.87 (0.19) in cases and 0.95 (0.11) in controls ($p = 0.002$). The

EQ-VAS mean (SD), which subjectively evaluates quality of life, was at 78 (17.6) in cases and 86.7 (9.7) in controls ($p < 0.001$).

Thus, outpatient cases had a significantly lower health-related quality of life than controls one year after SARS-CoV-2 infection.

3.3. The 5 Domains of EQ-5D-5L Score

Of the COVID-19 cases, 47.9% reported problems in at least one of the EQ-5D-5L dimensions compared with 35.8% of the controls, with 6.3% and 2.5% reporting severe or extreme problems, respectively.

The distribution of the EQ-5D-5L scores in the five domains showed a significant difference in pain or discomfort ($p < 0.001$) and daily activities ($p = 0.01$) (Figure 2).

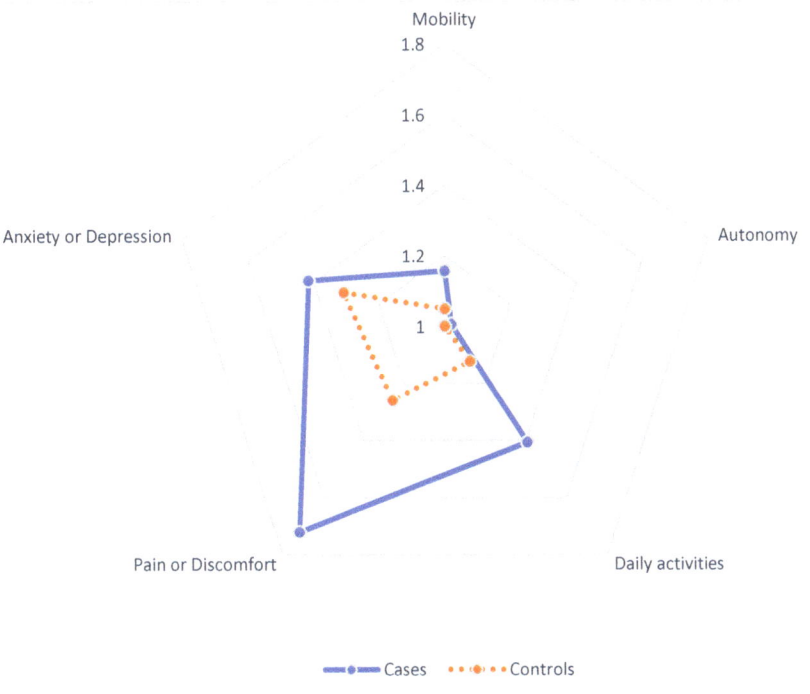

Figure 2. Each domain of EQ-5D-5L score.

Approximately 43% of the cases complained of a problem in the area of pain or discomfort compared to 21% of the controls. Regarding daily activities, approximately 23% of the cases complained of a problem compared to 6% of the controls.

However, there were no significant differences in autonomy, mobility, and anxiety or depression between the two groups. More than 20% of the patients in the two groups were complained of anxiety or depression.

4. Discussion

4.1. Main Outcome

The main objective of this study was to assess the long-term health-related quality of life in outpatients with COVID-19. One year after SARS-CoV-2 infection, outpatients cases had significantly lower health-related quality of life than controls with an EQ-5D-5L index mean of 0.87 and an EQ-EVA mean of 78; alteration was more intense in pain or discomfort and daily activities.

4.2. Comparison with Literature

These COVID-19 ambulatory patients may have an impaired quality of life after SARS-CoV-2 infection compared like initially hospitalised patients. In 2020, in France, the EQ-5D-5L index mean was 0.86, and the EQ-EVA mean was 70.3 among 120 patients more than 100 days after hospitalization [15]. However, this study included a few severe patients because those hospitalised directly in the ICU were excluded. Thus, the alteration in the quality of life post-COVID does not only concern hospitalised patients, but also ambulatory patients who should not be neglected.

Lower values are found in other countries, such as the United Kingdom [19], Norway [20], and Iran [14] with EQ-5D-5L index of 0.72, 0.69, and 0.61, respectively. However, the post-COVID evaluation period was much shorter (between 1 and 3 months), which could have influenced the quality of life. In the United Kingdom and Norway, these lower values can also be explained by the characteristics of patients who initially present with severity criteria (ICU admission). The lower EQ-5D-5L index value in Iran (middle-income country) compared to the UK and Norway (high-income country) may be due to better health services of rich countries rather than patient characteristics, such as age (average 58.4 years in Iran vs. 70.5 years in the UK) or disease severity (18% of patients in Iran vs. 32% in the UK in the ICU).

In ambulatory care, we also found lower values in Belgium [21]: the EQ-5D-5L index mean was 0.63 and the EQ-VAS mean was 51.3 less than 3 months after confirmed SARS-CoV-2 infection. These low values can be explained by the method of selection made from a Facebook group that included 1200 patients with persistent symptoms following an episode of COVID-19, which underestimates the quality of life in an ambulatory population. We also noted that the most affected areas were pain or discomfort, and daily activities, as we found in our study. This is more valuable as this "long COVID" population, which complains of persistent symptoms, is overrepresented here. Management of these patients should focus on the assessment of pain or discomfort, and daily activities.

4.3. Persistent Symptoms

The most frequently reported symptoms were fatigue (39.6%) and dyspnoea (24%), which was also found in other studies [15,19], and the presence of these symptoms one year after SARS-CoV-2 infection in outpatients was notable.

The prevalence of fatigue is consistent with previous outbreaks of SARS, H1N1, and Ebola, in which a large proportion of patients with fatigue were found eligible for a diagnosis of chronic fatigue syndrome/myalgic encephalomyelitis [22]. The prevalence of dyspnoea is comparable to that reported in a meta-analysis, in which 11% to 45% of SARS and MERS survivors suffered from dyspnoea for up to 12 months [23].

Fatigue and dyspnoea are likely to contribute to the reduced ability to perform daily activities observed in this cohort of COVID-19 outpatients.

4.4. Anxiety or Depression

Our results showed that more than one-fifth of the patients complained of anxiety or depression in both cases and controls, with no significant difference. Anxiety or depression probably do not explain the deterioration in quality of life observed in these cases. The presence of this problem in cases and controls can be explained by the impact of the COVID-19 pandemic on the mental health of the general population [24,25].

Therefore, caution is needed before categorising all patient's post-COVID complaints as "functional".

4.5. Determinants

Regarding the characteristics of the two groups, a significant difference was found in the cardiological history and obesity. All others characteristics didn't show a significant difference between the two groups. The statistical comparison with a control group rule out the influence of external factors on quality of life.

Biological tests were not available during the initial phase of the epidemic. According to the recommendations in force, they are mainly used in high-risk cases. This may explain the predominance of certain comorbidities among cases compared to controls.

This factors alone (cardiological history and obesity) probably do not explain the difference of quality of life between the two groups. Indeed, the previous SARS and MERS outbreaks, which used the SF-36 to measure health-related quality of life, showed significantly poor quality of life at 1 year, which is lower than the quality of life of those affected by chronic diseases (using normative data) [26]. The previous publications in 2020 and 2021 also showed a lower post-COVID quality of life in different populations of several countries. Thus, the impaired quality of life observed in outpatient cases likely reflects the impact of COVID-19.

5. Strengths and Limitations

There are many retrospective studies on the consequences of COVID-19, but few prospective cohorts and even fewer comparative prospective cohorts with long-term follow-ups. To our knowledge, this study is the first to show an alteration in the quality of life one year after infection with SARS-CoV-2 in an ambulatory population through a statistical comparison with an uninfected control group. This statistical comparison with a control group is fundamental to rule out the influence of external factors on quality of life, as our way of life has been upset by this pandemic (confinement, wearing a mask, social distancing, etc.).

The strength of our study lies in its multicentre and prospective nature. Cases were selected during the first wave based on a positive COVID test (PCR or CT scan) and not on suspicion of COVID, which limits the risk of selection bias. We used a reliable scale (EQ-5D-5L score) to assess quality of life because it is a commonly used instrument, validated in clinical research, and translated into French with reference values, allowing us to compare our results with other studies. This questionnaire is standardised and administered by a single contact, which limits measurement bias.

Our study had several limitations. We obtained a little less than half (43%) of the answers to the questionnaire, although corresponding to our initial estimate, which represents a high rate of inaccessible patients. Phone calls as a method of contact limited the ability to contact some participants such as people with dementia, speech difficulties, and non-French speakers. Our sample was not representative of the original population. In addition, the case population had more comorbidities (cardiological history and obesity) than the controls because of an initial sorting of the use of a PCR test according to the severity criteria. Thus, our results must be confirmed in larger cohorts to be able to be extrapolated to the general population.

This outpatient study only included patients over 18 years of age, while persistent symptoms were also described in the paediatric population [27].

Patients were infected during the first wave of the epidemic in 2020, but the virus is constantly gaining mutations, which can lead to changes in its internal characteristics, such as virulence or contagiousness [28], as well as in its clinical expression [29]: therefore, we can question the reproducibility of the results with the new variants.

6. Conclusions

This study is the first to show an alteration in the quality of life of COVID-19 outpatients after one year. This study suggests an impact of COVID-19 on the long-term quality of life of outpatients and hope to improve the management of long COVID. Appropriate guidance and community rehabilitation programs are required for outpatients with persistent symptoms of COVID-19. Research must continue to confirm these results in larger cohorts.

Author Contributions: All authors developed the protocol. P.C. and F.P.-L. extracted data. V.T., D.K. and B.B. were involved with synthesising the data, interpreting the findings and writing the first draft of the manuscript. All authors have read and agreed to the published version of the manuscript.

Funding: This research received no external funding.

Institutional Review Board Statement: The study was conducted in accordance with the Declaration of Helsinki, and approved by the French Institutional Review Board (protocol code 21.04172.000078).

Informed Consent Statement: Not applicable.

Data Availability Statement: The data presented in this study are available on reasonable request from the corresponding author.

Acknowledgments: We would like to acknowledge the valuable contributions of our Patients.

Conflicts of Interest: The authors declare no conflict of interest.

References

1. Public Health France. Available online: https://www.santepubliquefrance.fr/dossiers/coronavirus-covid-19/coronavirus-chiffres-cles-et-evolution-de-la-covid-19-en-france-et-dans-le-monde (accessed on 3 March 2021).
2. Yelin, D.; Wirtheim, E.; Vetter, P.; Kalil, A.C.; Bruchfeld, J.; Runold, M.; Guaraldi, G.; Mussini, C.; Gudiol, C.; Pujol, M.; et al. Long-term consequences of COVID-19: Research needs. *Lancet Infect. Dis.* **2020**, *20*, 1115–1117. [CrossRef]
3. Alwan, N.A. What Exactly is Mild COVID-19? Available online: https://blogs.bmj.com/bmj/2020/07/28/nisreen-a-alwan-what-exactly-is-mild-covid-19/ (accessed on 3 March 2021).
4. Paul Garner on Long Haul COVID-19—Don't Try to Dominate This Virus, Accommodate It. Available online: https://blogs.bmj.com/bmj/2020/09/04/paul-garner-on-long-haul-covid-19-dont-try-and-dominate-this-virus-accommodate-it/ (accessed on 3 March 2021).
5. Alwan, N.; Attree, E.; Blair, J.M.; Bogaert, D.; Bowen, M.-A.; Boyle, J.; Bradman, M.; Briggs, T.A.; Burns, S.; Campion, D.; et al. From doctors as patients: A manifesto for tackling persisting symptoms of covid-19. *BMJ* **2020**, *370*. [CrossRef] [PubMed]
6. Mahase, E. Covid-19: What do we know about "long covid"? *BMJ* **2020**, *370*, m2815. [CrossRef] [PubMed]
7. Ngai, J.C.; Ko, F.W.S.; Ng, S.; To, K.-W.; Tong, M.; Hui, D. The long-term impact of severe acute respiratory syndrome on pulmonary function, exercise capacity and health status. *Respirology* **2010**, *15*, 543–550. [CrossRef] [PubMed]
8. Carfi, A.; Bernabei, R.; Landi, F. For the Gemelli Against COVID-19 Post-Acute Care Study Group. Persistent Symptoms in Patients After Acute COVID-19. *JAMA* **2020**, *324*, 603. [CrossRef] [PubMed]
9. Huang, C.; Huang, L.; Wang, Y.; Li, X.; Ren, L.; Gu, X.; Kang, L.; Guo, L.; Liu, M.; Zhou, X.; et al. 6-month consequences of COVID-19 in patients discharged from hospital: A cohort study. *Lancet* **2021**, *397*, 220–232. [CrossRef]
10. Petersen, M.S.; Kristiansen, M.F.; Hanusson, K.D.; Danielsen, M.E.; Steig, B.; Gaini, S.; Strøm, M.; Weihe, P. Long COVID in the Faroe Islands: A Longitudinal Study Among Nonhospitalized Patients. *Clin. Infect. Dis.* **2020**, *73*, e4058–e4063. [CrossRef]
11. Ladds, E.; Rushforth, A.; Wieringa, S.; Taylor, S.; Rayner, C.; Husain, L.; Greenhalgh, T. Persistent symptoms after Covid-19: Qualitative study of 114 "long Covid" patients and draft quality principles for services. *BMC Health Serv. Res.* **2020**, *20*, 1144. [CrossRef]
12. Rubin, R. As Their Numbers Grow, COVID-19 "Long Haulers" Stump Experts. *JAMA* **2020**, *324*, 1381. [CrossRef]
13. Kingstone, T.; Taylor, A.K.; O'Donnell, C.A.; Atherton, H.; Blane, D.N.; Chew-Graham, C.A. Finding the 'right' GP: A qualitative study of the experiences of people with long-COVID. *BJGP Open* **2020**, *4*, 1143. [CrossRef]
14. Arab-Zozani, M.; Hashemi, F.; Safari, H.; Yousefi, M.; Ameri, H. Health-Related Quality of Life and its Associated Factors in COVID-19 Patients. *Osong Public Health Res. Perspect.* **2020**, *11*, 296–302. [CrossRef] [PubMed]
15. Garrigues, E.; Janvier, P.; Kherabi, Y.; Le Bot, A.; Hamon, A.; Gouze, H.; Doucet, L.; Berkani, S.; Oliosi, E.; Mallart, E.; et al. Post-discharge persistent symptoms and health-related quality of life after hospitalization for COVID-19. *J. Infect.* **2020**, *81*, e4–e6. [CrossRef]
16. Testa, M.A.; Simonson, D.C. Assessment of Quality-of-Life Outcomes. *N. Engl. J. Med.* **1996**, *334*, 835–840. [CrossRef]
17. EQ-5D. Available online: https://euroqol.org/ (accessed on 10 April 2021).
18. Logue, J.K.; Franko, N.M.; McCulloch, D.J.; McDonald, D.; Magedson, A.; Wolf, C.R.; Chu, H.Y. Sequelae in Adults at 6 Months After COVID-19 Infection. *JAMA Netw. Open* **2021**, *4*, e210830. [CrossRef] [PubMed]
19. Halpin, S.J.; McIvor, C.; Whyatt, G.; Adams, A.; Harvey, O.; McLean, L.; Walshaw, C.; Kemp, S.; Corrado, J.; Singh, R.; et al. Postdischarge symptoms and rehabilitation needs in survivors of COVID-19 infection: A cross-sectional evaluation. *J. Med. Virol.* **2021**, *93*, 1013–1022. [CrossRef]

20. Lerum, T.V.; Aaløkken, T.M.; Brønstad, E.; Aarli, B.; Ikdahl, E.; Lund, K.M.A.; Durheim, M.T.; Rodriguez, J.R.; Meltzer, C.; Tonby, K.; et al. Dyspnoea, lung function and CT findings 3 months after hospital admission for COVID-19. *Eur. Respir. J.* **2020**, *57*, 2003448. Available online: https://erj.ersjournals.com/content/early/2020/11/26/13993003.03448-2020.short (accessed on 5 April 2021). [CrossRef] [PubMed]
21. Meys, R.; Delbressine, J.M.; Goërtz, Y.M.J.; Vaes, A.W.; Machado, F.V.C.; Van Herck, M.; Burtin, C.; Posthuma, R.; Spaetgens, B.; Franssen, F.M.E.; et al. Generic and Respiratory-Specific Quality of Life in Non-Hospitalized Patients with COVID-19. *J. Clin. Med.* **2020**, *9*, 3993. [CrossRef] [PubMed]
22. Islam, M.F.; Cotler, J.; Jason, L.A. Post-viral fatigue and COVID-19: Lessons from past epidemics. *Fatigue Biomed. Health Behav.* **2020**, *8*, 61–69. [CrossRef]
23. Ahmed, H.; Patel, K.; Greenwood, D.; Halpin, S.; Lewthwaite, P.; Salawu, A.; Eyre, L.; Breen, A.; O'Connor, R.; Jones, A.; et al. Long-term clinical outcomes in survivors of severe acute respiratory syndrome and Middle East respiratory syndrome coronavirus outbreaks after hospitalisation or ICU admission: A systematic review and meta-analysis. *J. Rehabilitation Med.* **2020**, *52*, jrm00063. [CrossRef]
24. Ping, W.; Zheng, J.; Niu, X.; Guo, C.; Zhang, J.; Yang, H.; Shi, Y. Evaluation of health-related quality of life using EQ-5D in China during the COVID-19 pandemic. *PLoS ONE* **2020**, *15*, e0234850. [CrossRef]
25. Hay, J.W.; Gong, C.L.; Jiao, X.; Zawadzki, N.K.; Zawadzki, R.S.; Pickard, A.S.; Xie, F.; Crawford, S.A.; Gu, N.Y. A US Population Health Survey on the Impact of COVID-19 Using the EQ-5D-5L. *J. Gen. Intern. Med.* **2021**, *36*, 1292–1301. [CrossRef] [PubMed]
26. Tansey, C.M.; Louie, M.; Loeb, M.; Gold, W.L.; Muller, M.P.; De Jager, J.; Cameron, J.; Tomlinson, G.; Mazzulli, T.; Walmsley, S.; et al. One-Year Outcomes and Health Care Utilization in Survivors of Severe Acute Respiratory Syndrome. *Arch. Intern. Med.* **2007**, *167*, 1312–1320. [CrossRef] [PubMed]
27. Berg, S.K.; Nielsen, S.D.; Nygaard, U.; Bundgaard, H.; Palm, P.; Rotvig, C.; Christensen, A.V. Long COVID symptoms in SARS-CoV-2-positive adolescents and matched controls (LongCOVIDKidsDK): A national, cross-sectional study. *Lancet Child Adolesc. Health* **2022**, *6*, 240–248. [CrossRef]
28. Zhang, J.; Cai, Y.; Xiao, T.; Lu, J.; Peng, H.; Sterling, S.M.; Walsh, R.M., Jr.; Rits-Volloch, S.; Zhu, H.; Woosley, A.N.; et al. Structural impact on SARS-CoV-2 spike protein by D614G substitution. *Science* **2021**, *372*, 372–530. [CrossRef] [PubMed]
29. Bager, P.; Wohlfahrt, J.; Rasmussen, M.; Albertsen, M.; Krause, T.G. Hospitalisation associated with SARS-CoV-2 delta variant in Denmark. *Lancet Infect. Dis.* **2021**, *21*, 1351. [CrossRef]

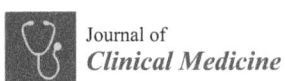

Article

Association of Clinical Features with Spike Glycoprotein Mutations in Iranian COVID-19 Patients

Shahrzad Ahangarzadeh [1], Alireza Yousefi [2], Mohammad Mehdi Ranjbar [2], Arezou Dabiri [3], Atefeh Zarepour [4], Mahmoud Sadeghi [5], Elham Heidari [5], Fariba Mazrui [5], Majid Hosseinzadeh [6], Behrooz Ataei [7], Ali Zarrabi [4], Laleh Shariati [8,9,*] and Shaghayegh Haghjooy Javanmard [3,*]

[1] Infectious Diseases and Tropical Medicine Research Center, Isfahan University of Medical Sciences, Isfahan 81746-73461, Iran
[2] Razi Vaccine and Serum Research Institute, Agricultural Research, Education, and Extension Organization (AREEO), Karaj 31585-854, Iran
[3] Applied Physiology Research Center, Cardiovascular Research Institute, Isfahan University of Medical Sciences, Isfahan 81746-73461, Iran
[4] Department of Biomedical Engineering, Faculty of Engineering and Natural Sciences, Istinye University, Istanbul 34396, Turkey
[5] Health Vice Chancellery of Isfahan Medical University, Isfahan University of Medical Sciences, Isfahan 81656-47194, Iran
[6] Department of Genetics and Molecular Biology, School of Medicine, Isfahan University of Medical Sciences, Isfahan 81746-73461, Iran
[7] Nosocomial Infection Research Center, Isfahan University of Medical Sciences, Isfahan 31379-23929, Iran
[8] Department of Biomaterials, Nanotechnology and Tissue Engineering, School of Advanced Technologies in Medicine, Isfahan University of Medical Sciences, Isfahan 81746-73461, Iran
[9] Biosensor Research Center, School of Advanced Technologies in Medicine, Isfahan University of Medical Sciences, Isfahan 81746-73461, Iran
* Correspondence: shariati_l59@yahoo.com (L.S.); shaghayegh.haghjoo@gmail.com (S.H.J.)

Abstract: Background: Mutations in spike glycoprotein, a critical protein of SARS-CoV-2, could directly impact pathogenicity and virulence. The D614G mutation, a non-synonymous mutation at position 614 of the spike glycoprotein, is a predominant variant circulating worldwide. This study investigated the occurrence of mutations in the crucial zone of the spike gene and the association of clinical symptoms with spike mutations in isolated viruses from Iranian patients infected with SARS-CoV-2 during the second and third waves of the COVID-19 epidemic in Isfahan, the third-largest city in Iran. Methods: The extracted RNA from 60 nasopharyngeal samples of COVID-19 patients were subjected to cDNA synthesis and RT-PCR (in three overlapping fragments). Each patient's reverse transcriptase polymerase chain reaction (RT-PCR) products were assembled and sequenced. Information and clinical features of all sixty patients were collected, summarized, and analyzed using the GENMOD procedure of SAS 9.4. Results: Analysis of 60 assembled sequences identified nine nonsynonymous mutations. The D614G mutation has the highest frequency among the amino acid changes. In our study, in 31 patients (51.66%), D614G mutation was determined. For all the studied symptoms, no significant relationship was observed with the incidence of D614G mutation. Conclusions: D614G, a common mutation among several of the variants of SARS-CoV-2, had the highest frequency among the studied sequences and its frequency increased significantly in the samples of the third wave compared to the samples of the second wave of the disease.

Keywords: COVID-19; clinical symptoms; spike glycoprotein; mutation; D614G

1. Introduction

A novel strain of coronavirus, SARS-CoV-2, suddenly appeared in Wuhan (China) in December 2019 and has outspread swiftly to the world. On 11 March 2020, WHO announced the rapidly spreading coronavirus disease as COVID-19, the fifth pandemic since the 1918 flu pandemic [1]. SARS-CoV-2 belongs to the betacoronavirus, and its genome encodes four structural proteins by four structural genes, spike (S), envelope (E), membrane (M), and nucleocapsid (N) genes [2]. The host range is controlled by multiple molecular interactions, including receptor interaction. Despite amino acid mutation in some key regions, the structure of the envelope spike (S) protein receptor-binding domain of SARS-CoV-2 is similar to that of SARS-CoV [3]. Immense structural investigations powerfully demonstrate that SARS-CoV-2 may use host receptor angiotensin-converting enzyme 2 (ACE2) to enter the cells [4], the same receptor that helps SARS-CoV to infect the airway epithelium and alveolar type 2 (AT2) pneumocytes, which are pulmonary cells that synthesize pulmonary surfactant [5]. In general, coronavirus's spike protein comprises two subunits: S1 and S2. The S1 subunit contains the N-terminal domain (NTD), receptor-binding domain (RBD), and subdomain 1 and 2 (SD1/2), which is responsible for binding to ACE2 receptor in target cells, and the S2 domain is responsible for cell membrane fusion during viral infection [6]. Consequently, this protein has an indispensable role in antigen-inducing potent immune response and is the main target for designing and developing vaccines and therapeutics [7]. Moreover, information on SARS-CoV-2 mutations, particularly mutations in surface proteins, such as spike proteins, is essential for estimating virus behavior in drug resistance, immune escape, and pathogenesis [8,9]. The D614G mutation, a non-synonymous mutation at position 614 of Spike glycoprotein, is a predominant variant circulating worldwide [10,11]. Many studies showed that this mutation is associated with higher infectivity [12], higher level of viral load in the upper respiratory tract [13], and higher fatality [14].

Clinical manifestations of 2019-nCoV infection are similar to SARS-CoV. At the onset of the disease, the most prevalent symptoms include fever, dry cough, dyspnea, chest pain, fatigue, and myalgia. Uncommon symptoms include headache, nasal congestion, dizziness, abdominal pain, diarrhea, nausea, and vomiting [15,16]. As the number of patients rises, there are concerns about accumulation of more severe and toxic viral variants. Drug and vaccine therapies can also cause specific and new mutations; therefore, tracing the characteristics of these variants, phylogeny, and at the same time, the demographic characteristics of the disease in different waves of COVID-19, are critical. This study investigated the occurrence and prevalence of mutation models in the crucial zone of the spike gene and the association of clinical symptoms with spike glycoprotein mutations in isolated viruses from Iranian patients infected with SARS-CoV-2 during the second and third waves of the COVID-19 epidemic in Isfahan, the third-largest city in Iran and the eighteenth most populous metropolis in the Middle East.

2. Material and Methods

2.1. Study Design and Participants

A total of 60 COVID-19 patients (30 samples belonged to the second wave and 30 to the third wave of the COVID-19 pandemic in the specialized clinics in Isfahan (Iran)) were considered to participate in this monocentric study from August to November 2020 in a prospective study. We chose RNA samples based on previous information of laboratory criteria (real-time PCR). SARS-CoV-2 infection was confirmed by reverse transcriptase real-time PCR. Then we contacted the patient and asked questions according to the questionnaire prepared for the symptoms of the disease. Clinical manifestations such as the presence or absence of fever or chills, shortness of breath, cough and sneezing, sore throat, runny nose, and nausea and vomiting are considered. Figure 1 presents the demographic and clinical characteristics of all study subjects. Also, to evaluate the relationship between the patient's sex with COVID-19 symptoms, patients were divided in two group: men and women. To investigate the relationship between age and COVID-19 symptoms, patients were divided into two groups according to age: $\leq$40 years and >40 years.

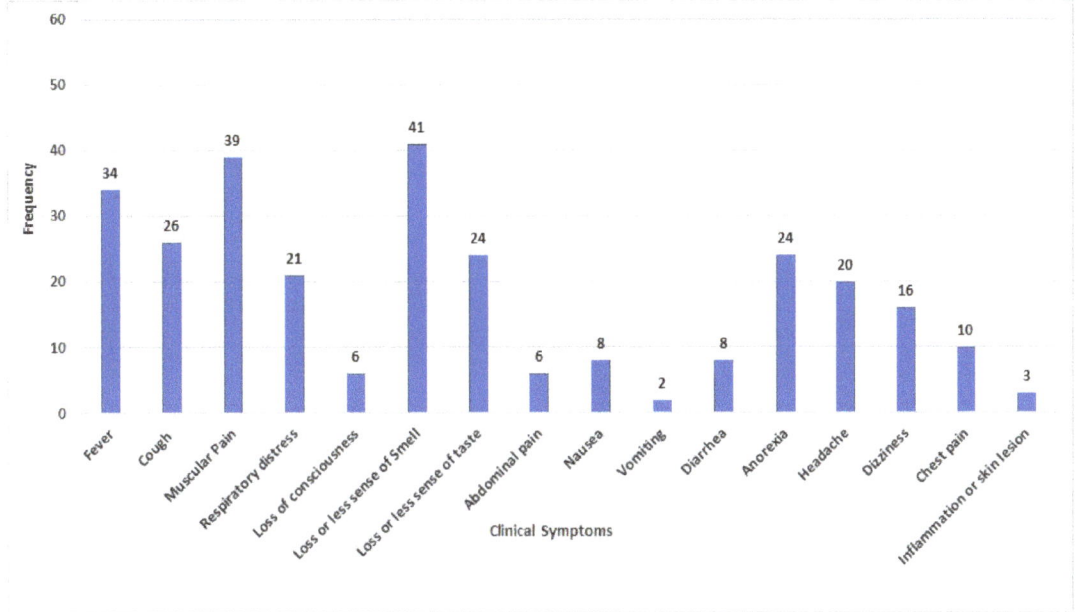

Figure 1. Frequency of clinical symptoms among 60 studied patients.

2.2. Reverse Transcription and RT-PCR

Five ng of each RNA sample, confirmed by a real-time PCR test, was used to synthesize the complementary DNA (with random hexamer primer) using the RevertAid First Strand cDNA Synthesis Kit (Biotechrabbit, Hennigsdorf, Germany), according to the manufacturer's protocol. Three pairs of primers were used to amplify three consecutive fragments of the spike gene sequence. The first fragment was amplified with F1 (TATCTTGGCAAACCACGCGA) and R1 (ACCAGCTGTCCAACCTGAAG) primers; the second fragment was amplified with F2 (CCCTCAGGGTTTTTCGGCTT), and R2 (CTGTGGATCACGGACAGCAT) primers, and the last fragment was amplified with F3 (CCAGCAACTGTTTGTGGACC) and R3 (GTGGCAAAACAGTAAGGCCG) primers. PCR reaction was performed in an Applied Biosystems ® GeneAmp ® PCR System according to the cycling program: 94 °C for 3.5 min, 94 °C for 40 s, 58/59/59.5 °C, respectively, for each fragment's primer for 45 s, and 72 °C for 2 min, 39 cycles, and a final extension step of 72 °C for 10 min.

2.3. Sequencing and Analysis

The final amplified fragments were prepared for sequencing using standard Sanger sequencing technology (GenFanavan Co., Tehran, Iran). To demonstrate and check the sequencing quality, we took advantage of Finch TV and Bioedit software (Geospiza Inc., Seattle, WA, USA). Final sequences were assembled from three overlapping sequence reads of each sample, and the authors submitted 100 assembled sequences (partial S gene sequences) to NCBI GenBank (Supplementary Table S1).

2.4. Mutation Detection

A multiple sequence alignment of all 100 sequences was performed to define the single nucleotide polymorphism (SNP) using CLUSTALW and the reference S gene sequence. Mutation at nucleotide and amino acid levels was analyzed using MEGA (Molecular

Evolutionary Genetics Analysis Platform) version X software [17]. Finally, the statistical analysis determined the relationship between clinical findings and genetic mutations.

2.5. Statistical Analysis

For statistical analysis, each patient's information was entered into SAS 9.4 (SAS Institute Inc., Cary, NC, USA) and analyzed using the GENMOD procedure. The data were analyzed using descriptive statistics, chi-square tests, independent *t*-tests, and one-way analysis of variance. A *p*-value < 0.05 was accepted as significant.

3. Results

3.1. Clinical Symptoms

The frequency of clinical features among all sixty patients was summarized. All patients participating in this study exhibited moderate to mild symptoms. As shown in Figure 1, symptoms such as loss of sense of smell, muscular pain, and fever were the most common among the patients.

3.2. Identified Single Nucleotide Mutations

Our sequencing results identified nine nonsynonymous mutations in at least five patients, resulting in amino acid changes in spike glycoprotein (Supplementary Table S1). Among these amino acid replacements, D111N, Q115H, E224K, and D228N were located in the NTD. Two mutations, D614G and Q675R, were in subdomains 1 and 2, and D820N, V826G, and D830N were on the S2 domain.

The most representative amino acid change was D614G. Its frequency was dramatically increased in patients selected from the third wave of the disease compared to patients chosen from the second wave (Figure 2).

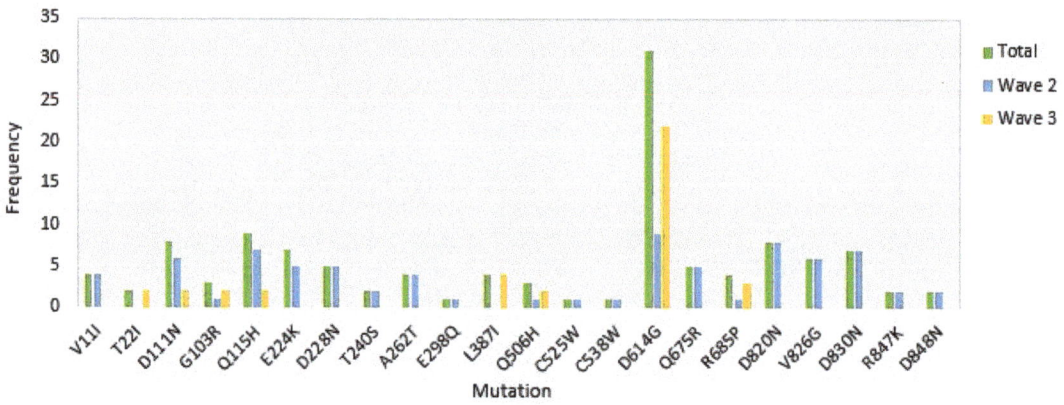

Figure 2. Frequency of amino acid replacements in sequences of spike glycoprotein among 60 sample sequences.

3.3. Statistical Analysis

Among the nine identified nonsynonymous mutations in this study, D614G is a vital mutation that causes structural and functional changes in the SARS-CoV-2 spike protein. First, the relationship between the D614G mutation and the incidence of COVID-19 symptoms in a total population of 60 people was investigated (Table 1). Then, the relationships between sex, age, and underlying disease history with the incidence of COVID-19 clinical symptoms were assessed.

Table 1. Statistical correlation between incidences of the clinical sings of the COVID-19 and mutation in D614G gene and their relevant *p* values.

	Incidence Rate	D614G Mutation	Wild Type	*p* Value
Total Number of Cases	60	51.66% (31/60)	48.33% (29/60)	NS
Fever	56.66% (34/60)	64.51% (20/31)	48.27% (14/29)	NS
Cough	43.33% (26/60)	51.61% (16/31)	34.48% (10/29)	NS
Muscular pain	65% (39/60)	74.19% (23/31)	55.17% (16/29)	NS
Respiratory distress	35% (21/60)	35.48% (11/31)	34.48% (10/29)	NS
Loss of consciousness	10% (6/60)	9.67% (3/31)	10.34% (3/29)	NS
Loss or less sense of smell	41.66% (25/60)	38.7% (12/31)	44.82% (13/29)	NS
Loss or less sense of taste	40% (24/60)	38.7% (12/31)	41.37% (12/29)	NS
Abdominal pain	10% (6/60)	9.67% (3/31)	10.34% (3/29)	NS
Nausea	13.33% (8/60)	19.34% (6/31)	6.89% (2/29)	NS
Vomiting	3.33% (2/60)	6.45% (2/31)	0% (0/29)	NS
Diarrhea	13.33% (8/60)	12.9% (4/31)	13.79% (4/29)	NS
Anorexia	40% (24/60)	45.16% (14/31)	34.48% (10/29)	NS
Headache	33.3% (20/60)	38.7% (12/31)	27.58% (8/29)	NS
Dizziness	26.6% (16/60)	29.03% (9/31)	24.13% (7/29)	NS
Chest pain	16.66% (10/60)	12.9% (4/31)	20.68% (6/29)	NS
Inflammation or skin lesion	5% (3/60)	3.22% (1/31)	6.89% (2/29)	NS

$p < 0.05$ = significant difference; NS = Non-significant ($p > 0.05$); $0.05 > p > 0.10$ = tendency.

Our study revealed D614G mutation in 31 patients (51.66%). The percentage of mutated and non-mutated individuals for each clinical sign was determined and then all data were compared statistically. No significant relationship was observed for all the studied symptoms with the incidence of D614G mutation.

It has been shown that 70% (42/60) of the studied patients were male, and 30% (18/60) were female at the time of sampling. Since, in this study, the collection of samples was random, the results showed that the prevalence of COVID-19 was statistically higher in men than women. There was no significant relationship between patients' sex and the incidence of symptoms in the study population (Supplementary Table S2).

Patients were divided into two groups according to age: ≤40 years and >40 years. After examining the relationship between symptoms and age, we found that in the studied patients, symptoms such as loss of sense of smell, headache, and chest pain were significantly higher in people ≤40 years (Supplementary Table S3).

4. Discussion

With the emergence of new varieties of SARS-CoV-2, controlling and combating this disease has become a global challenge [18]. The importance of the spike protein in the virulence and pathogenesis of the virus has been well identified in various studies [19]. Therefore, identifying and monitoring spike mutations and their effects on the function of the virus is essential for drug and vaccine design. Spike mutation could also directly impact spike interaction with neutralizing antibodies, leading to reinfection and even infection of fully vaccinated people [20,21].

Gender is one of the known factors in the severity of the SARS-CoV-2 disease, and men are more susceptible to the virus [22].

Different independent research has revealed that mutations in spike and other proteins of SARS-CoV-2 can potentially impact the clinical outcomes of affected patients [23–25].

Meta-analyses and observational studies have shown that mutations increase the risk of disease severity and death [24,25].

Therefore, different clinical outcomes may be associated with genetic mutations in SARS-CoV-2 spike glycoprotein. However, it is necessary to adjust for individual risk factors to establish such an association reliably. The most severe outcomes are expected to be associated with pre-existing diseases in affected persons. Age and comorbidities such as hypertension, obesity, cardiovascular disorders, immune suppression, smoking, and diabetes are more important predictors of severity, hospitalization, and mortality than SARS-CoV-2 mutations [26].

Some genome information of SARS-CoV-2 revealed that the mutation rate of SARS-CoV-2 is about 1~2 nucleotides/month [26]. A similar study in Jiangsu Province of China showed that more men were infected with the SARS-CoV-2 compared to women and its tendency was to younger ages. Also, the number of asymptomatic infected patients was more (predominantly in Alpha and Beta variants), but patients infected with Delta (17%) variant presented more severe clinical features. A total of 935 SNPs were detected in 165 SARS-CoV-2 samples, and missense mutation was the dominant mutation. They found that 20% of SNP changes occurred in the spike glycoprotein (S) gene as well as nine SNPs loci in S gene were significantly correlated with the severity of disease in patients [26,27]. It is worth mentioning that amino acid substitution of p.Asp614Gly was significantly positively correlated with the clinical severity of patients. In Jiangsu Province of China, the amino acid substitution of p.Ser316Thr and p.Lu484Lys were significantly negatively correlated with the course of the disease [27].

In Turkey, results clearly showed concordance between the variant distributions, the number of cases, and the timelines of different variant accumulations [28].

D614G is a vital mutation that causes structural changes, increasing the affinity of ACE2 and leading to functional changes in SARS-CoV-2 spike protein [29]. This mutation may affect the binding activity of the S1 domain and change the secondary structure of the protein [21,27]. Zhang and colleagues [12] showed that the D614G mutation can increase the infectivity of the virus by increasing virion spike density. Becerra-Flores et al. have reported that this mutation is associated with a higher fatality rate [14]. Vanderheiden et al. computationally simulated and analyzed the functional effects of mutation D614G and found that the D614 position has a critical role in transitions of spike glycoprotein between an open and closed state [30].

In our study, D614G was the most abundant mutation in Iranian samples (Supplementary Table S1). There was no significant relationship between disease symptoms and D614G mutation in this study. D614G also is common among several of the variants of SARS-CoV-2 and increases transmissibility and viral load [13,31]. Also, in India, the spike D614G mutation has become the most common variant since December 2019. Similarly, detected in Europe and the United States, it has dramatically increased the transmission ability of SARS-CoV-2 [32]. A study has reported that high prevalence of variant D614G in the spike in Costa Rica is similar to the rest of the world. This study also showed an increased detection of a spike T1117I mutation from March to November 2020 [33]. In another study by Molina-Mora in Costa Rica, the analysis of the mutation T1117I in spike showed a polyphyletic pattern along with the emergence of local lineages around the world. This mutation seems to have a significant role in higher affinity to molecules and scarce immunity changes [34].

Our study achieved important molecular epidemiological results on the correlation of clinical features (history) with mutation of SARS-CoV-2 in the center of Iran (Isfahan province). Also, there were limitations to our study. First, this is a monocentric study. Second, some of the samples had some errors and no complete history behind them, so larger numbers of samples are further needed to minimize the errors. Also, we excluded those samples with ambiguous history. Third, the correlation of mutation with the potential biological function of variants and demographic characteristics is required for further investigations.

Supplementary Materials: The following supporting information can be downloaded at: https://www.mdpi.com/article/10.3390/jcm11216315/s1, Table S1. Nonsynonymous mutations identified in the spike protein of SARS-CoV-2 isolated from COVID-19 patients in Isfahan, Iran compared with hCoV-19/Wuhan/WIV04/2019; Table S2. Association between patients' sex and COVID-19 symptoms in patients; Table S3. Association between age and COVID-19 symptoms in patients.

Author Contributions: S.A. and M.M.R. conceived and designed the experiments. L.S., S.H.J. and B.A. helped to design the study. A.Y. performed statistical analysis. M.S., E.H., F.M. and M.H. collected and prepared samples. S.A. and L.S. performed the experiments. L.S., M.M.R., A.Z. (Atefeh Zarepour) and A.D. were involved in the manuscript preparation. M.S., E.H., F.M., A.Z. (Ali Zarrabi) and M.H. were involved in writing—review and editing. All authors reviewed the manuscript. All authors have read and agreed to the published version of the manuscript.

Funding: The project was supported by Isfahan University of Medical Sciences [grant number: 198284].

Institutional Review Board Statement: The research related to human use has complied with all the relevant national regulations and institutional policies, follows the tenets of the Helsinki Declaration, and has been approved by the ethical committee of Isfahan University of Medical Sciences (IR.MUI.MED.REC.1398.734).

Informed Consent Statement: Written informed consent was obtained from patients prior to participation in this study.

Data Availability Statement: The data of this research would be available upon request to corresponding author, subjected to confirmation of Ethical Board Committee.

Acknowledgments: The authors would like to thank Isfahan University of Medical Sciences for kind supports.

Conflicts of Interest: Authors declare no conflict of interest and/or commercial products or companies.

References

1. Huang, Y.; Yang, C.; Xu, X.-F.; Xu, W.; Liu, S.-W. Structural and functional properties of SARS-CoV-2 spike protein: Potential antivirus drug development for COVID-19. *Acta Pharmacol. Sin.* **2020**, *41*, 1141–1149. [CrossRef] [PubMed]
2. Shereen, M.A.; Khan, S.; Kazmi, A.; Bashir, N.; Siddique, R. COVID-19 infection: Emergence, transmission, and characteristics of human coronaviruses. *J. Adv. Res.* **2020**, *24*, 91–98. [CrossRef] [PubMed]
3. Lu, R.; Zhao, X.; Li, J.; Niu, P.; Yang, B.; Wu, H.; Wang, W.; Song, H.; Huang, B.; Zhu, N. Genomic characterisation and epidemiology of 2019 novel coronavirus: Implications for virus origins and receptor binding. *Lancet* **2020**, *395*, 565–574. [CrossRef]
4. Wan, Y.; Shang, J.; Graham, R.; Baric, R.S.; Li, F. Receptor recognition by the novel coronavirus from Wuhan: An analysis based on decade-long structural studies of SARS coronavirus. *J. Virol.* **2020**, *94*, e00127-20. [CrossRef]
5. Li, W.; Moore, M.J.; Vasilieva, N.; Sui, J.; Wong, S.K.; Berne, M.A.; Somasundaran, M.; Sullivan, J.L.; Luzuriaga, K.; Greenough, T.C. Angiotensin-converting enzyme 2 is a functional receptor for the SARS coronavirus. *Nature* **2003**, *426*, 450–454. [CrossRef]
6. Xue, X.; Shi, J.; Xu, H.; Qin, Y.; Yang, Z.; Feng, S.; Liu, D.; Jian, L.; Hua, L.; Wang, Y. Dynamics of binding ability prediction between spike protein and human ACE2 reveals the adaptive strategy of SARS-CoV-2 in humans. *Sci. Rep.* **2021**, *11*, 3187. [CrossRef]
7. Verma, S.; Patil, V.M.; Gupta, M.K. Mutation informatics: SARS-CoV-2 receptor-binding domain of the spike protein. *Drug Discov. Today* **2022**, *27*, 103312. [CrossRef] [PubMed]
8. Zhou, W.; Xu, C.; Wang, P.; Anashkina, A.A.; Jiang, Q. Impact of mutations in SARS-COV-2 spike on viral infectivity and antigenicity. *Brief. Bioinform.* **2022**, *23*, bbab375. [CrossRef]
9. Mohammadi, E.; Shafiee, F.; Shahzamani, K.; Ranjbar, M.M.; Alibakhshi, A.; Ahangarzadeh, S.; Shariati, L.; Hooshmandi, S.; Ataei, B.; Javanmard, S.H. Novel and emerging mutations of SARS-CoV-2: Biomedical implications. *Biomed. Pharmacother.* **2021**, *139*, 111599. [CrossRef]
10. Huang, S.-W.; Miller, S.O.; Yen, C.-H.; Wang, S.-F. Impact of genetic variability in ACE2 expression on the evolutionary dynamics of SARS-CoV-2 spike D614G mutation. *Genes* **2020**, *12*, 16. [CrossRef]
11. Volz, E.; Hill, V.; McCrone, J.T.; Price, A.; Jorgensen, D.; O'Toole, Á.; Southgate, J.; Johnson, R.; Jackson, B.; Nascimento, F.F. Evaluating the effects of SARS-CoV-2 spike mutation D614G on transmissibility and pathogenicity. *Cell* **2021**, *184*, 64–75.e11. [CrossRef] [PubMed]
12. Zhang, L.; Jackson, C.B.; Mou, H.; Ojha, A.; Peng, H.; Quinlan, B.D.; Rangarajan, E.S.; Pan, A.; Vanderheiden, A.; Suthar, M.S. SARS-CoV-2 spike-protein D614G mutation increases virion spike density and infectivity. *Nat. Commun.* **2020**, *11*, 6013. [CrossRef] [PubMed]

13. Korber, B.; Fischer, W.M.; Gnanakaran, S.; Yoon, H.; Theiler, J.; Abfalterer, W.; Hengartner, N.; Giorgi, E.E.; Bhattacharya, T.; Foley, B. Tracking changes in SARS-CoV-2 spike: Evidence that D614G increases infectivity of the COVID-19 virus. *Cell* **2020**, *182*, 812–827.e819. [CrossRef]
14. Becerra-Flores, M.; Cardozo, T. SARS-CoV-2 viral spike G614 mutation exhibits higher case fatality rate. *Int. J. Clin. Pract.* **2020**, *74*, e13525. [CrossRef] [PubMed]
15. Wang, D.; Hu, B.; Hu, C.; Zhu, F.; Liu, X.; Zhang, J.; Wang, B.; Xiang, H.; Cheng, Z.; Xiong, Y. Clinical characteristics of 138 hospitalized patients with 2019 novel coronavirus–infected pneumonia in Wuhan, China. *JAMA* **2020**, *323*, 1061–1069. [CrossRef] [PubMed]
16. Huang, C.; Wang, Y.; Li, X.; Ren, L.; Zhao, J.; Hu, Y.; Zhang, L.; Fan, G.; Xu, J.; Gu, X. Clinical features of patients infected with 2019 novel coronavirus in Wuhan, China. *Lancet* **2020**, *395*, 497–506. [CrossRef]
17. Kumar, S.; Stecher, G.; Li, M.; Knyaz, C.; Tamura, K. MEGA X: Molecular evolutionary genetics analysis across computing platforms. *Mol. Biol. Evol.* **2018**, *35*, 1547–1549. [CrossRef]
18. Dimonte, S.; Babakir-Mina, M.; Taib Hama-Soor, S.A. Genetic Variation and Evolution of the 2019 Novel Coronavirus. *Public Health Genom.* **2021**, *24*, 54–66. [CrossRef]
19. Bano, I.; Sharif, M.; Alam, S. Genetic drift in the genome of SARS COV-2 and its global health concern. *J. Med. Virol.* **2022**, *94*, 88–98. [CrossRef]
20. Daniloski, Z.; Jordan, T.X.; Ilmain, J.K.; Guo, X.; Bhabha, G.; Sanjana, N.E. The Spike D614G mutation increases SARS-CoV-2 infection of multiple human cell types. *Elife* **2021**, *10*, e65365. [CrossRef]
21. Souza, P.F.; Mesquita, F.P.; Amaral, J.L.; Landim, P.G.; Lima, K.R.; Costa, M.B.; Farias, I.R.; Belém, M.O.; Pinto, Y.O.; Moreira, H.H. The spike glycoproteins of SARS-CoV-2: A review of how mutations of spike glycoproteins have driven the emergence of variants with high transmissibility and immune escape. *Int. J. Biol. Macromol.* **2022**, *208*, 105–125. [CrossRef] [PubMed]
22. Jin, J.-M.; Bai, P.; He, W.; Wu, F.; Liu, X.-F.; Han, D.-M.; Liu, S.; Yang, J.-K. Gender differences in patients with COVID-19: Focus on severity and mortality. *Front. Public Health* **2020**, *8*, 152. [CrossRef] [PubMed]
23. Mendiola-Pastrana, I.R.; López-Ortiz, E.; Río de la Loza-Zamora, J.G.; González, J.; Gómez-García, A.; López-Ortiz, G. SARS-CoV-2 variants and clinical outcomes: A systematic review. *Life* **2022**, *12*, 170. [CrossRef] [PubMed]
24. Patone, M.; Thomas, K.; Hatch, R.; San Tan, P.; Coupland, C.; Liao, W.; Mouncey, P.; Harrison, D.; Rowan, K.; Horby, P. Mortality and critical care unit admission associated with the SARS-CoV-2 lineage B.1.1.7 in England: An observational cohort study. *Lancet Infect. Dis.* **2021**, *21*, 1518–1528. [CrossRef]
25. Li, L.; Liu, Y.; Tang, X.; He, D. The disease severity and clinical outcomes of the SARS-CoV-2 variants of concern. *Front. Public Health* **2021**, *9*, 1929.
26. Wang, S.; Zou, X.; Li, Z.; Fu, J.; Fan, H.; Yu, H.; Deng, F.; Huang, H.; Peng, J.; Zhao, K. Analysis of Clinical Characteristics and Virus Strains Variation of Patients Infected With SARS-CoV-2 in Jiangsu Province—A Retrospective Study. *Front. Public Health* **2021**, *9*, 791600. [CrossRef]
27. Wang, C.; Zheng, Y.; Niu, Z.; Jiang, X.; Sun, Q. The virological impacts of SARS-CoV-2 D614G mutation. *J. Mol. Cell Biol.* **2021**, *13*, 712–720. [CrossRef]
28. Hatirnaz Ng, O.; Akyoney, S.; Sahin, I.; Soykam, H.O.; Bayram Akcapinar, G.; Ozdemir, O.; Kancagi, D.D.; Sir Karakus, G.; Yurtsever, B.; Kocagoz, A.S. Mutational landscape of SARS-CoV-2 genome in Turkey and impact of mutations on spike protein structure. *PLoS ONE* **2021**, *16*, e0260438. [CrossRef]
29. Jackson, C.B.; Zhang, L.; Farzan, M.; Choe, H. Functional importance of the D614G mutation in the SARS-CoV-2 spike protein. *Biochem. Biophys. Res. Commun.* **2021**, *538*, 108–115. [CrossRef]
30. Verkhivker, G.M.; Agajanian, S.; Oztas, D.Y.; Gupta, G. Landscape-Based Mutational Sensitivity Cartography and Network Community Analysis of the SARS-CoV-2 Spike Protein Structures: Quantifying Functional Effects of the Circulating D614G Variant. *ACS Omega* **2021**, *6*, 16216–16233. [CrossRef]
31. Prü, B.M. Variants of SARS CoV-2: Mutations, transmissibility, virulence, drug resistance, and antibody/vaccine sensitivity. *Front. Biosci.-Landmark* **2022**, *27*, 65. [CrossRef] [PubMed]
32. SeyedAlinaghi, S.; Mirzapour, P.; Dadras, O.; Pashaei, Z.; Karimi, A.; MohsseniPour, M.; Soleymanzadeh, M.; Barzegary, A.; Afsahi, A.M.; Vahedi, F. Characterization of SARS-CoV-2 different variants and related morbidity and mortality: A systematic review. *Eur. J. Med. Res.* **2021**, *26*, 51. [CrossRef]
33. Molina-Mora, J.A.; Cordero-Laurent, E.; Godínez, A.; Calderón-Osorno, M.; Brenes, H.; Soto-Garita, C.; Pérez-Corrales, C.; de Estudios, C.-C.C.I.; del SARS-CoV, G.; Rica, C. SARS-CoV-2 genomic surveillance in Costa Rica: Evidence of a divergent population and an increased detection of a spike T1117I mutation. *Infect. Genet. Evol.* **2021**, *92*, 104872. [CrossRef] [PubMed]
34. Molina-Mora, J.A. Insights into the mutation T1117I in the spike and the lineage B.1.1.389 of SARS-CoV-2 circulating in Costa Rica. *Gene Rep.* **2022**, *27*, 101554. [CrossRef] [PubMed]

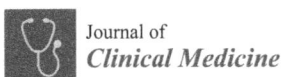

Article

Impact of COVID-19 Pandemic on Initiation of Immunosuppressive Treatment in Immune-Mediated Inflammatory Diseases in Austria: A Nationwide Retrospective Study

Maximilian Kutschera [1], Valentin Ritschl [2,3], Berthold Reichardt [4], Tanja Stamm [2,3,*], Hans Kiener [5], Harald Maier [6], Walter Reinisch [1], Bernhard Benka [7] and Gottfried Novacek [1]

1. Department of Internal Medicine III, Division of Gastroenterology and Hepatology, Medical University of Vienna, 1090 Vienna, Austria
2. Institute of Outcomes Research, Center for Medical Statistics, Informatics and Intelligent Systems, Medical University of Vienna, 1090 Vienna, Austria
3. Ludwig Boltzmann Institute for Arthritis and Rehabilitation, 1090 Vienna, Austria
4. Austrian Health Insurance Fund, 7000 Eisenstadt, Austria
5. Department of Internal Medicine III, Division of Rheumatology, Medical University of Vienna, 1090 Vienna, Austria
6. Department of Dermatology, Medical University of Vienna, 1090 Vienna, Austria
7. AGES—Austrian Agency for Health and Food Safety Ltd., Division of Public Health, 1220 Vienna, Austria
* Correspondence: tanja.stamm@meduniwien.ac.at; Tel.: +43-1-40400-16370

Citation: Kutschera, M.; Ritschl, V.; Reichardt, B.; Stamm, T.; Kiener, H.; Maier, H.; Reinisch, W.; Benka, B.; Novacek, G. Impact of COVID-19 Pandemic on Initiation of Immunosuppressive Treatment in Immune-Mediated Inflammatory Diseases in Austria: A Nationwide Retrospective Study. J. Clin. Med. 2022, 11, 5308. https://doi.org/10.3390/jcm11185308

Academic Editors: Francesco Pugliese, Francesco Alessandri and Giovanni Giordano

Received: 9 August 2022
Accepted: 3 September 2022
Published: 9 September 2022

Publisher's Note: MDPI stays neutral with regard to jurisdictional claims in published maps and institutional affiliations.

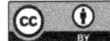

Copyright: © 2022 by the authors. Licensee MDPI, Basel, Switzerland. This article is an open access article distributed under the terms and conditions of the Creative Commons Attribution (CC BY) license (https://creativecommons.org/licenses/by/4.0/).

Abstract: Objective: Conventional immunosuppressive and advanced targeted therapies, including biological medications and small molecules, are a mainstay in the treatment of immune-mediated inflammatory diseases (IMID). However, the COVID-19 pandemic caused concerns over these drugs' safety regarding the risk and severity of SARS-CoV-2 infection. Thus, we aimed to assess the impact of the COVID-19 pandemic on the initiation of these treatments in 2020. Study Design and Setting: We conducted a population-based retrospective analysis of real-world data of the Austrian health insurance funds on the initiation of conventional immunosuppressive and advanced targeted therapies. The primary objective was to compare the initiation of these medications in the year 2020 with the period 2017 to 2019. Initiation rates of medication were calculated by comparing a certain unit of time with an average of the previous ones. Results: 95,573 patients were included. During the first lockdown in Austria in April 2020, there was a significant decrease in the initiations of conventional immunosuppressives and advanced targeted therapies compared to previous years ($p < 0.0001$). From May 2020 onwards, numbers rapidly re-achieved pre-lockdown levels despite higher SARS-CoV-2 infection rates and subsequent lockdown periods at the end of 2020. Independent from the impact of the COVID-19 pandemic, a continuous increase of starts of advanced targeted therapies and a continuous decrease of conventional immunosuppressants during the observation period were observed. Conclusions: In IMID patients, the COVID-19 pandemic led to a significant decrease of newly started conventional immunosuppressive and advanced targeted therapies only during the first lockdown in Austria.

Keywords: Immune-mediated inflammatory diseases; conventional immunosuppressive treatment; advanced targeted therapy; inflammatory bowel disease; rheumatoid arthritis; psoriasis

1. Introduction

In December 2019, the Coronavirus Disease 2019 (COVID-19), caused by the severe acute respiratory syndrome coronavirus type 2 (SARS-CoV-2), was first reported in Wuhan, China [1–3] from where it rapidly spread throughout the world, leading to a pandemic [4].

As of 30 June 2022, SARS-CoV-2 has affected around 560 million identified cases, with over six million confirmed deaths [5].

While most cases of COVID-19 are mild and have a favorable course, the disease can become severe, resulting in hospitalization, respiratory failure, or even death [6]. The most important reported risk factors for a severe course of COVID-19 are older age, cardiovascular and chronic pulmonary diseases, obesity, diabetes, and immune deficiency [7–9].

Conventional immunosuppressive and especially advanced targeted therapies (ADT), including biological medications and small molecules, are a mainstay in the medical treatment of immune-mediated inflammatory diseases (IMID), such as inflammatory bowel diseases (IBD), rheumatic diseases, and psoriasis, as well as less common dermatological inflammatory diseases [10–14]. These medications may be associated with a generally increased risk of infections, such as serious and opportunistic infections described in IBD patients treated with immune-suppressive regimens [15,16] Thus, the COVID-19 pandemic and the speed of its spread caused concerns over the safety of these drugs owing to the lack of evidence respective of risk and severity of infection with SARS-CoV-2. However, early expert consensus balanced out a potentially increased risk of severe COVID-19 by the benefits of continuation of an effective biological treatment, and it was recommended not to stop effective medication [17–20]. This management of continuation of effective maintenance therapy has also been described in the real-world setting [21].

Little is known about the initiation of conventional immunosuppressive therapies and ADT in IMID during the COVID-19 pandemic. Studies on IBD patients revealed that around 80% to 90% of patients needing to start any biological therapy received their treatment start regularly during the first lockdown [22,23]. On the one hand, pandemic mitigation strategies might have led to the cancelation or postponement of face-to-face meetings with new patients [22,23]. On the other hand, concerns about a potentially increased risk for severe COVID-19 might have contributed to a delay in initiating immunosuppressive and biological drugs. In particular, corticosteroids, methotrexate, azathioprine/6-mercaptopurine, JAK-inhibitors, and rituximab have been mentioned to be associated with an increased risk of severe COVID-19 outcomes [24–26]. However, this has not been described at the beginning of the pandemic. A survey among the European Alliance of Associations for Rheumatology countries revealed a delay between symptom onset and a first rheumatological visit as well as the postponement of treatment decisions during the first wave of the COVID-19 pandemic, which negatively impacted early treatment and treat-to-target strategies requiring tight control [27]. Such undertreatment could lead to flares and complications of the underlying inflammatory disease with subsequent hospitalizations. From a macro-level perspective, especially the initiation of new ADT could be an indicator for estimating undertreatment in patients with IMID.

Therefore, our nationwide study aimed to assess the number of newly started conventional immunosuppressive and advanced targeted therapies during the first waves of the COVID-19 pandemic in the year 2020 in Austria and to compare these data with the respective timeframe of previous years.

2. Materials and Methods

2.1. Design

Based on dispensing data from Austrian health insurance funds, we conducted a population-based retrospective analysis with a four-year observation period from 2017 to 2020. Dispensing data means that all data on prescribed medications picked up at the pharmacy and covered by the Austrian health insurance funds can be retrieved. Austrian health insurance funds cover 98% of all residents in Austria (8,755,124 persons in December 2020).

2.2. Participants and Data Extraction

Data from all patients with initiations of conventional immunosuppressive therapy, ADT, including biological medications and small molecules, and other disease-specific medications were included. The initiation of treatment was defined as all first prescriptions from 2017 to 2020. To fulfill this definition, no previous prescription of the same drug among the listed medications was allowed from the beginning of the previous year (in 2016) (for timeline of the study see Supplemental Figure S1). However, due to Austrian regulations, only patients who received their medications outside of a hospital could be included since treatment data of hospitalized patients were not available for our analysis. The diagnosis of the IMID could only be recorded in case of hospitalization during the observation period, so we examined new prescriptions of drugs approved and reimbursed for IMID in Austria, despite being unaware of the patients' exact diagnosis. To increase the number of known diagnoses, we assigned medications to a diagnosis of an IMID if the medication was approved only for that indication.

2.3. Objectives

The primary objective was to evaluate the impact of the COVID-19 pandemic on the initiation of conventional immunosuppressive therapy and ADT in the year 2020 compared to the period 2017 to 2019 in IMID in Austria. The secondary objective was to evaluate the course of initiation of these treatments in IMID in Austria during the observation period regardless of the COVID-19 pandemic.

The primary endpoint was the first prescription of conventional immunosuppressive therapy, ADT, and other medications for immune-mediated inflammatory diseases.

2.4. Data Analysis

The frequency of newly started conventional immunosuppressive therapy, ADT, and other specific medications was calculated for every month of 2020 and compared with monthly prescription rates of the three previous years (2017–2019). The medications used for this analysis were categorized and are listed in Table 1. Other specific medications without immunosuppressive effects were included as a possible sign of hindered contact between patients and physicians due to pandemic mitigation strategies.

Table 1. Advanced targeted therapies (biologics and small molecules) and conventional immunosuppressive medications, and other specific medications included in the analysis.

Biologics	TNF-Alpha Inhibitors	Adalimumab, Certolizumab Pegol, Etanercept, Golimumab, Infliximab
	Anti C5	eculizumab
	IL-1 inhibitors	anakinra, canakinumab
	IL-4 inhibitors	dupilumab
	IL-6 inhibitors	sarilumab, tocilizumab
	IL-17 Inhibitors	brodalumab, ixekizumab, secukinumab
	IL-23 inhibitors	guselkumab, risankizumab, tildrakizumab
	IL12/23 inhibitor	ustekinumab
	Anti-BAFF	belimumab
	B-cell depletion	rituximab
	integrin $\alpha_4\beta_7$ inhibitor	vedolizumab
	Co-Stimulation inhibitor	abatacept
Small molecules	PDE4 inhibitors	apremilast
	JAK-inhibitors	baricitinib, tofacitinib, upadacitinib
Conventional immunosuppressive medications		azathioprine, cyclosporine, leflunomide, mycophenolate mofetil, methotrexate
Others		sulfalazine, mesalazine

Re-identifying subjects by the Medical University of Vienna was impossible as only birth year, high-level region of residence (one of the nine Austrian counties), gender, and, if applicable, death year were included. Moreover, ethical approval was given by the ethics committee and internal review board of Vienna (EC No. 1330/2021).

2.5. Statistical Analysis

Data sets from 13 different health insurances were combined. Within this step, we adjusted for multiply insured individuals by combining their data. For categorical data, absolute and relative frequencies were calculated and depicted using bar charts. Metric variables were summarized by calculating the mean and standard deviation. This was done for the entire study sample and separately for subgroups.

Differences between groups were tested using Chi-2 tests (categorical data), *t*-tests, or Wilcoxon–Mann–Whitney tests (metric data). To balance the potential effects of oversampling, we assessed the clinical meaningfulness of significant differences. Medication categories were summarized where appropriate. Initiation rates of medication were calculated by comparing a certain unit of time (month, year) with an average of the previous ones. *p*-values below 0.05 were considered statistically significant. We used R (https://www.r-project.org, R version 4.2.1, accessed on 23 June 2022)) to perform the statistical analysis.

3. Results

3.1. Patients' Characteristics

We identified 95,573 patients with the start of at least one conventional immunosuppressive and/or advanced targeted therapy and/or other disease-specific medication from 2017 to 2020. Of these, 43,402 were male (45%; mean age 50.6 years; SD ± 18.1 years), and 52,171 were female (55%; mean age 53.4 years; SD ± 18.7 years). The diagnosis of IMID recorded in case of hospitalization was available in 9.7% of the patients (Table 2). In addition, in a total of 59.5% patients, we could assign diagnoses by using medications that were only approved for a single indication during the observation period (Supplementary Table S1). In the entire data set, 122,213 medications were started in the years 2017 to 2020. The number of starts of every medication is given in the supplemental material (Supplemental Table S2). The majority of the patients had only one treatment start (90,021; 94.2%), 3822 patients (4.0%) had two, 1500 patients (1.6%) had three, and 230 patients (0.2%) had four or more treatment starts with different medications.

Table 2. Diagnoses of immune-mediated inflammatory diseases in 9234 patients.

Diagnosis	n (%)
Crohn's disease; n (%)	3488 (37.8)
Ulcerative colitis; n (%)	2805 (30.4)
Rheumatoid arthritis; n (%)	1543 (16.7)
Plaque psoriasis; n (%)	629 (6.8)
Ankylosing spondylitis; n (%)	259 (2.8)
Hidradenitis suppurativa; n (%)	179 (1.9)
Childhood arthritis; n (%)	151 (1.6)
Uveitis; n (%)	112 (1.2)
Psoriatic arthritis; n (%)	35 (0.4)
Behçet–Krankheit; n (%)	33 (0.4)

3.2. Impact of the COVID-19 Pandemic on the Initiation of Conventional Immunosuppressive and Advanced Targeted Therapies

During the first lockdown in Austria in spring 2020 (week 12–week 20), there was a significant decrease in the overall initiation of conventional immunosuppressive therapies and ADT in April 2020 compared to previous years (all $p < 0.0001$, one sample Chi-2 tests) (Figure 1, Supplemental Figure S2). After the first lockdown, initial prescriptions of conventional immunosuppressive therapies and ADT re-achieved pre-lockdown levels despite higher infection rates with SARS-CoV-2 in the total population. In addition, in subsequent lockdown periods (second lockdown in Austria week 45–week 48; third lockdown week 53; Figure 2, the frequency of initiation of conventional immunosuppressive therapies and ADT did not decrease again (Figures 1 and 3). This was mainly observed for the starts for biologics which even exceeded the number of starts in the corresponding months of the previous years (Figure 1, Supplemental Figure S2).

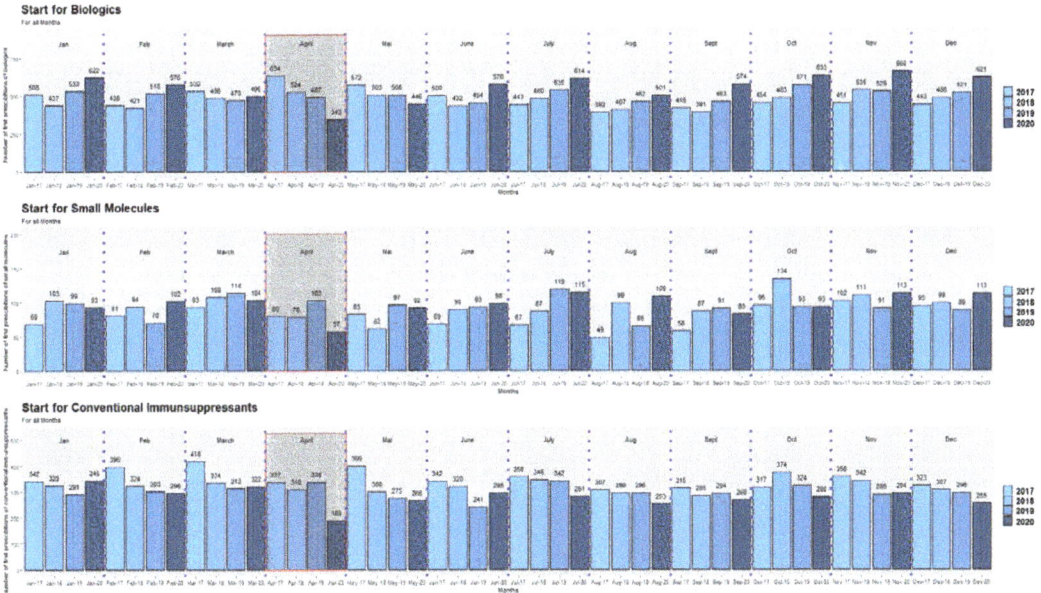

Figure 1. Starts of biological medications, small molecules, and conventional immunosuppressive medications in the period 2017–2020. The red rectangles mark the timeframe of a significant decrease of the initiation of biologics, small molecules as well as conventional immunosuppressants during the first lockdown (April 2020 compared to the corresponding timeframe of previous years). The scaling of the y-axis differs for the presentation of the three medication groups to demonstrate at best the decrease of the medication starts in April 2020.

We also investigated the initiation of mesalazine (Supplemental Figure S3), which was also significantly reduced in April 2020 during the first lockdown compared to the corresponding months of the previous years (both $p < 0.0001$). No mesalazine initiation changes occurred during subsequent lockdowns at the end of 2020.

3.3. Changes in the Initiation of Therapies during the Observation Period Independent from COVID-19

Independent from the COVID-19 pandemic, the number of initiations of different medication groups significantly changed during the observation period (2017–2020). We detected a continuous rise in the initiation of biological medications of 6.7% per year as well as of small molecules of 6.1% per year, respectively (calculated as compound annual growth rate, both $p < 0.0001$) (Figure 2). The starts of small molecules increased from

2017 to 2018 by 22.8% and stayed stable in the following years. In contrast, the start of immunosuppressive medications significantly decreased by 5.9% per year ($p < 0.0001$) (Figure 2), and mesalazine even by 6.1% per year ($p < 0.0001$) (Supplemental Figure S4).

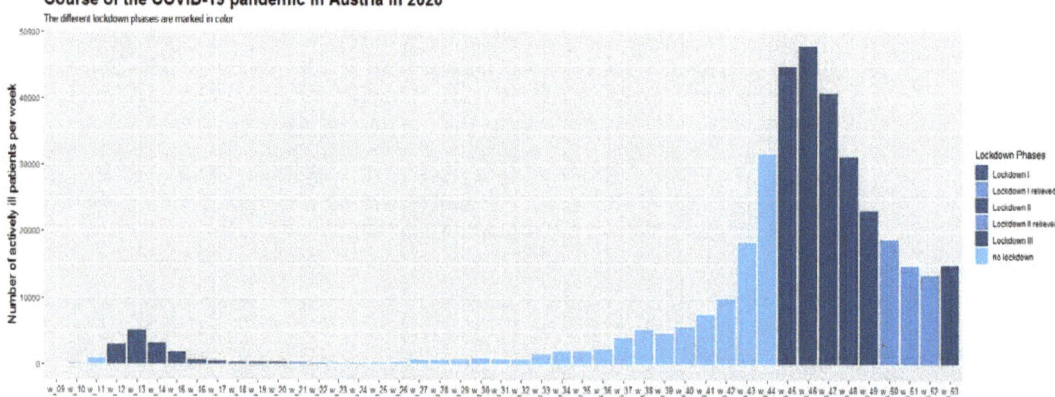

Figure 2. Positive COVID-19 cases by week in 2020 in Austria (first positive laboratory diagnosis).

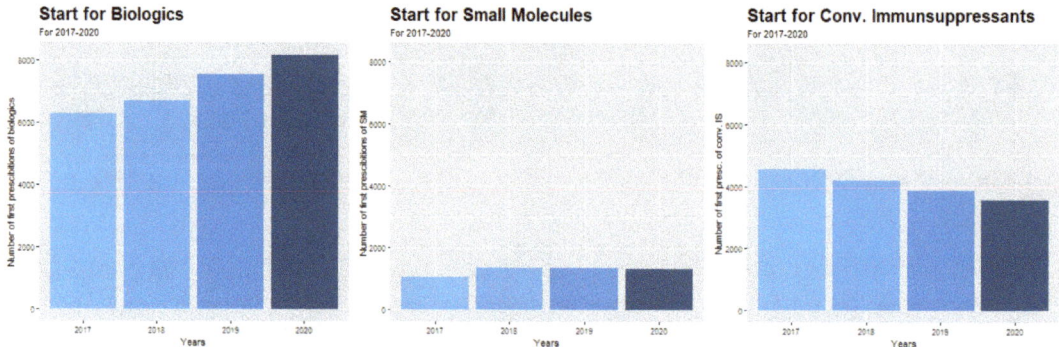

Figure 3. Annual starts for biological medications, small molecules, and conventional immunosuppressive medications in the period 2017–2020.

4. Discussion

Our nationwide study revealed that the COVID-19 pandemic led to a significant decrease in the initiation of conventional immunosuppressive and advanced targeted therapies in patients with immune-mediated inflammatory diseases, including inflammatory bowel diseases, during the first lockdown in 2020 in Austria. However, after that, the initiation of these substances rapidly re-achieved pre-lockdown levels despite much higher infection rates with SARS-CoV-2 and subsequent lockdown periods at the end of 2020.

Little has been reported about the initiation of conventional immunosuppressive medications and ADT during lockdown periods. An Italian web-based survey revealed that 79% to 92% of patients needing to start any intravenous or subcutaneous biological therapy, respectively, received their first administration regularly during the first lockdown [22]. Another study reported that biological therapy started as planned in 21 patients out of 25 (86%) [23]. However, as far as we are aware, no data have been published about either the initiation of other IMID-specific medications during the first lockdown period or about the initiation during subsequent lockdowns resulting from even higher infection rates.

That decrease in the initiation of therapy during the first lockdown seemed to be caused by the concern that conventional immunosuppressive medications and ADT could increase the risk of infection with SARS-CoV-2 and a more severe course of COVID 19 in case of an infection. However, for patients with immune-mediated inflammatory diseases, an increased risk of infection with SARS-CoV-2 and a more aggressive course has not been demonstrated in several later publications [28–32], though the literature also revealed partially conflicting results [33–36]. Some medications have been associated with an enhanced risk of severe COVID-19 outcomes. This has been described for corticosteroids, methotrexate, azathioprine/6-mercaptopurine, JAK-inhibitors, and rituximab, but not for the other in IMID broadly used biologics [20,37–40]. This gain in knowledge and subsequent recommendations of national and international scientific societies is likely to be mainly responsible for the lack of impact of high infection rates with SARS-CoV-2 and subsequent lockdowns on start of immunosuppressive and biological medications at the end of 2020 [41].

Another probable reason for the reduced initiations of immunosuppressive and biological medications might have been reduced contact between patients and physicians due to pandemic mitigation strategies, which might have led to the cancellation or postponement of face-to-face meetings [22,23]. This assumption might be confirmed by the fact that the number of starts with mesalazine, which does not seem to have any immunosuppressive effect, was also significantly reduced during the first lockdown, which might be a sign of reduced patient visits during the lockdown. Consistent with this observation, effects in other fields of patient care have been described. For example, it was reported that back in the spring of 2020, the pandemic led to a marked reduction in the number of people referred, diagnosed, and treated for colorectal cancer [20,42]. In addition, other countries also observed a significant decrease in IBD-related procedures during the first lockdown, especially in April 2020 [43].

We did not observe a decrease in immunosuppressive and biological treatments in the entire year 2020. This means that the start of the immunosuppressive and biological medications was only delayed for a short period.

Independent of any impact of the COVID-19 pandemic, our study revealed a continuous increase of starts of biological medications and small molecules during the observation period from 2017 to 2020. Other publications have reported similar findings over the last years [43–47]. Biosimilars led to overall reductions in health care expenses. On the other hand, the start of conventional immunosuppressive drugs decreased continuously during the same period. The increase in biological medications and small molecules could also be due to an increasing incidence and prevalence of immune-mediated inflammatory diseases. Still, corresponding data are not available for Austria. However, the decreasing number of starts of immunosuppressive medications that are already longer on the market suggests that it is more likely to shift to a more progressive treatment attitude according to recommendations of scientific organizations [48–51].

Interestingly, there was also a significant annual decrease in the start of mesalazine during the observation period. Mesalazine is only approved for inflammatory bowel diseases. It is a mainstay in treating mild to moderate ulcerative colitis but has low effectiveness in Crohn's disease. As we do not have any reason to believe that the prevalence of ulcerative colitis decreased within the last years in Austria, this finding is likely due to diminishing prescriptions for Crohn's disease [52]. As there has been a report that the usage of mesalazine could be associated with an increased risk of severe COVID-19 [25], this was still unknown at the time of the first wave of the pandemic and could not be confirmed later on [37]. Therefore, we assume that this had no influence on the prescription of mesalazine during the first wave of COVID-19.

The study has its strengths but also limitations. The data of the Austrian health insurance funds cover the majority (98%) of the Austrian population. Furthermore, we included all starts for immunosuppressive and biological treatments and small molecules, mainly in IBD, rheumatologic diseases, and psoriasis. However, only medications prescribed on an outpatient basis could be recorded since treatment data of hospitalized patients were not available for our analysis. This might have affected medications that are given intravenously, e.g., infliximab. Nevertheless, as some of these drugs were used off-label in patients with COVID-19, the presence of inpatient treatments might have been a bias and therefore, in the absence of inpatient treatment, there can be no prescriptions due to COVID-19 disease. However, we assume that the overall results are barely affected as the vast majority of patients are being prescribed ADT during ambulatory visits. In this analysis, we focused on prescribed first courses of ADT only. To determine the pattern of use of other medications, including for example corticosteroids or other medications such as budesonide and beclomethasone, would be an interesting further analysis. It would require a different dataset extracted also from the electronic health records with information on discontinuation, changes in dosing, patients not taking medications, etc. A further limitation is that we could not assign our findings to specific diagnoses since the diagnosis recorded in case of hospitalization was only available in around 10% of the patients. However, if we assigned medications to only approved indications, the percentage of available diagnoses would rise to approximately 60%. We considered comparing the number of initial courses of a drug to other substances to assess whether drugs with greater a priori safety, such as ustekinumab or vedolizumab, were prescribed more often compared to drugs which were considered to have a slightly higher risk of infection, such as TNF-alpha inhibitors. However, as the number of cases for each drug was too small, we could not provide for a reliable statement.

5. Conclusions

In summary, our study revealed a significant decrease in initiations of conventional immunosuppressive and advanced targeted therapies, including biological treatments and small molecules, during the first COVID-19 pandemic lockdown in April 2020. Concerns over an increased risk of infection with SARS-CoV-2 and a more severe course of COVID-19 in case of an infection and pandemic mitigation strategies with subsequent cancellation or postponement of face-to-face meetings appear to be the most important reasons for that finding. However, that decrease in initiations of medications was not observed during subsequent lockdown periods despite much higher infection rates. One can guess that this was also true in later periods with high infection rates in 2021 and at the beginning of 2022, encouraged by the availability of vaccinations against SARS-CoV-2 as the most effective option to prevent severe COVID-19. Independent of the impact of the COVID-19 pandemic, we observed a continuous increase in the start of biological medications and small molecules and a continuous decrease of conventional immunosuppressants during the observation period from 2017 to 2020.

Supplementary Materials: The following supporting information can be downloaded at: https://www.mdpi.com/article/10.3390/jcm11185308/s1, Table S1: Diagnoses of immune-mediated inflammatory diseases in 56,913 out of 95,573 patients; Table S2: Starts of medications during the observation period 2017 to 2020 (n = 122,213); Figure S1: Timeline of the study, Figure S2: Start of TNFα inhibitors in the period 2017–2020, Figure S3: Start of mesalazin (2017–2020), Figure S4: Annual start of mesalazine from 2017 to 2020.

Author Contributions: Conceptualization, M.K., V.R., B.R., T.S. and G.N.; Data curation, V.R. and B.R.; Formal analysis, V.R.; Investigation, M.K., H.K., H.M., B.B., and G.N.; Methodology, V.R. and T.S.; Software, V.R.; Supervision, T.S., H.K., W.R. and G.N.; Writing -original draft, M.K.; Writing – review and editing, B.R., T.S., H.K., H.M., W.R., B.B. and G.N. All authors have read and agreed to the published version of the manuscript.

Funding: This research received no specific grant from public, commercial, or non-for-profit funding agencies.

Institutional Review Board Statement: The study was conducted in accordance with the guidelines of the Declaration of Helsinki and approved by the ethics committee of the medical university of Vienna (Nr: 1330/2021, 12.05.2021).

Informed Consent Statement: Due to the retrospective style of this study and the anonymity of all patients, no informed consent was required by the ethics committee of the medical university of Vienna.

Data Availability Statement: The dataset and R code can be obtained from the corresponding author upon reasoned request.

Acknowledgments: The authors thank the members of the Pharmacoeconomics Advisory Council of the Austrian Social Health Insurance Funds for providing the data. The authors wish to convey their gratitude to Karin Allmer for quality assurance with the database query, and to Ludwig Weissengruber for the organisational support in data acquisition and generation.

Conflicts of Interest: MK: no conflict of interest. VR: no conflict of interest. BR: no conflict of interest. TS: has received grant/research support from AbbVie and Roche, has been a consultant for AbbVie and Sanofi Genzyme, and has been a paid speaker for AbbVie, Novartis, Roche, Sanofi, and Takeda. HK: no conflict of interest. HM: received fees as a lecturer and author for Bayer AG, as a lecturer for PelPharma Handels GmbH, and author for La Roche Posay Laboratoire Dermatologique. Furthermore, he worked as a consultant for Philips Austria GmbH Consumer Lifestyle, and Moser Medical Group kosmetische Haarchirurgie GmbH. WR: received fees from Abbvie, Algernon, Amgen, AM Pharma, AMT, AOP Orphan, Arena Pharmaceuticals, Astellas, Astra Zeneca, Avaxia, Roland Berger GmbH, Bioclinica, Biogen IDEC, Boehringer-Ingelheim, Bristol-Myers Squibb, Calyx, Cellerix, Chemocentryx, Celgene, Centocor, Celltrion, Covance, Danone Austria, DSM, Elan, Eli Lilly, Ernest & Young, Falk Pharma GmbH, Ferring, Galapagos, Gatehouse Bio Inc., Genentech, Gilead, Grünenthal, ICON, Index Pharma, Inova, Intrinsic Imaging, Janssen, Johnson & Johnson, Kyowa Hakko Kirin Pharma, Landos Biopharma, Lipid Therapeutics, LivaNova, Mallinckrodt, Medahead, MedImmune, Millenium, Mitsubishi Tanabe Pharma Corporation, MSD, Nash Pharmaceuticals, Nestle, Nippon Kayaku, Novartis, Ocera, OMass, Otsuka, Parexel, PDL, Periconsulting, Pharmacosmos, Philip Morris Institute, Pfizer, Procter & Gamble, Prometheus, Protagonist, Provention, Quell Therapeutics, Robarts Clinical Trial, Sandoz, Schering-Plough, Second Genome, Seres Therapeutics, Setpointmedical, Sigmoid, Sublimity, Takeda, Teva Pharma, Therakos, Theravance, Tigenix, UCB, Vifor, Zealand, Zyngenia, and 4SC. BB: Bernhard Benka is an employee of the company Austrian Agency for Health and Food Safety Ltd. GN: has received consulting fees from AbbVie, MSD, Takeda, Janssen, Sandoz, Pfizer, Astro Pharma, Falk Pharma, Ferring, Gilead, Galapagos and Vifor.

Conference Presentation: This work was presented in part as a poster at the annual congress of the European Crohn's Colitis Organization, February 2020, and the annual congress of the Austrian society of gastroenterology and hepatology, September 2022.

Abbreviations

ADT	advanced targeted therapies
IMID	immune-mediated inflammatory diseases
IBD	inflammatory bowel diseases
RA	rheumatoid arthritis
PA	psoriatic arthritis
SM	small molecules

References

1. Huang, C.; Wang, Y.; Li, X.; Ren, L.; Zhao, J.; Hu, Y.; Zhang, L.; Fan, G.; Xu, J.; Gu, X.; et al. Clinical features of patients infected with 2019 novel coronavirus in Wuhan, China. *Lancet* **2020**, *395*, 497–506. [CrossRef]
2. Lu, R.; Zhao, X.; Li, J.; Niu, P.; Yang, B.; Wu, H.; Wang, W.; Song, H.; Huang, B.; Zhu, N.; et al. Genomic characterization and epidemiology of 2019 novel coronavirus: Implications for virus origins and receptor binding. *Lancet* **2020**, *395*, 565–574. [CrossRef]
3. Zhu, N.; Zhang, D.; Wang, W.; Li, X.; Yabg, B.; Song, J.; Zhao, X.; Huang, B.; Shi, W.; Lu, R.; et al. China Novel Coronavirus Investigating and Research Team. A novel coronavirus from patients with Pneumonia in China, 2019. *N. Engl. J. Med.* **2020**, *382*, 727–733. [CrossRef] [PubMed]
4. Morens, D.M.; Daszak, P.; Taubenberger, J.K. Escaping Pandora's box—Another novel coronavirus. *N. Engl. J. Med.* **2020**, *382*, 1293–1295. [CrossRef]
5. Available online: https://coronavirus.jhu.edu/map.html (accessed on 31 July 2022).
6. Guan, W.J.; Ni, Z.Y.; Hu, Y.; Liang, W.; Ou, C.; He, J.; Liu, L.; Shan, H.; Lei, C.; Hui, D.; et al. China Medical Treatment Expert Group for Covid-19. Clinical characteristics of coronavirus disease 2019 in China. *N. Engl. J. Med.* **2020**, *382*, 1708–1720. [CrossRef]

7. Vygen-Bonnet, S.; Koch, J.; Bogdan, C.; Harder, T.; Heininger, U.; Kling, K.; Littmann, M.; Meerpohl, J.; Meyer, H.; Mertens, T.; et al. Beschluss und wissenschaftliche begründung der Ständigen Impfkommission (STIKO) für die COVID-19-Impfempfehlung. *Epid. Bull.* **2021**, *2*, 3–63.
8. Mayerhöfer, T.; Klein, S.; Peer, A.; Perschinka, F.; Lehner, G.; Hasslacher, J.; Bellmann, R.; Gasteiger, L.; Mittermayr, M.; Exchertzhuber, S.; et al. Changes in characteristics and outcomes of critically ill COVID-19 patients in Tyrol (Austria) over 1 year. *Wien. Klin. Wochenschr.* **2021**, *133*, 1237–1247. [CrossRef]
9. Gao, Y.; Ding, M.; Dong, X.; Zhang, J.; Azkur, A.; Azkur, D.; Gan, H.; Sun, Y.; Fu, W.; Li, W.; et al. Risk factors for severe and critically ill COVID-19 patients: A review. *Allergy* **2021**, *76*, 428–455. [CrossRef]
10. Gomollón, F.; Dignass, A.; Annese, V.; Tilg, H.; Assche, G.; Lindsay, J.; Peyrin-Biroulet, L.; Cullen, G.; Daperno, M.; Kucharzik, T.; et al. 3rd European Evidence-based Consensus on the diagnosis and Management of Crohn's Disease 2016: Part 1: Diagnosis and Medical Treatment. *J. Crohn's Colitis* **2017**, *11*, 3–25. [CrossRef]
11. Harbord, M.; Eliakim, R.; Bettenworth, D.; Karmiris, K.; Katsanos, K.; Kopylov, U.; Kucharzik, T.; Molnár, T.; Raine, T.; Sebastian, S.; et al. Third European Evidence-based Consensus on Diagnosis and Management of Ulcerative Colitis. Part 2: Current Management. *J. Crohn's Colitis* **2017**, *11*, 769–784. [CrossRef]
12. Aletaha, D.; Smolen, J.S. Diagnosis and management of rheumatoid arthritis: A review. *JAMA* **2018**, *320*, 1360–1372. [CrossRef] [PubMed]
13. Ighani, A.; Partridge, A.; Shear, N.; Lynde, C.; Gulliver, W.; Sibbald, C.; Fleming, P. Comparison of management guidelines for moderate-to-severe plaque psoriasis: A review of phototherapy, systemic therapies, and biologic agents. *J. Cutan. Med. Surg.* **2019**, *23*, 204–221. [CrossRef] [PubMed]
14. Verstockt, B.; Ferrante, M.; Vermeire, S.; Van Assche, G. New treatment options for inflammatory bowel diseases. *J. Gastroenterol.* **2018**, *53*, 585–590. [CrossRef] [PubMed]
15. Kirchgesner, J.; Lemaitre, M.; Carrat, F.; Zureik, M.; Carbonnel, F.; Dray-Spira, R. Risk of serious and opportunistic infections associated with treatment of inflammatory bowel diseases. *Gastroenterology* **2018**, *155*, 337–346.e10. [CrossRef]
16. Kirchgesner, J.; Deai, R.; Beaugerie, L.; Schneeweiss, S.; Kim, S. Risk of serious infections with vedolizumab versus tumor necrosis factor antagonists in patients with inflammatory bowel disease. *Clin. Gastroenterol. Hepatol.* **2022**, *20*, 314–324. [CrossRef]
17. Restellini, S.; Pittet, V. Inflammatory Bowel Disease and COVID-19. ECCO Letter. Published 30 September 2020. Available online: https://ecco-ibd.eu/publications/ecco-news/item/inflammatory-bowel-disease-and-covid-19.html (accessed on 31 July 2022).
18. Alunno, A.; Najm, A.; Machado, P.; Bertheussen, H.; Burmester, G.; Carubbi, F.; De Mraco, G.; Giacomelli, R.; Hermine, O.; Isaacs, J.; et al. EULAR points to consider on pathophysiology and use of Immunomodulatory therapies in COVID-19. *Ann. Rheum. Dis.* **2021**, *80*, 698–706. [CrossRef] [PubMed]
19. COVID-19 Clinical Guidance for Adult Patients with Rheumatic Diseases, Developed by the ACR COVID-19 Clinical Guidance Task Force. Available online: https://www.rheumatology.org/Portals/0/Files/ACR-COVID-19-Clinical-Guidance-Summary-Patients-with-Rheumatic-Diseases.pdf (accessed on 31 July 2022).
20. Lin, S.; Lau, L.; Chanchlani, L.; Kennedy, N.; Ng, S. Recent advances in clinical practice: Management of inflammatory bowel disease during the COVID-19 pandemic. *Gut* **2022**, *71*, 1426–1439. [CrossRef] [PubMed]
21. Scaldaferri, F.; Pugliese, D.; Privitera, G.; Onali, S.; Lopetuso, L.; Rizzati, G.; Settanni, C.; Pizzoferrato, M.; Schiavoni, E.; Turchini, L.; et al. Impact of COVID-19 pandemic on the daily management of biotechnological therapy in inflammatory bowel disease patients: Reorganisational response in a high-volume Italian inflammatory bowel disease centre. *United Eur. Gastroenterol. J.* **2020**, *8*, 775–781. [CrossRef]
22. Saibeni, S.; Scucchi, L.; Dragoni, G.; Bezzio, C.; Miranda, A.; Ribaldone, D.; Bertani, A.; Bossa, F.; Allocca, M.; Buda, D.; et al. Activities related to inflammatory bowel disease management during and after the coronavirus disease 2019 lockdown in Italy: How to maintain standards of care. *United Eur. Gastroenterol. J.* **2020**, *8*, 1228–1235. [CrossRef]
23. Allocca, M.; Fiorino, G.; Furfaro, F.; Gilardi, D.; Radice, S.; D'Amico, F.; Zilli, A.; Danese, S. Maintaining the Quality Standards of Care for Inflammatory Bowel Disease Patients during the COVID-19 pandemic. *Clin. Gastroenterol. Hepatol.* **2020**, *18*, 1882–1883. [CrossRef]
24. Shintaro, A.; Shadi, H.; Dejan, M.; Sakuraba, A. Prevalence and Clinical outcomes of COVID-19 in patients with autoimmune diseases: A systematic review and meta-analysis. *Ann. Rheum. Dis.* **2021**, *80*, 384–391.
25. Ungaro, C.; Brenner, E.; Gearry, R.; Kaplan, G.; Kissous-Hung, M.; Lewis, J.; Ng, S.; Rahier, J.; Reinisch, W.; Steinwurz, F.; et al. Effect of IBD medications on COVID-19 outcomes: Results from an international registry. *Gut* **2021**, *70*, 725–732. [CrossRef] [PubMed]
26. Bachiller-Corral, J.; Boteanu, A.; Garcia-Villanueva, M.; Puente, C.; Revenga, M.; Diaz-Miguel, M.; Rodriguez-Garcia, A.; Morell-Hita, J.; Valero, M.; Larena, C.; et al. Risk of severe COVID-19 infection in patients with inflammatory rheumatic diseases. *J. Rheumatol.* **2021**, *48*, 1098–1102. [CrossRef] [PubMed]
27. Dejaco, C.; Alunno, A.; Bijlsma, J.; Boonen, A.; Combe, B.; Finckh, A.; Machado, P.; Padjen, I.; Sivera, F.; Stamm, T.; et al. Influence of COVID-19 pandemic on decisions for the management of people with inflammatory rheumatic and musculoskeletal diseases: A survey among EULAR countries. *Ann. Rheum. Dis.* **2020**, *80*, 518–526. [CrossRef]
28. Ansarin, K.; Taghizadieh, A.; Safiri, S.; Mahdavi, A.; Ranjbar, S.; Teymouri, S.; Maleki, M.; Khabbazi, A. COVID-19 outcomes in patients with systemic autoimmune diseases treated with immunomodulatory drugs. *Ann. Rheum. Dis.* Online ahead of print. 2020. [CrossRef]

29. Emmi, G.; Bettiol, A.; Mattioli, I.; Silvestri, E.; Di Scala, G.; Urban, M.; Vaglio, A.; Prisco, D. SARS-CoV-2 infection among patients with systemic autoimmune diseases. *Autoimmun. Rev.* **2020**, *19*, 102575. [CrossRef]
30. Fredi, M.; Cavazzana, I.; Moschetti, L.; Andreoli, L.; Franceschini, F. COVID-19 in patients with rheumatic diseases in northern Italy: A single-centre observa- tional and case-control study. *Lancet Rheumatol.* **2020**, *2*, e549–e556. [CrossRef]
31. Liu, M.; Gao, Y.; Zhang, Y.; Shi, S.; Chen, Y.; Tian, J. The association between severe or dead COVID-19 and autoimmune diseases: A systematic review and meta-analysis. *J. Infect.* **2020**, *81*, e93–e95. [CrossRef]
32. Macaluso, F.S.; Orlando, A. COVID-19 in patients with inflamma- tory bowel disease: A systematic review of clinical data. *Digest. Liver Dis.* **2020**, *52*, 1222–1227. [CrossRef]
33. D'Silva, K.M.; Serling-Boyd, N.; Wallwork, R.; Hsu, T.; Fu, X.; Gravallese, E.; Choi, H.; Sparks, J.; Wallace, Z. Clinical characteristics and outcomes of patients with coronavirus disease 2019 (COVID-19) and rheumatic disease: A comparative cohort study from a US hot spot. *Ann. Rheum. Dis.* **2020**, *79*, 1156–1162. [CrossRef]
34. Gianfrancesco, M.; Hyrich, K.L.; Al-Adely, S.; Carmona, L.; Danila, M.; Gossec, L.; Izadi, Z.; Jacobsohn, L.; Katz, P.; Lawson-Tovey, S.; et al. Characteristics associated with hospitalisation for COVID-19 in people with rheumatic disease: Data from the COVID-19 Global Rheuma- tology Alliance physician-reported registry. *Ann. Rheum. Dis.* **2020**, *79*, 859–866. [CrossRef]
35. Pablos, J.L.; Galindo, M.; Carmona, L.; Lledó, A.; Retuerto, M.; Blanco, R.; Gonzalez-Gay, M.; Martinez-Lopez, D.; Castrejón, I.; Alvaro-Gracia, J.; et al. Clinical outcomes of hospitalised patients with COVID-19 and chronic inflammatory and autoimmune rheumatic diseases: A multicentric matched cohort study. *Ann. Rheum. Dis.* **2020**, *79*, 1544–1549. [CrossRef] [PubMed]
36. Bower, H.; Frisell, T.; Giuseppe, D.; Delcoigne, B.; Alenius, G.M.; Baecklund, E.; Chatzidionysiou, K.; Feltelius, N.; Forsblad-d'Elia, H.; Kastbom, A.; et al. Effects oft he COVID-19 pandemic on patients with inflammatory joint diseases in Sweden: From infection severity to impact on care provision. *RMD Open* **2021**, *7*, e001987. [CrossRef]
37. Ungaro, R.C.; Brenner, E.; Agrawal, M.; Zhang, X.; Kappelman, M.; Colombel, J.F. Impact of medications on COVID-19 outcomes in inflammatory bowel disease: Analysis of more than 6000 patients from an international registry. *Gastroenterology* **2022**, *162*, 316–319. [CrossRef]
38. Kridin, K.; Schonmann, Y.; Bitan, D.; Damiani, G.; Peretz, A.; Weinstein, O.; Cohen, A. Coronavirus disease 2019 (COVID-19)-associated hospitalization and mortality in patitnets with psoriasis: A population-based study. *Am. J. Clin. Dermatol.* **2021**, *22*, 709–718. [CrossRef] [PubMed]
39. Izadi, Z.; Brenner, E.; Mahil, S.; Dand, N.; Yiu, Z.; Yates, M.; Ungaro, R.; Zhang, X.; Agrawal, M.; Colombel, J.F. Association between tumor necrosis factor inhibitors and the risk of hopitalisation or death among patients with immune-mediated inflammatory disesase and COVID-19. *JAMA Netw. Open* **2021**, *4*, e2129639. [CrossRef] [PubMed]
40. Regierer, A.C.; Hasseli, R.; Schäfer, M.; Hoyer, B.; Krause, A.; Lorenz, H.M.; Pfeil, A.; Richter, J.; Schmeiser, T.; Schulze-Koops, H.; et al. TNFi is associated with positive outcome, but JAKi and rituximab are associated with negative outcomes of SARS-CoV-2 infection in patients with RMD. *RMD Open* **2021**, *7*, e001896. [CrossRef]
41. Magro, F.; Rahier, J.-F.; Abreu, C.; MacMahon, E.; Hart, A.; Van der Woude, C.; Gordon, H.; Adamina, M.; Viget, N.; Vavricka, S.; et al. Inflammatory Bowel Disease Management During the COVID-19 Outbreak: The Ten Do's and Don'ts from the ECCO-COVID Taskforce. *J. Crohn's Colitis* **2020**, *14* (Suppl. S3), S798–S806. [CrossRef]
42. Morris, E.; Goldacre, R.; Spata, E.; Mafham, M.; Finan, P.; Shelton, J.; Richards, M.; Spencer, K.; Emberson, J.; Hollings, S.; et al. Impact of the COVID-19 pandemic on the detection and management of colorectal cancer in England: A population-based study. *Lancet Gastroenterol. Hepatol.* **2021**, *6*, 199–208. [CrossRef]
43. Groen, M.; Derks, M.; Kuijpers, C.; Nagtegaal, I.; Hoentjen, F. Reduction in Inflammatory Bowel Disease Healthcare during the Coronavirus Disease 2019 Pandemic: A nationwide retrospective cohort study. *Gastroenterology* **2021**, *160*, 935–937. [CrossRef]
44. Mendelsohn, A.; Nam, Y.; Marshall, J.; McDermott, C.; Kochar, B.; Kappelman, M.; Brown, J.; Lockhart, C. Utilization patterns and characteristics of users of biologic anti-inflammatory agents in a large, US commercially insured population. *Pharmacol. Res. Perspect.* **2021**, *9*, e00708. [CrossRef]
45. Han, J.; Lee, J.; Han, K.; Seo, H.; Bang, C.; Park, Y.; Lee, J.; Park, Y. Epidemiology and medication trends in patients with Psoriasis: A nationwide population-based Cohort Study from Korea. *Acta Derm. Venereol.* **2018**, *98*, 396–400. [CrossRef] [PubMed]
46. Sánchez-Piedra, C.; Sueiro-Delgado, D.; García-González, J.; Ros-Vilamajo, I.; Prior-Español, A.; Moreno-Ramos, M.; Garcia-Magallon, B.; Calvo-Gutiérrez, J.; Perez-Vera, Y.; Martín-Domenech, R.; et al. Changes in the use patterns of bDMARDs in patients with rheumatic diseases over the past 13 years. *Sci. Rep.* **2021**, *11*, 15051. [CrossRef] [PubMed]
47. Alulis, S.; Vadstrup, K.; Borsi, A.; Nielsen, A.; Jørgensen, T.; Qvist, N.; Munkholm, P. Treatment patterns for biologics in ulcerative colitis and Crohn's disease: A Danish nationwide register study from 2003 to 2015. *Scand. J. Gastroenterol.* **2020**, *55*, 265–271. [CrossRef] [PubMed]
48. Torres, J.; Bonovas, S.; Doherty, G.; Kucharzik, T.; Gisbert, J.; Raine, T.; Adamina, M.; Armuzzi, A.; Bachmann, O.; Bager, P.; et al. on behalf of the European Crohn's and Colitis Organisation [ECCO], ECCO Guidelines on Therapeutics in Crohn's Disease: Medical Treatment. *J. Crohn's Colitis* **2020**, *14*, 4–22. [CrossRef]
49. Raine, T.; Bonovas, S.; Burisch, J.; Kucharzik, T.; Adamina, M.; Annese, V.; Bachmann, O.; Bettenworth, D.; Chaparro, M.; Czuber-Dochan, W.; et al. ECCO Guidelines on Therapeutics in Ulcerative Colitis: Medical Treatment. *J. Crohn's Colitis* **2022**, *16*, 2–17. [CrossRef]

50. Alunno, A.; Najm, A.; Machado, P.M.; Bertheussen, H.; Burmester, G.R.; Carubbi, F.; De Marco, G.; Giacomelli, R.; Hermine, O.; Isaacs, J.; et al. 2021 update of the EULAR points to consider on the use of immunomodulatory therapies in COVID-19. *Ann. Rheum. Dis.* **2022**, *81*, 34–40. [CrossRef]
51. Menter, A.; Strober, B.E.; Kaplan, D.H.; Kivelevitch, D.; Prater, E.; Stoff, B.; Armstrong, A.; Connor, C.; Cordoro, K.; Davis, D.; et al. Joint AAD-NPF guidelines of care for the management and treatment of psoriasis with biologics. *J. Am. Acad Dermatol.* **2019**, *80*, 1029–1072. [CrossRef]
52. Alatab, S.; Sepanlou, S.; Ikuta, K.; Vahedi, H.; Bisignano, C.; Safiri, S.; Sadeghi, A.; Nixon, M.; Abdoli, A.; Abolhassani, H.; et al. on behalf of the GBD 2017 Inflammatory Bowel Disease Collaborators. The global, regional, and national burden of inflammatory bowel disease in 195 countries and territories, 1990–2017: A systematic analysis for the global burden of disease study 2017. *Lancet Gastroenterol. Hepatol.* **2020**, *5*, 17–30. [CrossRef]

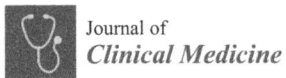

Review

Endocrinological Involvement in Children and Adolescents Affected by COVID-19: A Narrative Review

Valeria Calcaterra [1,2,*,†], Veronica Maria Tagi [2,†], Raffaella De Santis [2], Andrea Biuso [2], Silvia Taranto [2], Enza D'Auria [2] and Gianvincenzo Zuccotti [2,3]

1. Department of Internal Medicine and Therapeutics, University of Pavia, 27100 Pavia, Italy
2. Department of Pediatrics, Vittore Buzzi Children's Hospital, 20154 Milan, Italy; veronica.tagi@gmail.com (V.M.T.); raffaella.desantis@unimi.it (R.D.S.); andreabiuso@gmail.com (A.B.); silvia.taranto@unimi.it (S.T.); enza.dauria@unimi.it (E.D.); gianvincenzo.zuccotti@unimi.it (G.Z.)
3. Department of Biomedical and Clinical Sciences, University of Milan, 20122 Milan, Italy
* Correspondence: valeria.calcaterra@unipv.it
† These authors contributed equally to this work.

Abstract: Since the advent of the severe acute respiratory syndrome coronavirus 2 (SARS-CoV-2) pandemic, an increased incidence of several endocrinological anomalies in acute-phase and/or long-term complications has been described. The aim of this review is to provide a broad overview of the available literature regarding changes in the worldwide epidemiology of endocrinological involvement in children since December 2019 and to report the evidence supporting its association with coronavirus disease 2019 (COVID-19). Although little is known regarding the involvement of endocrine organs during COVID-19 in children, the current evidence in adults and epidemiological studies on the pediatric population suggest the presence of a causal association between the virus and endocrinopathies. Untreated transient thyroid dysfunction, sick euthyroid syndrome, nonthyroidal illness syndrome, and hypothalamic–pituitary–adrenal (HPA) axis and central precocious puberty have been observed in children in acute infection and/or during multisystem inflammatory syndrome development. Furthermore, a higher frequency of ketoacidosis at onset in children with a new diagnosis of type 1 diabetes is reported in the literature. Although the direct association between COVID-19 and endocrinological involvement has not been confirmed yet, data on the development of different endocrinopathies in children, both during acute infection and as a result of its long-term complications, have been reported. This information is of primary importance to guide the management of patients with previous or current COVID-19.

Keywords: SARS-CoV-2; COVID-19; thyroid disease; adrenal glands; hypothalamus; hypophysis; precocious puberty; gonad; diabetes; children; adolescents

1. Introduction

Early after the first description of severe acute respiratory syndrome coronavirus 2 (SARS-CoV-2), there was strong evidence of a milder clinical presentation of the infection in most children, with 90% of cases being asymptomatic, mild, or moderate [1]. The prevalence of severe coronavirus disease 2019 (COVID-19) in children also remained low after the spread of new variants with greater transmissibility, like delta and omicron [2]. These findings have been attributed to several immunological mechanisms distinguishing children from adults, including a higher production of interferons at the mucosal surface, which rapidly alert the immune system at the first sign of infection [3]; a faster innate immune response due to their mostly untrained T cells, which are more likely to respond to novel viruses; and expression of acquired specific antibodies or memory cells through previous exposure to the endemic coronaviruses that commonly circulate among infants [4].

Citation: Calcaterra, V.; Tagi, V.M.; De Santis, R.; Biuso, A.; Taranto, S.; D'Auria, E.; Zuccotti, G. Endocrinological Involvement in Children and Adolescents Affected by COVID-19: A Narrative Review. *J. Clin. Med.* **2023**, *12*, 5248. https://doi.org/10.3390/jcm12165248

Academic Editors: Francesco Pugliese, Francesco Alessandri and Giovanni Giordano

Received: 27 May 2023
Revised: 5 August 2023
Accepted: 10 August 2023
Published: 11 August 2023

Copyright: © 2023 by the authors. Licensee MDPI, Basel, Switzerland. This article is an open access article distributed under the terms and conditions of the Creative Commons Attribution (CC BY) license (https://creativecommons.org/licenses/by/4.0/).

Despite their less severe manifestations in the acute phase, two main long-term complications of COVID-19 have been reported in children: multisystem inflammatory syndrome in children (MIS-C) and long COVID.

MIS-C is a serious and potentially fatal complication involving the cardiovascular system and other organs such as the stomach, liver, and intestines, with an estimated incidence of 316 every 1,000,000 children infected with SARS-CoV-2 before the availability of vaccines [5]. Since the symptoms typically begin four to six weeks after the initial infection, it has been hypothesized that the virus remains in children's gut, causing an irritation in its mucosa. For this reason, viral antigens manage to pass through the gut's barrier to circulation, reaching other organs and triggering a major inflammatory response [6].

Long COVID is a heterogeneous multisystemic condition characterized by the persistence of signs and symptoms that occur three months from the onset of COVID-19 and last at least two months and cannot be explained by an alternative diagnosis [7]

Lopez-Leon et al. [8] conducted a systematic review, showing a prevalence of long COVID in pediatric patients of 25.24%. The most frequently reported symptoms were mood alterations (16.50%), fatigue (9.66%), sleep disorders (8.42%), headache (7.84%), and respiratory symptoms (7.62%). Similar to adults, the detected risk factors for the development of long COVID in children are older age, female sex, severe COVID-19, overweight/obesity, comorbid allergic diseases, and other long-term comorbidities [8]. No guidelines exist to address long COVID diagnosis and management. The underlying pathogenetic mechanisms and correct management of these patients have not yet been defined [8].

SARS-CoV-2 is known to interact with the host cells through its spike protein by binding to the membrane enzyme angiotensin converting enzyme 2 (ACE2). Once the virus enters the cells, the STAT3/NF-kB pathway is activated, causing the production of proinflammatory cytokines and chemokines, which leads to a systemic hyperinflammation known as "cytokine storm" [9].

ACE2 is not expressed only by the lung cells: it is ubiquitarian, which explains the multiorgan impairment typically observed in COVID-19 [10].

Endocrine tissues express ACE2 as well, especially at the level of the thyroid, ovaries and testis, and this may be responsible for the endocrinological involvement during SARS-CoV-2 infection [11,12]. Since the advent of the pandemic, there has been increases in the incidence of several endocrinological anomalies and in the severity of their manifestations in both adults and children [13].

The aim of this narrative review is to provide an overview of the available literature regarding the epidemiology of the endocrinological involvement in children since December 2019 and to report the evidence supporting its association with COVID-19. To revise data on the endocrine disorders during SARS-CoV-2 infection, it is useful to define adequate pediatric long-term monitoring.

2. Materials and Methods

A narrative review on the potential connections between SARS-CoV-2 infection and endocrinological impairment in children was performed. We conducted an extensive literature search on PubMed and Embase, with language restricted to English only and publication dates between 2019 and present time (1 May 2023), divided by different organs or systems. We included in our review all types of articles (original article, review, met-analysis, case report, case series, and clinical practice guideline) regarding children aged 1–18 years with a proven ongoing or previous SARS-CoV-2 infection or diagnosis of MIS-C who experienced an impairment of one or more of the main endocrine organs or systems involved in children with COVID19: thyroid, adrenal glands, hypothalamus–pituitary system, gonads and pancreas. Articles focusing only on adults were excluded from our review. The list of keywords used for each analyzed endocrine system or organ and the respective type and number of articles found are summarized in Table 1. Starting from a total of 424 papers screened by title/abstract, the authors reviewed the full texts of relevant articles (*n* = 190).

Table 1. List of keywords used in our literature search categorized by endocrine system or organ and respective type and number of articles found.

Endocrine System or Organ	Keywords	Number of Suitable Articles (Total Number)	Type of Article
Thyroid	"thyroid" OR "hyperthyroidism" OR "hypothyroidism" OR "thyroiditis" AND "coronavirus disease 2019" OR "COVID-19" OR "SARS-CoV-2" OR "MIS-C" OR "multisystem inflammatory syndrome" AND "children" OR "adolescents"	12 (33)	1 cross-sectional study 3 cohort studies 1 case control study 1 retrospective case note review 1 cross-sectional chart review 2 narrative reviews 3 case reports
Adrenal glands	"adrenal insufficiency" OR "hypercortisolism" AND "coronavirus disease 2019" OR "COVID-19" OR "SARS-CoV-2" OR "MIS-C" OR "multisystem inflammatory syndrome" AND "children" OR "adolescents"	10 (10)	2 narrative reviews 2 single-center or multicenter cohort studies 1 cross-sectional study 1 clinical practice guideline 4 case reports
Hypothalamus-pituitary system	"hypothalamus" OR "pituitary" OR "Hypopituitarism" OR "hypophysitis" OR "growth hormone" OR "central precocious puberty" AND "coronavirus disease 2019" OR "COVID-19" OR "SARS-CoV-2" OR "MIS-C" OR "multisystem inflammatory syndrome" AND "children" OR "adolescents"	34 (96)	4 cross-sectional studies 1 case control study 17 retrospective studies 9 reviews 3 case reports
Gonads	"puberty" OR "central precocious puberty" AND "coronavirus disease 2019" OR "COVID-19" OR "SARS-CoV-2" OR "MIS-C" OR "multisystem inflammatory syndrome" AND "children" OR "adolescents"	32 (32)	5 narrative reviews 1 cohort study 6 cross-sectional studies 20 case-control studies
Pancreas	"type 1 diabetes" OR "juvenile onset diabetes" OR "insulin-dependent diabetes" OR "T1D" AND "coronavirus disease 2019" OR "COVID-19" OR "SARS-CoV-2" OR "MIS-C" OR "multisystem inflammatory syndrome" AND "children" OR "adolescents"	102 (253)	2 meta-analyses 6 narrative reviews 72 cohort studies 9 cross-sectional studies 2 case-control studies 11 case reports or case series

3. Thyroid

Very limited studies and reports describe the association between SARS-CoV-2 infection and thyroid disease in pediatric subjects [14,15]. McCowan et al. [14] conducted a study on 244 children with anomalies in thyroid function, either hypothyroidism or hyperthyroidism, in a tertiary pediatric endocrine center in the United Kingdom before and after COVID-19 to identify any change in their presentation. Despite an unchanged rate of thyroid dysfunction before and after the pandemic, they observed an increase in the number of cases of untreated transient thyroid dysfunction. They speculated that this finding may be due to the development of thyroiditis secondary to SARS-CoV-2 infection, which regressed before requiring treatment [14].

A retrospective chart analysis on 233 children screened for TSH level in New York did not find any significant difference in the frequency of TSH abnormalities prior and after the pandemic started. However, it is unknown who had a prior COVID-19 infection or who received anti-SARS-CoV-2 vaccination among them [16].

A cross-sectional analytical study assessed the levels of free thyroxine (fT4), fT3, TSH and inflammatory markers, especially interleukin-6 (IL-6), in hospitalized children and adults with moderate-to-severe COVID-19 infection [17]. In total, 67.7% of all patients and 78% of the pediatric population had an abnormal thyroid profile, with sick euthyroid syndrome, which is characterized by low fT3 levels with normal TSH levels, associated with a systemic illness, being the most frequent. This status was associated with a significantly higher risk of death and severe inflammation (detected using high IL-6 levels), highlighting the importance of monitoring thyroid function test results in patients with severe COVID-19 infection [17]. The higher reported incidence of thyroid dysfunction in comparison to other studies, where most analyzed patients presented with mild COVID-19, suggests a correlation of the severity of the disease with thyroid gland impairment [15,18]. In line with these data, a retrospective study on pediatric patients referred to our center and diagnosed with MIS-C revealed that more than 90% of patients exhibited nonthyroidal illness syndrome (NTIS), defined as any abnormality in thyroid function (TF) tests (FT3, FT4, and TSH) in the presence of critical illness and absence of a pre-existing hormonal abnormality [19]. Among the NTIS laboratory profile variants, an isolated decrease in the level of fT3 was the most common [19]. Concordant data were obtained from a subsequent prospective cohort study on a population of 43 children and adolescents with MIS-C, where 79% of patients presented low FT3 levels, which, in 10 cases, was associated with abnormal values of fT4 and/or TSH. Twenty months later, a restoration of TH balance was observed in 100% of patients [20].

The association of MIS-C with thyroid disfunction was also studied in another cohort of 46 children and an aged-matched control group. Also in this case, NTIS was reported in 97.2% of MIS-C cases. Moreover, the FT3 levels were lower in patients with MIS-C who were admitted to the ICU with worse clinical presentations [21].

Although the available data regarding the involvement of thyroid function during COVID-19 infection in childhood are still limited, the current evidence supports the theory that the virus plays a certain role in thyroid dysfunction, which is transitory in most cases. Therefore, given the heterogeneity of dysthyroid manifestations, it would be useful to routinely assess thyroid function indices in patients with a COVID-19 infection, especially if they present with moderate to severe disease signs and MIS-C in order to start, when needed, the appropriate treatment as soon as possible [13].

It has been hypothesized that SARS-CoV-2 may enter the thyroid cells via ACE2 and transmembrane serine protease (2TMPRSS2), which is highly expressed in this gland [22,23]. It is well known that viral-infections-related thyroiditis causes preformed colloid release and consequently impairs raised thyroid hormone concentrations. Furthermore, COVID-19 may destroy follicular cells through an autoimmune mechanism [24]. Indeed, virus-induced cytokine storm is characterized by hyperactivity of the Th1/Th17 immune response with overexpression of proinflammatory cytokines, such as IL-6, which has been demonstrated to be strongly associated with thyroiditis [25]. The latter has been tested in adult populations, assessing patients' thyroid antibody status. A study conducted in India revealed positivity of anti-TPO antibodies in 13.6% of the participants [26]. A similar frequency was observed in a large group of European patients, 23.6% of whom were seropositive for at least one thyroid autoantibody [27]. Regarding this hypothesis, Flokas et al. [28] reported an interesting case of a 14-year-old girl with vitiligo who was hospitalized for hypotensive shock following COVID-19 infection, initially treated as MIS-C and afterward discovered to be autoimmune thyroiditis and primary adrenal insufficiency. The concomitance of these autoimmune conditions led to the diagnosis of autoimmune polyglandular syndrome 2 (APS2) [28]. The role of COVID-19 in the ethiopathogenesis of APS2 is unclear, but it might be the trigger of the rapid progression of both adrenal insufficiency and hypothyroidism [28].

A third potential mechanism is a selective transient pituitary dysregulation, secondary either to the direct cytotoxic effect of the virus on the hypophysis and an indirect effect of the cytokine storm that would induce NTIS [29–32].

It must be also taken into account that the COVID-19 pandemic reduced the general population's access to health services worldwide, and this could have had an impact on the severity of thyroid disease at diagnosis in adults [33], as also suggested by a study conducted in the United Kingdom, where nearly 1/3 of children with trisomy 21 did not receive the recommended annual TSH screening in 2020, in comparison with 3% in 2015 [34].

4. Adrenal Glands

COVID-19 infection in children has been associated with adrenal gland involvement. As reported, the infection can cause primary adrenal insufficiency, mediated by the activation of cytokines, such as IL-6 and toll-like receptors (TLR), and secondary failure due to glucocorticoids, one of the main treatments for children affected by MIS-C. A retrospective study conducted in a tertiary pediatric hospital in the U.K. collected data from a population of more than 100 children with MIS-C; prolonged and high-dose steroid therapy is often used in severe MIS-C and it can cause hypothalamic–pituitary–adrenal (HPA) axis suppression [35]. A case of an 11-year-old Turkish boy with adrenal insufficiency during MIS-C is reported in the literature; adrenal function was still impaired at a 4-month follow-up [36]. Flokas et al. [28] reported the case of a 14-year-old girl with vitiligo, with new-onset of autoimmune polyglandular syndrome type 2 (hypothyroidism and primary adrenal insufficiency) shortly after SARS-CoV-2 infection. The authors concluded that it would be prudent to monitor autoimmune conditions triggered by SARS-CoV-2 infection, especially in patients with previous autoimmune diseases [28].

On the other hand, patients who already suffer from primary or secondary adrenal insufficiency have an increased vulnerability to infections, including to COVID-19; SARS-CoV-2 infection could trigger a potential life-threatening condition such as an adrenal crisis due to an increased demand of glucocorticoids, both in adults and children. Close monitoring of these patients is then recommended. In particular, in cases of mild to moderate infection, clinical practice guidelines recommend to double or triple the usual daily hydrocortisone dose; in cases of severe infection or profuse vomiting, medical evaluation is mandatory to initiate parenteral administration of glucocorticoids. Only close monitoring is recommended in asymptomatic patients [37]. A multicentric study, conducted in 12 centers in 8 European countries between January 2020 and December 2021, reported data from 64 patients (13 of those children) with adrenal insufficiency and acute SARS-CoV-2 infection; the clinical outcome in this population appeared good with appropriate glucocorticoid dose adjustments [38].

Even if there is evidence in the literature that the population with adrenal insufficiency is at higher risk of SARS-CoV-2 infection, which can lead to adrenal crisis, data are still conflicting regarding the more severe clinical course of the COVID-19 disease in these patients. Banull et at. [39] conducted a retrospective study, collecting data of 390 pediatric patients, concluding that children with a pre-existing endocrine condition, such as diabetes mellitus, adrenal insufficiency, or hypothyroidism, can have a more severe clinical presentation in case of SARS-CoV-2 infection, with a higher risk of hospitalization and/or intensive care unit admission. Chien et al. [40] reported a case of a 17-year-old boy with a positive test for SARS-CoV-2, fever, and neurological symptoms (altered mental status, seizures), with a history of surgical resection of a craniopharyngioma; a prompt hydrocortisone dose rapidly resolved neurological symptoms. The authors concluded that early recognition and treatment with corticosteroids can prevent long-term consequences, especially in patients with brain tumors or Addison's disease. An Italian study also reported the case of a 9-year-old child infected with SARS-CoV-2 with a history of suprasellar nongerminomatous germ cell tumor, diabetes insipidus, and hypothalamic-pituitary failure [41].

Also, children may suffer from tertiary adrenal insufficiency due to chronic treatment with corticosteroids for other medical conditions and subsequent iatrogenic immune impairment, with an increased risk of SARS-CoV-2 infection and more severe clinical course [37]. So, endogenous conditions leading to hypercortisolism, such as Cushing syndrome, may also represent a risk factor for SARS-CoV-2 infection and a severe course of the disease. There are no available data in the literature on the association between COVID-19 and hypercortisolism in children. Furthermore, it is important to consider that chronic cortisol excess leads not only to immune impairment but also to comorbidities (hypertension, obesity, and hyperglycemia), which are associated with a higher risk of severe COVID-19 disease.

To summarize, SARS-CoV-2 infection may be responsible, in children, for both direct and indirect HPA axis alteration due to glucocorticoids treatment in case of MIS-C. On the other hand, children who already have an impairment of adrenal function, insufficiency or hypercortisolism need careful monitoring in case of COVID-19 disease.

5. Hypothalamic–Pituitary Involvement

In the literature, there are very limited data about the association between SARS-CoV-2 and the hypothalamic–pituitary axis in children and adolescents.

As with its predecessors, SARS-CoV-2 may enter the central nervous system through the olfactory bulb, reaching hypothalamus and hypophysis [41], which constitute putative targets for this virus due to the expression of ACE-2 receptors and TMPRSS2 on the surfaces of hypothalamic and pituitary cells [42–44].

Different injury mechanisms regarding COVID-19 infection and the hypothalamic–pituitary axis have been hypothesized in the literature: direct hypothalamic injury induced by the virus itself, reversible immune-mediated hypophysitis, molecular mimicry between specific virus sequences and ACTH with subsequent cross-reaction, massive cytokine production that reduces ACTH release, decreasing its effect on adrenal tissue [44–50].

5.1. Pituitary Gland Involvement of SARS-CoV-2 Virus

One of the few cases reported in the literature of a potential involvement of hypophysis by SARS-CoV-2 in children is for a 4-year-old girl with a rapid-onset obesity with hypothalamic dysfunction, hypoventilation, and autonomic dysregulation (ROHHAD)-syndrome-like phenotype after COVID-19 infection: she developed electrolyte alterations (hypernatremia and hyperchloremia), hypocorticism and hypothyroidism, central hypoventilation, bulimia, and progressive obesity with metabolic disimpairment. The MRI of the brain showed mild posthypoxic changes, and the condition was resolved with nonsteroidal anti-inflammatory drugs and monthly courses of intravenous immunoglobulin [51].

The second case of the involvement of hypophysis of the virus concerns an 18-year-old previously healthy girl who presented with symptomatic lymphocytic hypophysitis three weeks after COVID-19 (the first ever reported in the literature). She complained of acute onset headache and dizziness for 5 days. This condition was documented with a brain MRI and treated with methylprednisolone 250 mg IV every 6 h on days 1–3; on day 3, they observed symptomatic clinical improvement with a significant decrease in the intensity of the headaches [52].

5.2. SARS-CoV-2 Infection in Children with Pre-Existing Hypothalamic–Pituitary Axis Dysfunction

There is no evidence that children affected by hypopituitarism present a higher risk of contracting COVID-19 infection or experiencing a severe disease course, not even patients affected by secondary adrenal insufficiency [40,53].

As evidence of this, R. Gaudino et al. [40] reported the case of a 9-year-old boy with SARS-CoV-2 and a recent diagnosis of suprasellar nongerminomatous germ cell tumor, also suffering from diabetes insipidus and hypothalamic–pituitary failure, who remained asymptomatic for the duration of the infection without requiring any change in his habitual replacement therapy.

What has emerged in these years, however, is that patients affected by hypopituitarism and secondary adrenal insufficiency potentially have a higher risk of undergoing adrenal crisis during the SARS-CoV-2 infection, as with any other infection [13].

5.3. Growth Hormone (GH) Release and Precocious Puberty during SARS-CoV-2 Pandemic

During COVID-19, we have also witnessed two opposing phenomena: a reduction in pediatric GH deficiency and an increase in central precocious puberty (CPP) diagnoses [54].

Regarding tests investigating pediatric GH deficiency, Peinkhofer et al. [54] detected a striking reduction (−35%) in tests performed in 2020 compared with 2019, in contrast with the trend of previous years, which consisted of an in increase in referrals for growth issues. Some hypotheses postulated to explain this phenomenon are that both pediatricians and families had less opportunity to detect short stature and delayed growth because of fewer well-child visits and fewer chances to compare their children with classmates; moreover, some appointments were probably cancelled during pandemic due to the tendency to avoid hospitals [54].

Regarding CPP diagnoses, COVID-19 infection in children has been associated with several endocrine disorders.

Many retrospective and cross-sectional studies have reported a significant increase during the pandemic in central CPP diagnoses and in pubertal progression rate in patients already diagnosed with CPP compared with the prepandemic period [54–80].

The first retrospective study reporting an increase in CPP diagnoses and a faster rate of pubertal progression during the first lockdown (March–July 2020), compared with the same period in the previous five years, was conducted by Stagi et al. [76]. The first hypothesis was that BMI increase and electronic device overuse were both significantly higher in the pandemic group [76]. In following retrospective Italian studies, no significant differences in BMI increase were found in patients diagnosed with CPP during the pandemic [54,79,80], but Umano et al. reported sleep disturbances as a frequent comorbidity [80].

The same trend was reported all over the world. In a retrospective study by Fu et al., the data from 22 medical institutions in China showed that 4281 female patients were diagnosed with new-onset precocious puberty between February and May 2020, five times more than observed in the same period in 2018 and three times more than observed in the same period in 2019; the authors also reported weight and BMI were significantly higher in the 2020 group [70]. All the studies cited above reported the same increase in CPP diagnoses, especially in women, and a faster rate of pubertal progression, but a correlation with a BMI increase during the pandemic was not always found.

Many authors then tried to explain this new trend. SARS-CoV-2 infection may have direct and indirect effects on puberty. Focusing on direct effects, three main possible mechanisms have been considered, but they need to be investigated further as they are still poorly understood: direct inflammation of the olfactory bulb, which shares a common embryogenic origin with the hypothalamic GnRH neurons; blood–brain barrier disruption; and cytokine storm [81]. The indirect effects of SARS-CoV-2 probably played a more significant role in this outbreak of CPP diagnoses, and they consist of physical and psychosocial changes due to lockdown and social distancing during the pandemic. Among the social effects, stress fear and anxiety linked to social distancing and lack of physical activity, family mourning, and the worldwide burden of pandemic might have played a fundamental role. In fact, these psychological conditions may activate GABA A receptors and consequently the stress pathways responsible for puberty onset [82]. Regarding physical changes, reductions in physical activity, increased BMI, and glucose and insulin metabolism alterations have been widely reported in children and adolescents during the pandemic, and obesity has been associated with the secular trend in puberty anticipation [83]. Also, even hyperinsulinemia not associated with obesity has been correlated with precocious puberty, since insulin resistance may be responsible for an increased bioavailability of sex hormones [84]. Other factors that may be associated with this trend include increased screen time due to online school classes and a reduction in outdoor activities, vitamin D deficiency [85] (which has already been associated with precocious puberty, especially in girls), and sleep disorders [86].

Two recent retrospective studies help us to better understand the correlation between CPP and SARS-CoV-2 infection. The first one, conducted by Goffredo et al., showed that children with precocious puberty presented lower bone age advancement and higher levels of 17-hydroxyprogesterone than those observed prelockdown. These findings strongly suggest the influence of newly emerged environmental factors on pubertal development, although no study has been able to demonstrate a single cause–effect association until now [58].

The second one [68] registered the number of girls with suspected precocious puberty and the relative percentage of rapidly progressive CPP from 2019 to 2022. The authors found a significant increase in both of these diagnoses during 2020 compared with 2019 and a gradual decrease in the same diagnoses in 2021 and 2022, concurrent with the progressive resumption of daily activities. These findings suggest, once again, that radical lifestyle changes and the consequent stress due to the COVID-19 lockdown that children and adolescents underwent might have been crucial in regulating pubertal timing during the pandemic [68].

To summarize, the direct effect of SARS-CoV-2 infection on CPP onset remains unclear, but physical and psychological aspects related to the pandemic may have triggered a GnRH pulsatile secretion, leading to CPP.

6. Diabetes

The association between COVID-19 infection and type 1 diabetes (T1D) in children has been extensively studied in the last three years. However, the available data regarding the trend of incidence of newly diagnosed T1D during the COVID-19 pandemic are conflicting [87,88].

Several studies report a clear increase in the incidence of T1D since the beginning of the worldwide spread of the SARS-CoV-2 virus [89–113]. According to a meta-analysis by Rahmati et al. [114], the global new-onset of childhood T1D rate in 2020 was 32.39 per 100,000 children, clearly higher in comparison with 2019 (19.73 per 100,000 children) [114]. In a cohort study in seven U.S. centers, T1D was reported in 781,419 children and adolescents aged 0–17 years with laboratory-confirmed COVID-19 [115]. However, most of the above-mentioned studies did not find a direct cause–effect link between COVID-19 infection and T1D onset [89–111].

A case–control study conducted on children and adults with and without T1D in Colorado, USA, showed no difference in the prevalence of SARS-CoV-2 antibodies in the two groups during 2020 [116]. Similar results were reported in a study conducted on subjects aged <16 years in Belgium, in whom SARS-CoV-2 serology was tested within the first month from diabetes onset [117]. Conversely, other centers have reported a previous coronavirus infection or precise exposure to the virus in most of their patients newly diagnosed with T1DM [112,113].

In agreement with these studies, the CDC analyzed IQVIA healthcare data from March 2020 to February 2021 and estimated diabetes incidence among patients aged <18 years with proven COVID-19 infection. This incidence was found to be significantly higher than the incidence of T1D in children without COVID-19 (hazard ratio = 2.66, 95% CI = 1.98–3.56) [118,119].

Given the present data, it has been also hypothesized that SARS-CoV-2 might stimulate the autoimmune system, especially for pancreatic autoimmunity, therefore triggering the onset of T1D [113,114].

Other authors did not find any change in the incidence of T1D during the pandemic [119–124], but rather a change in the seasonal pattern, as suggested by the data from the Worldwide SWEET Registry [122]. In fact, in 2020, a shift in the seasonality of T1D incidence, with more cases in the summer months, was observed [122]. This may have been due to the hygiene measures and social distancing adopted during the lockdown, which may have further reduced the prevalence of viral infections in the winter/spring season, decreasing the impact of viral triggers for T1D onset in potentially susceptible subjects [122].

Some studies describe a decreased incidence of T1D after the beginning of the pandemic [125,126]. A possible explanation for this finding, in addition to the increased protection measures against COVID-19, which reduced the risk of contracting the most common viral forms, is the increased expression of CD8 + lymphocytes in T1D, which may protect these patients against infections [125,127].

Data about the prevalence of diabetic ketoacidosis (DKA) are much more concordant in the literature. Several cohort studies [91,93,98,102,106,123,126–163] and two meta-analyses [114,164] report increases in DKA frequency and DKA severity at diagnosis among newly diagnosed T1D patients. A multicenter study, involving 13 national diabetes registries (Australia, Austria, Czechia, Denmark, Germany, Italy, Luxembourg, New Zealand, Norway, Slovenia, Sweden, the USA (Colorado), and Wales) compared the observed DKA prevalence in children and adolescents in 2020 and 2021 to predictions based on trends over the prepandemic years 2006–2019. The pre-existing increase in the prevalence of DKA at diagnosis of T1D in children and adolescents from 2006 to 2019 was exacerbated in 2020 and 2021 [165].

To better study the association between SARS-CoV-2 and DKA prevalence at T1D onset, Kamrath et al. [166] calculated the relative risk (RR) of DKA at diagnosis of T1D during the year 2020 to assess whether it was associated with the regional incidence of COVID-19 cases and deaths. The applied multivariable mixed-effects log-binomial model revealed a significant association between the regional weekly incidences of COVID-19 cases and COVID-19-related deaths and the corresponding rates of ketoacidosis at diagnosis of T1D during the first half of the year 2020 [166].

Only a few centers did not observe a significant difference between the prepandemic and postpandemic era [94,105,108,167]. This finding has been attributed to increased parental supervision during the pandemic, which might have prevented severe disease decompensation in some cases [167].

Some authors have attributed the higher frequency of DKA to delayed diagnosis and initiation of insulin replacement therapy [168,169]. It has been suggested that elevated HbA1c at diagnosis of T1D, beyond an increase in the prevalence of DKA at onset, may be the consequence of a delay in diagnosis and insulin treatment initiation secondary to the pandemic difficulties [136]. Moreover, a retrospective cohort study on seven U.S. centers observed the highest frequency of DKA among T1D diabetes during COVID-19 surges in non-Hispanic Black patients, bringing attention to the problem of reduced access to health care during the pandemic by patients who are victims of health inequities [115].

To better understand the association between SARS-CoV-2 infection and DKA, a retrospective study compared insulin-mediated tissue glucose disposal (TGD) during standardized therapy for DKA in all children with pre-existing T1D with or without COVID-19. The median TGD was 46% lower among patients with COVID-19 infection in comparison with those without the infection. These results suggest that SARS-CoV-2 is associated with greater insulin resistance in DKA among patients affected by T1D, leading to the hypothesis that COVID-19 causes a metabolic impairment beyond factors that typically contribute to pediatric DKA [170].

To summarize, although the literature is discordant, the evidence of a potential role of SARS-CoV-2 in T1D onset and DKA frequency in newly diagnosed and known T1D diabetes is quite consistent, which deserves further investigation to understand the underlying responsible mechanisms. It is well known that some viral infections, especially rubella, Coxsackie, mumps, enterovirus, and the Epstein–Barr virus, represent important environmental risk factors for the development of T1D [171,172]. Since the start of the SARS-CoV-2 pandemic, attention has been paid on this novel virus as a further infective cause in the development and progression of T1D [173]. In fact, beyond the organizational problems related to the lockdown and the decreased access to health services during the pandemic [174], some biological mechanisms have been hypothesized to contribute to its pathogenesis [175].

Two main mechanisms are known to be responsible for the damage caused to pancreatic cells by different viruses. The first one is the direct cytolysis of virally infected cells; the second one is an autoimmune reaction [176]. The role of COVID-19 still needs to be clarified; however, pancreatic cell damage seems to occur, especially in patients with severe SARS-CoV-2 infection [174,177–180]. Nevertheless, the presence of the virus has been demonstrated only in the pancreas of deceased patients [181,182]. Rubino et al. [177] suggested that SARS-CoV-2 may bind to its cellular entry ACE-2 receptors, even in the pancreatic beta cells, where these cells are abundant, leading to pancreatic beta cell destruction. Another theory that could explain the association between SARS-CoV-2 and T1D development and the worse presentation at onset is virus-induced aberrant immune response, which may attack the pancreatic islet cells, mimicking the pathogenesis of insulin-dependent diabetes mellitus [183]. Indeed, cytokine storm, commonly found in COVID-19, may impair β-cell insulin secretion and glucose control [184]. However, the latter hypothesis was tested by Rewers et al. [185] by measuring autoantibodies to insulin, glutamic acid decarboxylase, islet antigen 2, and zinc transporter 8 autoantibodies in children both with and without previous COVID-19 infection, defined by the presence of antibodies to both SARS-CoV-2 receptor binding domain and nucleocapsid proteins. No association of SARS-CoV-2 infection with autoimmunity related to the development of T1D was observed in 50.000 youths from different populations in Colorado and Bavaria [185].

Another recently advanced hypothesis is that SARS-CoV-2 may cause T1D through the interferon-α-activated latent ribonuclease (RNaseL) signaling pathway [186]. Excessive RNaseL activity may lead to the degradation of both pathogen and host RNA, leading to cellular damage. This activity is regulated by phosphodiesterases such as PDE12. PDE12 expression has been shown to be decreased in individuals with recently diagnosed T1D. This seems to have a protective effect against viral infections, upregulating RNaseL activity; however, a potential side effect is a trigger of beta-cell damage [186].

MIS-C, as a severe complication of SARS-CoV-2 in children, may also be responsible for the pathogenesis of insulin resistance (IR). An exploratory study analyzed the glycemic patterns of 30 normal-weight children affected by MIS-C, showing a high prevalence of IR and glycemic fluctuation [187]. Data on the persistence of IR have been also described [188]. These evidence suggest that regular glucose monitoring of both fasting and postprandial glucose levels should be performed in patients with MIS-C.

7. Limits in the Scope of the Study

As mentioned in the Materials and Methods, our narrative review has some limits due to the selection method of the articles. Language was restricted to English only to ensure authors' complete understanding of the articles analyzed. Furthermore, to standardize the search, it was decided to use PubMed and Embase as databases. We are aware that this selection may have resulted in the exclusion of some documents reporting different results from those shown. The above-mentioned factors, together with the relatively small number of available articles in the literature, represent a limit in the scope of our study.

8. Conclusions

Although little is known regarding the involvement of the endocrine system during COVID-19 in children; the current evidence in adults and epidemiological studies on the pediatric population suggest the presence of a causal association between the virus and endocrinopathies.

The available data support the hypothesis that SARS-CoV-2 is responsible for transitory thyroid dysfunction. Thus, it would be a good practice to assess thyroid function markers in children affected with COVID-19 infection, especially if with moderate or severe manifestations and MIS-C.

Furthermore, the virus might affect the HPA axis in both direct and indirect ways due to glucocorticoids treatment in case of MIS-C. Also, it is recommended to pay special attention to children with known impairment of adrenal function who experience SARS-CoV-2 infection, because they may present with a more severe clinical picture than healthy children.

The hypothalamic–pituitary axis may also be affected in different ways: a case of ROHHAD-syndrome-like presentation and a case of hypophysitis after COVID-19 infection have been reported in children. Moreover, an increase in CPP incidence has been observed since the advent of the COVID-19 pandemic. The direct effect of the virus in the pathogenesis of CPP is still unclear; however, it has been suggested that its related physical and psychological aspects may act as triggers of GnRH pulsatile secretion.

Regarding T1D, despite some discordant evidence, many cohort studies support the role of SARS-CoV-2 in T1D onset and DKA frequency in newly diagnosed and known T1D diabetes. It has been suggested that this association is due to the combined direct effects of the virus on pancreatic cells, the indirect effects of the virus through its consequent inflammatory response, and delayed diagnoses secondary to the healthcare difficulties encountered worldwide. An association between IR and MIS-C should be also considered.

In conclusion, although data regarding the relationship between COVID-19 and endocrinological involvement in pediatric patients are limited, they suggest the correlation between SARS-CoV-2 infection and impairment in different organs in this population, as more extensively reported in adults Therefore, further studies are needed to clarify the role of SARS-CoV-2 infection in the development of different endocrinopathies in children, both during acute infection and as a result of its long-term complications. Moreover, health institutions should be aware of this likely association and highlight endocrine involvement in this population of interest. This information is of primary importance to guide the management of patients with previous or current COVID-19.

Author Contributions: Conceptualization, V.C., V.M.T. and G.Z.; methodology, V.C., V.M.T., R.D.S., A.B., S.T., E.D. and G.Z.; writing—original draft preparation, V.C., V.M.T., R.D.S., A.B. and S.T.; writing—review and editing, V.C., V.M.T., R.D.S., A.B., S.T., E.D. and G.Z.; supervision, V.C. and G.Z.; All authors have read and agreed to the published version of the manuscript.

Funding: The project received contributions from (1) HORIZON-HLTH-2021-CORONA-01 CoVICIS project number 101046041; (2) Bando Cariplo Networking ricerca e formazione post-COVID protocol number 2021-4490.

Institutional Review Board Statement: Not applicable.

Informed Consent Statement: Not applicable.

Data Availability Statement: Not applicable.

Conflicts of Interest: The authors declare no conflict of interest.

References

1. Guan, W.-J.; Ni, Z.-Y.; Hu, Y.; Liang, W.-H.; Ou, C.-Q.; He, J.-X.; Liu, L.; Shan, H.; Lei, C.-L.; Hui, D.S.C.; et al. China Medical Treatment Expert Group for Covid-19 Clinical Characteristics of Coronavirus Disease 2019 in China. *N. Engl. J. Med.* **2020**, *382*, 1708–1720.
2. Brodin, P. SARS-CoV-2 infections in children: Understanding diverse outcomes. *Immunity* **2022**, *55*, 201–209.
3. Solomon, M.D.; Escobar, G.J.; Lu, Y.; Schlessinger, D.; Steinman, J.B.; Steinman, L.; Lee, C.; Liu, V.X. Risk of severe COVID-19 infection among adults with prior exposure to children. *Proc. Natl. Acad. Sci. USA* **2022**, *119*, e2204141119.
4. Mallapaty, S. Kids and covid: Why young immune systems are still on top. *Nature* **2021**, *597*, 166–168.
5. Payne, A.B.; Gilani, Z.; Godfred-Cato, S.; Belay, E.D.; Feldstein, L.R.; Patel, M.M.; Randolph, A.G.; Newhams, M.; Thomas, D.; Magleby, R.; et al. MIS-C Incidence Authorship Group. Incidence of multisystem inflammatory syndrome in children among US persons infected with SARS-CoV-2. *JAMA Netw. Open* **2021**, *4*, e2116420.
6. Noval Rivas, M.; Porritt, R.A.; Cheng, M.H.; Bahar, I.; Arditi, M. Multisystem inflammatory syndrome in children and long covid: The SARS-CoV-2 viral superantigen hypothesis. *Front. Immunol.* **2022**, *13*, 941009.
7. Soriano, J.B.; Murthy, S.; Marshall, J.C.; Relan, P.; Diaz, J.V.; WHO Clinical Case Definition Working Group on Post-COVID-19 Condition. A clinical case definition of post-COVID-19 condition by a Delphi consensus. *Lancet Infect. Dis.* **2022**, *22*, e102–e107.

8. Lopez-Leon, S.; Wegman-Ostrosky, T.; Ayuzo Del Valle, N.C.; Perelman, C.; Sepulveda, R.; Rebolledo, P.A.; Cuapio, A.; Villapol, S. Long-COVID in children and adolescents: A systematic review and meta-analyses. *Sci. Rep.* **2022**, *12*, 9950.
9. Ashraf, U.M.; Abokor, A.A.; Edwards, J.M.; Waigi, E.W.; Royfman, R.S.; Hasan, S.A.; Smedlund, K.B.; Hardy, A.M.G.; Chakravarti, R.; Koch, L.G. SARS-CoV-2, ACE2 expression, and systemic organ invasion. *Physiol. Genom.* **2021**, *53*, 51–60.
10. Li, M.Y.; Li, L.; Zhang, Y.; Wang, X.S. Expression of the SARS-CoV-2 cell receptor gene ACE2 in a wide variety of human tissues. *Infect. Dis. Poverty* **2020**, *9*, 45.
11. Rotondi, M.; Coperchini, F.; Ricci, G.; Denegri, M.; Croce, L.; Ngnitejeu, S.T.; Villani, L.; Magri, F.; Latrofa, F.; Chiovato, L. Detection of SARS-CoV-2 receptor ACE-2 mRNA in thyroid cells: A clue for COVID-19-related subacute thyroiditis. *J. Endocrinol. Investig.* **2021**, *44*, 1085–1090.
12. Lazartigues, E.; Qadir, M.M.F.; Mauvais-Jarvis, F. Endocrine significance of SARS-CoV-2's reliance on ACE2. *Endocrinology* **2020**, *161*, bqaa108.
13. Gnocchi, M.; D'Alvano, T.; Lattanzi, C.; Messina, G.; Petraroli, M.; Patianna, V.D.; Esposito, S.; Street, M.E. Current evidence on the impact of the COVID-19 pandemic on paediatric endocrine conditions. *Front. Endocrinol.* **2022**, *13*, 913334. [CrossRef]
14. McCowan, R.; Wild, E.; Lucas-Herald, A.K.; McNeilly, J.; Mason, A.; Wong, S.C.; Ahmed, S.F.; Shaikh, M.G. The effect of COVID-19 on the presentation of thyroid disease in children. *Front. Endocrinol.* **2022**, *13*, 1014533. [CrossRef]
15. Seo, J.Y. Pediatric Endocrinology of Post-Pandemic Era. *Chonnam Med. J.* **2021**, *57*, 103–107.
16. Shidid, S.; Kohlhoff, S.; Smith-Norowitz, T.A. Thyroid stimulating hormone levels in children before and during the coronavirus disease-19 pandemic. *Health Sci. Rep.* **2022**, *5*, e579.
17. Dabas, A.; Singh, H.; Goswami, B.; Kumar, K.; Dubey, A.; Jhamb, U.; Yadav, S.; Garg, S. Thyroid Dysfunction in COVID-19. *Indian. J. Endocrinol. Metab.* **2021**, *25*, 198–201.
18. Lui, D.T.W.; Lee, C.H.; Chow, W.S.; Lee, A.C.H.; Tam, A.R.; Fong, C.H.Y.; Law, C.Y.; Leung, E.K.H.; To, K.K.W.; Tan, K.C.B.; et al. Thyroid dysfunction in relation to immune profile, disease status, and outcome in 191 patients with COVID-19. *J. Clin. Endocrinol. Metab.* **2021**, *106*, e926–e935.
19. Calcaterra, V.; Biganzoli, G.; Dilillo, D.; Mannarino, S.; Fiori, L.; Pelizzo, G.; Zoia, E.; Fabiano, V.; Carlucci, P.; Camporesi, A.; et al. Non-thyroidal illness syndrome and SARS-CoV-2-associated multisystem inflammatory syndrome in children. *J. Endocrinol. Investig.* **2022**, *45*, 199–208.
20. Calcaterra, V.; Zuccotti, G. Letter to the Editor: Changes in Thyroid Function in Children with Multisystem Inflammatory Syndrome Related to COVID-19 Observed over a 1-Year Follow-Up Period. *Thyroid* **2023**, *33*, 650–652.
21. Elvan-Tüz, A.; Ayrancı, I.; Ekemen-Keleş, Y.; Karakoyun, I.; Çatlı, G.; Kara-Aksay, A.; Karadağ-Öncel, E.; Dündar, B.N.; Yılmaz, D. Are Thyroid Functions Affected in Multisystem Inflammatory Syndrome in Children? *J. Clin. Res. Pediatr. Endocrinol.* **2022**, *14*, 402–408.
22. Hikmet, F.; Méar, L.; Edvinsson, Å.; Micke, P.; Uhlén, M.; Lindskog, C. The protein expression profile of ACE2 in human tissues. *Mol. Syst. Biol.* **2020**, *16*, e9610. [CrossRef]
23. Allam, M.M.; El-Zawawy, H.T.; Ahmed, S.M.; Aly Abdelhamid, M. Thyroid disease and covid-19 infection: Case series. *Clin. Case. Rep.* **2021**, *9*, e04225.
24. Bogusławska, J.; Godlewska, M.; Gajda, E.; Piekiełko-Witkowska, A. Cellular and molecular basis of thyroid autoimmunity. *Eur. Thyr. J.* **2022**, *11*, R1–R16.
25. Lania, A.; Sandri, M.T.; Cellini, M.; Mirani, M.; Lavezzi, E.; Mazziotti, G. Thyrotoxicosis in patients with COVID-19: The THYRCOV study. *Eur. J. Endocrinol.* **2020**, *183*, 381–387.
26. Ganie, M.A.; Charoo, B.A.; Sahar, T.; Bhat, M.H.; Ali, S.A.; Niyaz, M.; Sidana, S.; Yaseen, A. Thyroid Function, Urinary Iodine, and Thyroid Antibody Status Among the Tribal Population of Kashmir Valley: Data from Endemic Zone of a Sub-Himalayan Region. *Front. Public Health* **2020**, *8*, 555840.
27. Haller-Kikkatalo, K.; Alnek, K.; Metspalu, A.; Mihailov, E.; Metsküla, K.; Kisand, K.; Pisarev, H.; Salumets, A.; Uibo, R. Demographic associations for autoantibodies in disease-free individuals of a European population. *Sci. Rep.* **2017**, *7*, 44846.
28. Flokas, M.E.; Bustamante, V.H.; Kanakatti Shankar, R. New-Onset Primary Adrenal Insufficiency and Autoimmune Hypothyroidism in a Pediatric Patient Presenting with MIS-C. *Horm. Res. Paediatr.* **2022**, *95*, 397–401.
29. Chen, W.; Tian, Y.; Li, Z.; Zhu, J.; Wei, T.; Lei, J. Potential interaction between SARS-CoV-2 and thyroid: A Review. *Endocrinology* **2021**, *162*, bqab004.
30. Piticchio, T.; Le Moli, R.; Tumino, D.; Frasca, F. Relationship between betacoronaviruses and the endocrine system: A new key to understand the COVID-19 pandemic—A comprehensive review. *J. Endocrinol. Investig.* **2021**, *44*, 1553–1570.
31. Croce, L.; Gangemi, D.; Ancona, G.; Liboà, F.; Bendotti, G.; Minelli, L.; Chiovato, L. The cytokine storm and thyroid hormone changes in COVID-19. *J. Endocrinol. Investig.* **2021**, *44*, 891–904.
32. Kumari, K.; Chainy, G.B.N.; Subudhi, U. Prospective role of thyroid disorders in monitoring COVID-19 pandemic. *Heliyon* **2020**, *6*, e05712.
33. Medas, F.; Dobrinja, C.; Al-Suhaimi, E.A.; Altmeier, J.; Anajar, S.; Arikan, A.E.; Azaryan, I.; Bains, L.; Basili, G.; Bolukbasi, H.; et al. Effect of the COVID-19 pandemic on surgery for indeterminate thyroid nodules (THYCOVID): A retrospective, international, multicentre, cross-sectional study. *Lancet Diabetes Endocrinol.* **2023**, *11*, 402–413. [CrossRef]
34. Puri, S.; McLelland, B.; Bryce, N. 1651 the impact of covid-19 on thyroid surveillance offered to children with down syndrome. *Abstracts* **2021**, *106*, A444.

35. McGlacken-Byrne, S.M.; Johnson, M.; Penner, J.; du Pré, P.; Katugampola, H. Characterising approaches to steroid therapy in paediatric multisystem inflammatory syndrome temporally associated with SARS-CoV-2. *J. Paediatr. Child. Health* **2023**, *59*, 890–894. [CrossRef]
36. Kilci, F.; Yetimakman, A.F.; Jones, J.H.; Çizmecioğlu, F.M. A case of adrenal insufficiency during multisystem inflammatory syndrome in children. *Clin. Pediatr. Endocrinol.* **2022**, *31*, 163–167.
37. Arlt, W.; Baldeweg, S.E.; Pearce, S.H.S.; Simpson, H.L. Endocrinology in the time of COVID-19: Management of adrenal insufficiency. *Eur. J. Endocrinol.* **2020**, *183*, G25–G32.
38. Nowotny, H.F.; Bryce, J.; Ali, S.R.; Giordano, R.; Baronio, F.; Chifu, I.; Tschaidse, L.; Cools, M.; van den Akker, E.L.; Falhammar, H.; et al. Outcome of COVID-19 infections in patients with adrenal insufficiency and excess. *Endocr. Connect.* **2023**, *12*, e220416.
39. Banull, N.R.; Reich, P.J.; Anka, C.; May, J.; Wharton, K.; Kallogjeri, D.; Shimony, H.; Arbeláez, A.M. Association between Endocrine Disorders and Severe COVID-19 Disease in Pediatric Patients. *Horm. Res. Paediatr.* **2022**, *95*, 331–338.
40. Chien, T.C.; Chien, M.M.; Liu, T.L.; Chang, H.; Tsai, M.L.; Tseng, S.H.; Ho, W.L.; Su, Y.Y.; Lin, H.C.; Lu, J.H.; et al. Adrenal Crisis Mimicking COVID-19 Encephalopathy in a Teenager with Craniopharyngioma. *Children* **2022**, *9*, 1238.
41. Gaudino, R.; Orlandi, V.; Cavarzere, P.; Chinello, M.; Antoniazzi, F.; Cesaro, S.; Piacentini, G. Case Report: SARS-CoV-2 Infection in a Child With Suprasellar Tumor and Hypothalamic-Pituitary Failure. *Front. Endocrinol.* **2021**, *12*, 596654.
42. Han, T.; Kang, J.; Li, G.; Ge, J.; Gu, J. Analysis of 2019-nCoV receptor ACE2 expression in different tissues and its significance study. *Ann. Transl. Med.* **2020**, *8*, 1077.
43. Finsterer, J.; Scorza, F.A. The pituitary gland in SARS-CoV-2 infections, vaccinations, and post-COVID syndrome. *Clinics* **2022**, *78*, 100157.
44. Pal, R. COVID-19, hypothalamo-pituitary-adrenal axis and clinical implications. *Endocrine* **2020**, *68*, 251–252.
45. Siejka, A.; Barabutis, N. Adrenal insufficiency in the COVID-19 era. *Am. J. Physiol. Endocrinol. Metab.* **2021**, *320*, E784–E785.
46. Leow, M.K.S.; Kwek, D.S.K.; Ng, A.W.K.; Ong, K.C.; Kaw, G.J.L.; Lee, L.S.U. Hypocortisolism in survivors of severe acute respiratory syndrome (SARS). *Clin. Endocrinol.* **2005**, *63*, 197–202.
47. Wheatland, R. Molecular mimicry of ACTH in SARS—Implications for corticosteroid treatment and prophylaxis. *Med. Hypotheses* **2004**, *63*, 855–862.
48. Bateman, A.; Singh, A.; Kral, T.; Solomon, S. The immune-hypothalamic-pituitary-adrenal axis. *Endocr. Rev.* **1989**, *10*, 92–112.
49. Soni, A.; Pepper, G.M.; Wyrwinski, P.M.; Ramirez, N.E.; Simon, R.; Pina, T.; Gruenspan, H.; Vaca, C.E. Adrenal insufficiency occurring during septic shock: Incidence, outcome, and relationship to peripheral cytokine levels. *Am. J. Med.* **1995**, *98*, 266–271.
50. Guarner, J.; Paddock, C.D.; Bartlett, J.; Zaki, S.R. Adrenal gland hemorrhage in patients with fatal bacterial infections. *Mod. Pathol.* **2008**, *21*, 1113–1120.
51. Artamonova, I.N.; Petrova, N.A.; Lyubimova, N.A.; Kolbina, N.Y.; Bryzzhin, A.V.; Borodin, A.V.; Levko, T.A.; Mamaeva, E.A.; Pervunina, T.M.; Vasichkina, E.S.; et al. Case Report: COVID-19-Associated ROHHAD-Like Syndrome. *Front. Pediatr.* **2022**, *10*, 854367.
52. Joshi, M.; Gunawardena, S.; Goenka, A.; Ey, E.; Kumar, G. Post COVID-19 Lymphocytic Hypophysitis: A Rare Presentation. *Child. Neurol. Open* **2022**, *9*, 2329048X221103051.
53. Improving the Clinical Care of Children and Adolescents with Endocrine Conditions, including Diabetes, through Research and Education ESPE Patient Leaflet Information on COVID-19 and Pediatric Endocrine Diseases. Available online: https://www.ecdc.europa.eu/en/publications- (accessed on 15 May 2023).
54. Peinkhofer, M.; Bossini, B.; Penco, A.; Giangreco, M.; Pellegrin, M.C.; Vidonis, V.; Vittori, G.; Grassi, N.; Faleschini, E.; Barbi, E.; et al. Reduction in pediatric growth hormone deficiency and increase in central precocious puberty diagnoses during COVID 19 pandemics. *Ital. J. Pediatr.* **2022**, *48*, 49.
55. Arcari, A.J.; Rodríguez Azrak, M.S.; Boulgourdjian, E.M.; Costanzo, M.; Guercio, G.V.; Gryngarten, M.G. Precocious puberty in relation to the COVID-19 pandemic. A survey among Argentine pediatric endocrinologists. *Arch. Argent. Pediatr.* **2023**, *121*, e202202767.
56. Chen, Y.; Chen, J.; Tang, Y.; Zhang, Q.; Wang, Y.; Li, Q.; Li, X.; Weng, Z.; Huang, J.; Wang, X.; et al. Difference of Precocious Puberty Between Before and During the COVID-19 Pandemic: A Cross-Sectional Study Among Shanghai School-Aged Girls. *Front. Endocrinol.* **2022**, *13*, 349.
57. Elbarbary, N.S.; dos Santos, T.J.; de Beaufort, C.; Wiltshire, E.; Pulungan, A.; Scaramuzza, A.E. The Challenges of Managing Pediatric Diabetes and Other Endocrine Disorders During the COVID-19 Pandemic: Results from an International Cross-Sectional Electronic Survey. *Front. Endocrinol.* **2021**, *12*, 1447.
58. Goffredo, M.; Pilotta, A.; Parissenti, I.; Forino, C.; Tomasi, C.; Goffredo, P.; Buzi, F.; Badolato, R. Early onset of puberty during COVID-19 pandemic lockdown: Experience from two Pediatric Endocrinology Italian Centers. *J. Pediatr. Endocrinol. Metab.* **2023**, *36*, 290–298.
59. Yesiltepe Mutlu, G.; Eviz, E.; Haliloglu, B.; Kirmizibekmez, H.; Dursun, F.; Ozalkak, S.; Cayir, A.; Sacli, B.Y.; Ozbek, M.N.; Demirbilek, H.; et al. The effects of the covid-19 pandemic on puberty: A cross-sectional, multicenter study from Turkey. *Ital. J. Pediatr.* **2022**, *48*, 144.
60. Oliveira Neto, C.P.; Azulay, R.S.; Almeida, A.G.F.P.; Tavares, M.; Vaz, L.H.G.; Leal, I.R.L.; Gama, M.E.A.; Ribeiro, M.R.C.; Nascimento, G.C.; Magalhães, M.; et al. Differences in Puberty of Girls before and during the COVID-19 Pandemic. *Int. J. Environ. Res. Public Health* **2022**, *19*, 4733.

61. Sun, H.; Qian, Y.; Wan, N.; Liu, L. Differential diagnosis of precocious puberty in girls during the COVID-19 pandemic: A pilot study. *BMC Pediatr.* **2023**, *23*, 185.
62. Chioma, L.; Bizzarri, C.; Verzani, M.; Fava, D.; Salerno, M.; Capalbo, D.; Guzzetti, C.; Penta, L.; Di Luigi, L.; Di Iorgi, N.; et al. Sedentary lifestyle and precocious puberty in girls during the COVID-19 pandemic: An Italian experience. *Endocr. Connect.* **2022**, *11*, e210650.
63. Acar, S.; Özkan, B. Increased frequency of idiopathic central precocious puberty in girls during the COVID-19 pandemic: Preliminary results of a tertiary center study. *J. Pediatr. Endocrinol. Metab.* **2022**, *35*, 249–251.
64. Acinikli, K.Y.; Erbaş, İ.M.; Besci, Ö.; Demir, K.; Abacı, A.; Böber, E. Has the Frequency of Precocious Puberty and Rapidly Progressive Early Puberty Increased in Girls During the COVID-19 Pandemic? *J. Clin. Res. Pediatr. Endocrinol.* **2022**, *14*, 302.
65. Baby, M.; Ilkowitz, J.; Cheema Brar, P. Impacts of the COVID-19 pandemic on the diagnosis of idiopathic central precocious puberty in pediatric females in New York City. *J. Pediatr. Endocrinol. Metab.* **2023**, *36*, 517–522. [CrossRef]
66. Barberi, C.; Di Natale, V.; Assirelli, V.; Bernardini, L.; Candela, E.; Cassio, A. Implicating factors in the increase in cases of central precocious puberty (CPP) during the COVID-19 pandemic: Experience of a tertiary centre of pediatric endocrinology and review of the literature. *Front. Endocrinol.* **2022**, *13*, 3064.
67. Benedetto, M.; Riveros, V.; Eymann, A.; Terrasa, S.; Alonso, G. Analysis of the incidence of central precocious puberty treated with gonadotropin-releasing hormone analogs. Impact of the COVID-19 pandemic. *Arch. Argent. Pediatr.* **2023**, *121*, e202202849.
68. Chioma, L.; Chiarito, M.; Bottaro, G.; Paone, L.; Todisco, T.; Bizzarri, C.; Cappa, M. COVID-19 pandemic phases and female precocious puberty: The experience of the past 4 years (2019 through 2022) in an Italian tertiary center. *Front. Endocrinol.* **2023**, *14*, 533.
69. Choi, K.H.; Park, S.C. An increasing tendency of precocious puberty among Korean children from the perspective of COVID-19 pandemic effect. *Front. Pediatr.* **2022**, *10*, 1451.
70. Fu, D.; Li, T.; Zhang, Y.; Wang, H.; Wu, X.; Chen, Y.; Cao, B.; Wei, H. Analysis of the Incidence and Risk Factors of Precocious Puberty in Girls during the COVID-19 Pandemic. *Int. J. Endocrinol.* **2022**, *2022*, 9229153.
71. Geniuk, N.; De Jesús Suárez Mozo, M.; Pose, M.N.; Vidaurreta, S. Rapidly progressive precocious puberty during the COVID-19 lockdown. *Arch. Argent. Pediatr.* **2023**, *121*, e202202840.
72. Ariza Jimenez, A.B.; Aguilar Gomez-Cardenas, F.J.; de la Camara Moraño, C. Likely impact of COVID-19 on referrals to pediatric endocrinology: Increased incidence of precocious puberty in a third-level hospital. *Endocrinol. Diabetes. Nutr.* **2022**, *69*, 542–544.
73. Higuchi, S.; Matsubara, K.; Higuchi, S.; Matsubara, K.; Watanabe, Y.; Kitayama, K.; Yamada, Y.; Yorifuji, T. Clinical Pediatric Endocrinology Increased incidence of central precocious puberty during the coronavirus disease (COVID-19) pandemic at a single center in the Osaka Metropolitan Area of Japan. *Clin. Pediatr. Endocrinol.* **2023**, *32*, 58–64.
74. Mondkar, S.A.; Oza, C.; Khadilkar, V.; Shah, N.; Gondhalekar, K.; Kajale, N.; Khadilkar, A. Impact of COVID-19 lockdown on idiopathic central precocious puberty—Experience from an Indian centre. *J. Pediatr. Endocrinol. Metab.* **2022**, *35*, 895–900.
75. Orman, B.; Esen, S.; Keskin, M.; Şahin, N.M.; Savaş-Erdeve, Ş.; Çetinkaya, S. Status of Central Precocious Puberty Cases at the Onset of Coronavirus Disease 2019 Pandemic: A Single-Center Experience. *Turkish. Arch. Pediatr.* **2022**, *57*, 349.
76. Stagi, S.; De Masi, S.; Bencini, E.; Losi, S.; Paci, S.; Parpagnoli, M.; Ricci, F.; Ciofi, D.; Azzari, C. Increased incidence of precocious and accelerated puberty in females during and after the Italian lockdown for the coronavirus 2019 (COVID-19) pandemic. *Ital. J. Pediatr.* **2020**, *46*, 165.
77. Trujillo, M.V.; Rungvivatjarus, T.; Klein, K.O. Incidence of central precocious puberty more than doubled during COVID-19 pandemic: Single-center retrospective review in the United States. *Front. Pediatr.* **2022**, *10*, 1007730.
78. Turrizziani Colonna, A.; Curatola, A.; Sodero, G.; Lazzareschi, I.; Cammisa, I.; Cipolla, C. Central precocious puberty in children after COVID-19 outbreak: A single-center retrospective study. *Minerva Pediatr.* **2022**. ahead of print. [CrossRef]
79. Verzani, M.; Bizzarri, C.; Chioma, L.; Bottaro, G.; Pedicelli, S.; Cappa, M. Impact of COVID-19 pandemic lockdown on early onset of puberty: Experience of an Italian tertiary center. *Ital. J. Pediatr.* **2021**, *47*, 52.
80. Umano, G.R.; Maddaluno, I.; Riccio, S.; Lanzaro, F.; Antignani, R.; Giuliano, M.; Luongo, C.; Festa, A.; Miraglia del Giudice, E.; Grandone, A. Central precocious puberty during COVID-19 pandemic and sleep disturbance: An exploratory study. *Ital. J. Pediatr.* **2022**, *48*, 60.
81. Prosperi, S.; Chiarelli, F. Early and precocious puberty during the COVID-19 pandemic. *Front. Endocrinol.* **2023**, *13*, 3537.
82. Smith, S.S.; Aoki, C.; Shen, H. Puberty, steroids and GABAA receptor plasticity. *Psychoneuroendocrinology* **2009**, *34*, S91–S103.
83. Abou El Ella, S.S.; Barseem, N.F.; Tawfik, M.A.; Ahmed, A.F. BMI relationship to the onset of puberty: Assessment of growth parameters and sexual maturity changes in Egyptian children and adolescents of both sexes. *J. Pediatr. Endocrinol. Metab.* **2020**, *33*, 121–128.
84. Nokoff, N.; Thurston, J.; Hilkin, A.; Pyle, L.; Zeitler, P.S.; Nadeau, K.J.; Santoro, N.; Kelsey, M.M. Sex Differences in Effects of Obesity on Reproductive Hormones and Glucose Metabolism in Early Puberty. *J. Clin. Endocrinol. Metab.* **2019**, *104*, 4390.
85. Liu, S.; Zhu, X.; Wang, Y.; Yan, S.; Li, D.; Cui, W. The association between vitamin D levels and precocious puberty: A meta-analysis. *J. Pediatr. Endocrinol. Metab.* **2020**, *33*, 427–429.
86. Street, M.E.; Sartori, C.; Catellani, C.; Righi, B. Precocious Puberty and Covid-19 Into Perspective: Potential Increased Frequency, Possible Causes, and a Potential Emergency to Be Addressed. *Front. Pediatr.* **2021**, *9*, 978.
87. Zucchini, S.; Scozzarella, A.; Maltoni, G. Multiple influences of the COVID-19 pandemic on children with diabetes: Changes in epidemiology, metabolic control and medical care. *World J. Diabetes* **2023**, *14*, 198–208.

88. Karavanaki, K.; Rodolaki, K.; Soldatou, A.; Karanasios, S.; Kakleas, K. Covid-19 infection in children and adolescents and its association with type 1 diabetes mellitus (T1d) presentation and management. *Endocrine* **2023**, *80*, 237–252.
89. Miller, A.; Joseph, S.; Badran, A.; Umpaichitra, V.; Bargman, R.; Chin, V.L. Increased Rates of Hospitalized Children with Type 1 and Type 2 Diabetes Mellitus in Central Brooklyn during the COVID-19 Pandemic. *Int. J. Pediatr.* **2023**, *2023*, 4580809.
90. Farakla, I.; Lagousi, T.; Miligkos, M.; Nicolaides, N.C.; Vasilakis, I.A.; Mpinou, M.; Dolianiti, M.; Katechaki, E.; Taliou, A.; Spoulou, V.; et al. Stress hyperglycemia, Diabetes mellitus and COVID-19 infection: The impact on newly diagnosed type 1 diabetes. *Front. Clin. Diabetes Healthc.* **2022**, *3*, 818945.
91. Knip, M.; Parviainen, A.; Turtinen, M.; But, A.; Härkönen, T.; Hepojoki, J.; Sironen, T.; Iheozor-Ejiofor, R.; Uğurlu, H.; Saksela, K.; et al. Finnish Pediatric Diabetes Register. SARS-CoV-2 and type 1 diabetes in children in Finland: An observational study. *Lancet Diabetes Endocrinol.* **2023**, *11*, 251–260.
92. Gesuita, R.; Rabbone, I.; Marconi, V.; De Sanctis, L.; Marino, M.; Tiberi, V.; Iannilli, A.; Tinti, D.; Favella, L.; Giorda, C. Trends and cyclic variation in the incidence of childhood type 1 diabetes in two Italian regions over 33 years and during the COVID-19 pandemic. *Diabetes Obes. Metab.* **2023**, *25*, 1698–1703.
93. Baechle, C.; Eckert, A.; Kamrath, C.; Neu, A.; Manuwald, U.; Thiele-Schmitz, S.; Weidler, O.; Knauer-Fischer, S.; Rosenbauer, J.; Holl, R.W. Incidence and presentation of new-onset type 1 diabetes in children and adolescents from Germany during the COVID-19 pandemic 2020 and 2021: Current data from the DPV Registry. *Diabetes Res. Clin. Pract.* **2023**, *197*, 110559.
94. Hernández Herrero, M.; Terradas Mercader, P.; Latorre Martinez, E.; Feliu Rovira, A.; Rodríguez Zaragoza, N.; Parada Ricart, E. New diagnoses of type 1 diabetes mellitus in children during the COVID-19 pandemic Regional multicenter study in Spain. *Endocrinol. Diabetes Nutr.* **2022**, *69*, 709–714.
95. van den Boom, L.; Kostev, K.; Kuss, O.; Rathmann, W.; Rosenbauer, J. Type 1 diabetes incidence in children and adolescents during the COVID-19 pandemic in Germany. *Diabetes Res Clin. Pract.* **2022**, *193*, 110146.
96. Ansar, A.; Livett, T.; Beaton, W.; Carrel, A.L.; Bekx, M.T. Sharp Rise in New-Onset Pediatric Diabetes During the COVID-19 Pandemic. *WMJ* **2022**, *121*, 177–180.
97. Raicevic, M.; Samardzic, M.; Soldatovic, I.; Curovic Popovic, N.; Vukovic, R. Trends in nationwide incidence of pediatric type 1 diabetes in Montenegro during the last 30 years. *Front. Endocrinol.* **2022**, *13*, 991533.
98. Vorgučin, I.; Savin, M.; Stanković, Đ.; Miljković, D.; Ilić, T.; Simić, D.; Vrebalov, M.; Milanović, B.; Barišić, N.; Stojanović, V.; et al. Incidence of Type 1 Diabetes Mellitus and Characteristics of Diabetic Ketoacidosis in Children and Adolescents during the First Two Years of the COVID-19 Pandemic in Vojvodina. *Medicina* **2022**, *58*, 1013.
99. Cinek, O.; Slavenko, M.; Pomahačová, R.; Venháčová, P.; Petruželková, L.; Škvor, J.; Neumann, D.; Vosáhlo, J.; Konečná, P.; Kocourková, K.; et al. Type 1 diabetes incidence increased during the COVID-19 pandemic years 2020-2021 in Czechia: Results from a large population-based pediatric register. *Pediatr. Diabetes* **2022**, *23*, 956–960.
100. Schiaffini, R.; Deodati, A.; Rapini, N.; Pampanini, V.; Cianfarani, S. Increased incidence of childhood type 1 diabetes during the COVID-19 pandemic. Figures from an Italian tertiary care center. *J. Diabetes* **2022**, *14*, 562–563.
101. McKeigue, P.M.; McGurnaghan, S.; Blackbourn, L.; Bath, L.E.; McAllister, D.A.; Caparrotta, T.M.; Wild, S.H.; Wood, S.N.; Stockton, D.; Colhoun, H.M. Relation of Incident Type 1 Diabetes to Recent COVID-19 Infection: Cohort Study Using e-Health Record Linkage in Scotland. *Diabetes Care* **2023**, *46*, 921–928.
102. Lah Tomulić, K.; Matko, L.; Verbić, A.; Milardović, A.; Severinski, S.; Kolić, I.; Baraba Dekanić, K.; Šerifi, S.; Butorac Ahel, I. Epidemiologic Characteristics of Children with Diabetic Ketoacidosis Treated in a Pediatric Intensive Care Unit in a 10-Year-Period: Single Centre Experience in Croatia. *Medicina* **2022**, *58*, 638.
103. Passanisi, S.; Salzano, G.; Aloe, M.; Bombaci, B.; Citriniti, F.; De Berardinis, F.; De Marco, R.; Lazzaro, N.; Lia, M.C.; Lia, R.; et al. Increasing trend of type 1 diabetes incidence in the pediatric population of the Calabria region in 2019–2021. *Ital. J. Pediatr.* **2022**, *48*, 66.
104. Rosenberg, K. Increase in Type 1 Diabetes Incidence in Children During COVID-19. *Am. J. Nurs.* **2022**, *122*, 49.
105. Donbaloğlu, Z.; Tuhan, H.; Tural Kara, T.; Bedel, A.; Barsal Çetiner, E.; Singin, B.; Parlak, M. The Examination of the Relationship Between COVID-19 and New-Onset Type 1 Diabetes Mellitus in Children. *Turk. Arch. Pediatr.* **2022**, *57*, 222–227.
106. Abdou, M.; Hassan, M.M.; Hassanein, S.A.; Elsebaie, E.H.; Shamma, R.A. Presentations, Complications, and Challenges Encountered During Management of Type 1 Diabetes in Egyptian Children During COVID-19 Pandemic: A Single-Center Experience. *Front. Endocrinol.* **2022**, *13*, 814991.
107. Kamrath, C.; Rosenbauer, J.; Eckert, A.J.; Siedler, K.; Bartelt, H.; Klose, D.; Sindichakis, M.; Herrlinger, S.; Lahn, V.; Holl, R.W. Incidence of Type 1 Diabetes in Children and Adolescents During the COVID-19 Pandemic in Germany: Results from the DPV Registry. *Diabetes Care* **2022**, *45*, 1762–1771.
108. Nóvoa-Medina, Y.; Pavlovic-Nesic, S.; González-Martín, J.M.; Hernández-Betancor, A.; López, S.; Domínguez-García, A.; Quinteiro-Domínguez, S.; Cabrera, M.; De La Cuesta, A.; Caballero-Fernández, E.; et al. Role of the SARS-CoV-2 virus in the appearance of new onset type 1 diabetes mellitus in children in Gran Canaria, Spain. *J. Pediatr. Endocrinol. Metab.* **2022**, *35*, 393–397.
109. Vlad, A.; Serban, V.; Timar, R.; Sima, A.; Botea, V.; Albai, O.; Timar, B.; Vlad, M. Increased Incidence of Type 1 Diabetes during the COVID-19 Pandemic in Romanian Children. *Medicina* **2021**, *57*, 973.
110. Unsworth, R.; Wallace, S.; Oliver, N.S.; Yeung, S.; Kshirsagar, A.; Naidu, H.; Kwong, R.M.W.; Kumar, P.; Logan, K.M. New-Onset Type 1 Diabetes in Children During COVID-19: Multicenter Regional Findings in the U.K. *Diabetes Care* **2020**, *43*, e170–e171.

111. Nri-Ezedi, C.A.; Ulasi, T.O.; Okeke, K.N.; Okonkwo, I.T.; Echendu, S.T.; Agu, N.V.; Nwaneli, E.I. A surge of type 1 diabetes mellitus among Nigerian children during the Covid-19 pandemic. *Ann. Ib. Postgrad. Med.* **2022**, *20*, 58–64.
112. Herczeg, V.; Luczay, A.; Ténai, N.; Czine, G.; Tóth-Heyn, P. Anti-SARS-CoV-2 Seropositivity Among Children with Newly Diagnosed Type 1 Diabetes Mellitus: A Case-Control Study. *Indian Pediatr.* **2022**, *59*, 809–810.
113. Denina, M.; Trada, M.; Tinti, D.; Funiciello, E.; Novara, C.; Moretto, M.; Rosati, S.; Garazzino, S.; Bondone, C.; De Sanctis, L. Increase in newly diagnosed type 1 diabetes and serological evidence of recent SARS-CoV-2 infection: Is there a connection? *Front. Med.* **2022**, *9*, 927099.
114. Rahmati, M.; Keshvari, M.; Mirnasuri, S.; Yon, D.K.; Lee, S.W.; Il Shin, J.; Smith, L. The global impact of COVID-19 pandemic on the incidence of pediatric new-onset type 1 diabetes and ketoacidosis: A systematic review and meta-analysis. *J. Med. Virol.* **2022**, *94*, 5112–5127.
115. Lavik, A.R.; Ebekozien, O.; Noor, N.; Alonso, G.T.; Polsky, S.; Blackman, S.M.; Chen, J.; Corathers, S.D.; Demeterco-Berggren, C.; Gallagher, M.P.; et al. Trends in Type 1 Diabetic Ketoacidosis During COVID-19 Surges at 7 US Centers: Highest Burden on non-Hispanic Black Patients. *J. Clin. Endocrinol. Metab.* **2022**, *107*, 1948–1955.
116. Jia, X.; Gesualdo, P.; Geno Rasmussen, C.; Alkanani, A.A.; He, L.; Dong, F.; Rewers, M.J.; Michels, A.W.; Yu, L. Prevalence of SARS-CoV-2 Antibodies in Children and Adults with Type 1 Diabetes. *Diabetes. Technol. Ther.* **2021**, *23*, 517–521.
117. Messaaoui, A.; Hajselova, L.; Tenoutasse, S. Anti-SARS-CoV-2 antibodies in new-onset type 1 diabetes in children during pandemic in Belgium. *J. Pediatr. Endocrinol. Metab.* **2021**, *34*, 1319–1322.
118. Kompaniyets, L.; Bull-Otterson, L.; Boehmer, T.K.; Baca, S.; Alvarez, P.; Hong, K.; Hsu, J.; Harris, A.M.; Gundlapalli, A.V.; Saydah, S. Post-COVID-19 Symptoms and Conditions Among Children and Adolescents—United States, March 1, 2020–January 31, 2022. *MMWR Morb. Mortal. Wkly. Rep.* **2022**, *71*, 993–999.
119. Barrett, C.E.; Koyama, A.K.; Alvarez, P.; Chow, W.; Lundeen, E.A.; Perrine, C.G.; Pavkov, M.E.; Rolka, D.B.; Wiltz, J.L.; Bull-Otterson, L.; et al. Risk for newly diagnosed diabetes >30 days after SARS-CoV-2 infection among persons aged <18 years—United states, March 1, 2020–June 28, 2021. *MMWR Morb. Mortal. Wkly. Rep.* **2022**, *71*, 59–65.
120. Noorzae, R.; Junker, T.G.; Hviid, A.P.; Wohlfahrt, J.; Olsen, S.F. Risk of Type 1 Diabetes in Children Is Not Increased After SARS-CoV-2 Infection: A Nationwide Prospective Study in Denmark. *Diabetes Care* **2023**, *46*, 1261–1264.
121. Matsuda, F.; Itonaga, T.; Maeda, M.; Ihara, K. Long-term trends of pediatric type 1 diabetes incidence in Japan before and after the COVID-19 pandemic. *Sci. Rep.* **2023**, *13*, 5803.
122. Reschke, F.; Lanzinger, S.; Herczeg, V.; Prahalad, P.; Schiaffini, R.; Mul, D.; Clapin, H.; Zabeen, B.; Pelicand, J.; Phillip, M.; et al. The COVID-19 Pandemic Affects Seasonality, With Increasing Cases of New-Onset Type 1 Diabetes in Children, From the Worldwide SWEET Registry. *Diabetes Care* **2022**, *45*, 2594–2601.
123. Ata, A.; Jalilova, A.; Kırkgöz, T.; Işıklar, H.; Demir, G.; Altınok, Y.A.; Özkan, B.; Zeytinlioğlu, A.; Darcan, Ş.; Özen, S.; et al. Does COVID-19 predispose patients to type 1 diabetes mellitus? *Clin. Pediatr. Endocrinol.* **2022**, *31*, 33–37.
124. Tittel, S.R.; Rosenbauer, J.; Kamrath, C.; Ziegler, J.; Reschke, F.; Hammersen, J.; Mönkemöller, K.; Pappa, A.; Kapellen, T.; Holl, R.W. Did the COVID-19 lockdown affect the incidence of pediatric type 1 diabetes in Germany? *Diabetes Care* **2020**, *43*, e172–e173.
125. Pitocco, D.; Tartaglione, L.; Viti, L.; Di Leo, M.; Manto, A.; Caputo, S.; Pontecorvi, A. Lack of type 1 diabetes involvement in SARS-COV-2 population: Only a particular coincidence? *Diabetes Res. Clin. Pract.* **2020**, *164*, 108220.
126. Alassaf, A.; Gharaibeh, L.; Ibrahim, S.; Daher, A.; Irsheid, A.; Albaramki, J.; Odeh, R. Effect of COVID-19 pandemic on presentation and referral patterns of newly diagnosed children with type 1 diabetes in a developing country. *J. Pediatr. Endocrinol. Metab.* **2022**, *35*, 859–866.
127. Bombaci, B.; Passanisi, S.; Sorrenti, L.; Salzano, G.; Lombardo, F. Examining the associations between COVID-19 infection and pediatric type 1 diabetes. *Expert. Rev. Clin. Immunol.* **2023**, *19*, 489–497.
128. d'Annunzio, G.; Bassi, M.; De Rose, E.L.; Lezzi, M.; Minuto, N.; Calevo, M.G.; Gaiero, A.; Fichera, G.; Borea, R.; Maghnie, M. Increased Frequency of Diabetic Ketoacidosis: The Link With COVID-19 Pandemic. *Front. Clin. Diabetes Healthc.* **2022**, *3*, 846827.
129. Rivero-Martín, M.J.; Rivas-Mercado, C.M.; Ceñal-González-Fierro, M.J.; López-Barrena, N.; Lara-Orejas, E.; Alonso-Martín, D.; Alfaro-Iznaola, C.; Alcázar-Villar, M.J.; Sánchez-Escudero, V.; González-Vergaz, A. Severity of new-onset type 1 diabetes in children and adolescents during the coronavirus-19 disease pandemic. *Endocrinol. Diabetes. Nutr.* **2022**, *69*, 810–815.
130. Varol, F.; Ozyilmaz, L.G.B.; Sahin, E.G.; Can, Y.Y.; Altas, U.; Cam, H. Does the severity of diabetic ketoacidosis in children with type 1 diabetes change during the COVID-19 pandemic? A single-center experience from a pediatric intensive care unit. *N. Clin. Istanb.* **2022**, *9*, 429–435.
131. Leiva-Gea, I.; Fernández, C.A.; Cardona-Hernandez, R.; Lozano, M.F.; Bahíllo-Curieses, P.; Arroyo-Díez, J.; León, M.C.; Martín-Frías, M.; Barreiro, S.C.; Delgado, A.M.; et al. Increased Presentation of Diabetic Ketoacidosis and Changes in Age and Month of Type 1 Diabetes at Onset during the COVID-19 Pandemic in Spain. *J. Clin. Med.* **2022**, *11*, 4338.
132. Kiral, E.; Kirel, B.; Havan, M.; Keskin, M.; Karaoglan, M.; Yildirim, A.; Kangin, M.; Talay, M.N.; Urun, T.; Altug, U.; et al. Increased Severe Cases and New-Onset Type 1 Diabetes Among Children Presenting with Diabetic Ketoacidosis During First Year of COVID-19 Pandemic in Turkey. *Front. Pediatr.* **2022**, *10*, 926013.
133. Cherubini, V.; Marino, M.; Scaramuzza, A.E.; Tiberi, V.; Bobbio, A.; Delvecchio, M.; Piccinno, E.; Ortolani, F.; Innaurato, S.; Felappi, B.; et al. The Silent Epidemic of Diabetic Ketoacidosis at Diagnosis of Type 1 Diabetes in Children and Adolescents in Italy During the COVID-19 Pandemic in 2020. *Front. Endocrinol.* **2022**, *13*, 878634.

134. Pietrzak, I.; Michalak, A.; Seget, S.; Bednarska, M.; Beń-Skowronek, I.; Bossowski, A.; Chobot, A.; Dżygało, K.; Głowińska-Olszewska, B.; Górnicka, M.; et al. Diabetic ketoacidosis incidence among children with new-onset type 1 diabetes in Poland and its association with COVID-19 outbreak-Two-year cross-sectional national observation by PolPeDiab Study Group. *Pediatr. Diabetes* **2022**, *23*, 944–955. [CrossRef]
135. Lee, Y.; Kim, M.; Oh, K.; Kang, E.; Rhie, Y.-J.; Lee, J.; Hong, Y.H.; Shin, Y.-L.; Kim, J.H. Comparison of Initial Presentation of Pediatric Diabetes Before and During the Coronavirus Disease 2019 Pandemic Era. *J. Korean Med. Sci.* **2022**, *37*, e176. [CrossRef]
136. Kamrath, C.; Rosenbauer, J.; Eckert, A.J.; Ohlenschläger, U.; Sydlik, C.; Nellen-Hellmuth, N.; Holl, R.W. Glycated hemoglobin at diagnosis of type 1 diabetes and at follow-up in children and adolescents during the COVID-19 pandemic in Germany. *Pediatr. Diabetes* **2022**, *23*, 749–753.
137. Kaya, G.; Cimbek, E.A.; Yeşilbaş, O.; Bostan, Y.E.; Karagüzel, G. A Long-Term Comparison of Presenting Characteristics of Children with Newly Diagnosed Type 1 Diabetes Before and During the COVID-19 Pandemic. *J. Clin. Res. Pediatr. Endocrinol.* **2022**, *14*, 267–274.
138. Nagl, K.; Waldhör, T.; Hofer, S.E.; Fritsch, M.; Meraner, D.; Prchla, C.; Rami-Merhar, B.; Fröhlich-Reiterer, E. Alarming Increase of Ketoacidosis Prevalence at Type 1 Diabetes-Onset in Austria-Results from a Nationwide Registry. *Front. Pediatr.* **2022**, *10*, 820156.
139. Chambers, M.A.; Mecham, C.; Arreola, E.V.; Sinha, M. Increase in the Number of Pediatric New-Onset Diabetes and Diabetic Ketoacidosis Cases During the COVID-19 Pandemic. *Endocr. Pract.* **2022**, *28*, 479–485.
140. Mastromauro, C.; Blasetti, A.; Primavera, M.; Ceglie, L.; Mohn, A.; Chiarelli, F.; Giannini, C. Peculiar characteristics of new-onset Type 1 Diabetes during COVID-19 pandemic. *Ital. J. Pediatr.* **2022**, *48*, 26.
141. Gottesman, B.L.; Yu, J.; Tanaka, C.; Longhurst, C.A.; Kim, J.J. Incidence of New-Onset Type 1 Diabetes Among US Children During the COVID-19 Global Pandemic. *JAMA Pediatr.* **2022**, *176*, 414–415.
142. Luciano, T.M.; Halah, M.P.; Sarti, M.T.A.; Floriano, V.G.; da Fonseca, B.A.L.; Del Roio Liberatore, R., Jr.; Antonini, S.R. DKA and new-onset type 1 diabetes in Brazilian children and adolescents during the COVID-19 pandemic. *Arch. Endocrinol. Metab.* **2022**, *66*, 88–91.
143. Goldman, S.; Pinhas-Hamiel, O.; Weinberg, A.; Auerbach, A.; German, A.; Haim, A.; Zung, A.; Brener, A.; Strich, D.; Azoulay, E.; et al. Alarming increase in ketoacidosis in children and adolescents with newly diagnosed type 1 diabetes during the first wave of the COVID-19 pandemic in Israel. *Pediatr Diabetes* **2022**, *23*, 10–18.
144. Al-Abdulrazzaq, D.; Alkandari, A.; Alhusaini, F.; Alenazi, N.; Gujral, U.P.; Narayan, K.M.V.; Al-Kandari, H.; CODeR Group. Higher rates of diabetic ketoacidosis and admission to the paediatric intensive care unit among newly diagnosed children with type 1 diabetes in Kuwait during the COVID-19 pandemic. *Diabetes Metab. Res. Rev.* **2022**, *38*, e3506.
145. Kostopoulou, E.; Eliopoulou, M.I.; Rojas Gil, A.P.; Chrysis, D. Impact of COVID-19 on new-onset type 1 diabetes mellitus—A one-year prospective study. *Eur. Rev. Med. Pharmacol. Sci.* **2021**, *25*, 5928–5935.
146. Lee, M.S.; Lee, R.; Ko, C.W.; Moon, J.E. Increase in blood glucose level and incidence of diabetic ketoacidosis in children with type 1 diabetes mellitus in the Daegu-Gyeongbuk area during the coronavirus disease 2019 (COVID-19) pandemic: A retrospective cross-sectional study. *J. Yeungnam Med. Sci.* **2022**, *39*, 46–52.
147. Mameli, C.; Scaramuzza, A.; Macedoni, M.; Marano, G.; Frontino, G.; Luconi, E.; Pelliccia, C.; Felappi, B.; Guerraggio, L.P.; Spiri, D.; et al. Type 1 diabetes onset in Lombardy region, Italy, during the COVID-19 pandemic: The double-wave occurrence. *eClinicalMedicine* **2021**, *39*, 101067.
148. Alexandre, M.I.; Henriques, A.R.; Cavaco, D.; Rodrigues, L.; Costa, S.; Robalo, B.; Pereira, C.; Sampaio, M.L. New-Onset Type 1 Diabetes in Children and COVID-19. *Acta. Med. Port.* **2021**, *34*, 642–643. [CrossRef]
149. Dilek, S.Ö.; Gürbüz, F.; Turan, İ.; Celiloğlu, C.; Yüksel, B. Changes in the presentation of newly diagnosed type 1 diabetes in children during the COVID-19 pandemic in a tertiary center in Southern Turkey. *J. Pediatr. Endocrinol. Metab.* **2021**, *34*, 1303–1309.
150. Bogale, K.T.; Urban, V.; Schaefer, E.; Bangalore Krishna, K. The Impact of COVID-19 Pandemic on Prevalence of Diabetic Ketoacidosis at Diagnosis of Type 1 Diabetes: A Single-Centre Study in Central Pennsylvania. *Endocrinol. Diabetes Metab.* **2021**, *4*, e00235.
151. McGlacken-Byrne, S.M.; Drew, S.E.V.; Turner, K.; Peters, C.; Amin, R. The SARS-CoV-2 pandemic is associated with increased severity of presentation of childhood onset type 1 diabetes mellitus: A multi-centre study of the first COVID-19 wave. *Diabet Med.* **2021**, *38*, e14640.
152. Boboc, A.A.; Novac, C.N.; Ilie, M.T.; Ieșanu, M.I.; Galoș, F.; Bălgrădean, M.; Berghea, E.C.; Ionescu, M.D. The Impact of SARS-CoV-2 Pandemic on the New Cases of T1DM in Children. A Single-Centre Cohort Study. *J. Pers. Med.* **2021**, *11*, 551.
153. Ng, S.M.; Woodger, K.; Regan, F.; Soni, A.; Wright, N.; Agwu, J.C.; Williams, E.; Timmis, A.; Kershaw, M.; Moudiotis, C.; et al. Presentation of newly diagnosed type 1 diabetes in children and young people during COVID-19: A national UK survey. *BMJ Paediatr. Open* **2020**, *4*, e000884. [CrossRef]
154. Sellers, E.A.C.; Pacaud, D. Diabetic ketoacidosis at presentation of type 1 diabetes in children in Canada during the COVID-19 pandemic. *Paediatr. Child. Health* **2021**, *26*, 208–209.
155. Salmi, H.; Heinonen, S.; Hästbacka, J.; Lääperi, M.; Rautiainen, P.; Miettinen, P.J.; Vapalahti, O.; Hepojoki, J.; Knip, M. New-onset type 1 diabetes in Finnish children during the COVID-19 pandemic. *Arch. Dis. Child.* **2022**, *107*, 180–185. [CrossRef]
156. Sherif, E.M.; Elhenawy, Y.I.; Matter, R.M.; Aly, H.H.; Thabet, R.A.; Fereig, Y.A. Clinical characteristics and outcome of hospitalized children and adolescent patients with type 1 diabetes during the COVID-19 pandemic: Data from a single center surveillance study in Egypt. *J. Pediatr. Endocrinol. Metab.* **2021**, *34*, 925–936.

157. Alaqeel, A.; Aljuraibah, F.; Alsuhaibani, M.; Huneif, M.; Alsaheel, A.; Al Dubayee, M.; Alsaedi, A.; Bakkar, A.; Alnahari, A.; Taha, A.; et al. The Impact of COVID-19 Pandemic Lockdown on the Incidence of New-Onset Type 1 Diabetes and Ketoacidosis Among Saudi Children. *Front. Endocrinol.* **2021**, *12*, 669302. [CrossRef]
158. Ho, J.; Rosolowsky, E.; Pacaud, D.; Huang, C.; Lemay, J.; Brockman, N.; Rath, M.; Doulla, M. Diabetic ketoacidosis at type 1 diabetes diagnosis in children during the COVID-19 pandemic. *Pediatr. Diabetes* **2021**, *22*, 552–557. [CrossRef]
159. Jacob, R.; Weiser, G.; Krupik, D.; Takagi, D.; Peled, S.; Pines, N.; Hashavya, S.; Gur-Soferman, H.; Gamsu, S.; Kaplan, O.; et al. Diabetic Ketoacidosis at Emergency Department Presentation During the First Months of the SARS-CoV-2 Pandemic in Israel: A Multicenter Cross-Sectional Study. *Diabetes Ther.* **2021**, *12*, 1569–1574.
160. Dżygało, K.; Nowaczyk, J.; Szwilling, A.; Kowalska, A. Increased frequency of severe diabetic ketoacidosis at type 1 diabetes onset among children during COVID-19 pandemic lockdown: An observational cohort study. *Pediatr. Endocrinol. Diabetes Metab.* **2020**, *26*, 167–175.
161. Boddu, S.K.; Aurangabadkar, G.; Kuchay, M.S. New onset diabetes, type 1 diabetes and COVID-19. *Diabetes Metab. Syndr.* **2020**, *14*, 2211–2217.
162. Güemes, M.; Storch-de-Gracia, P.; Enriquez, S.V.; Martín-Rivada, Á.; Brabin, A.G.; Argente, J. Severity in pediatric type 1 diabetes mellitus debut during the COVID-19 pandemic. *J. Pediatr. Endocrinol. Metab.* **2020**, *33*, 1601–1603.
163. Kamrath, C.; Mönkemöller, K.; Biester, T.; Rohrer, T.R.; Warncke, K.; Hammersen, J.; Holl, R.W. Ketoacidosis in Children and Adolescents with Newly Diagnosed Type 1 Diabetes During the COVID-19 Pandemic in Germany. *JAMA* **2020**, *324*, 801–804.
164. Elgenidy, A.; Awad, A.K.; Saad, K.; Atef, M.; El-Leithy, H.H.; Obiedallah, A.A.; Hammad, E.M.; Ahmad, F.A.; Ali, A.M.; Dailah, H.G.; et al. Incidence of diabetic ketoacidosis during COVID-19 pandemic: A meta-analysis of 124,597 children with diabetes. *Pediatr. Res.* **2023**, *93*, 1149–1160.
165. Birkebaek, N.H.; Kamrath, C.; Grimsmann, J.M.; Aakesson, K.; Cherubini, V.; Dovc, K.; de Beaufort, C.; Alonso, G.T.; Gregory, J.W.; White, M.; et al. Impact of the COVID-19 pandemic on long-term trends in the prevalence of diabetic ketoacidosis at diagnosis of paediatric type 1 diabetes: An international multicentre study based on data from 13 national diabetes registries. *Lancet Diabetes Endocrinol.* **2022**, *10*, 786–794. [CrossRef]
166. Kamrath, C.; Rosenbauer, J.; Eckert, A.J.; Pappa, A.; Reschke, F.; Rohrer, T.R.; Mönkemöller, K.; Wurm, M.; Hake, K.; Raile, K.; et al. Incidence of COVID-19 and Risk of Diabetic Ketoacidosis in New-Onset Type 1 Diabetes. *Pediatrics* **2021**, *148*, e2021050856.
167. Nowak, Z.; Gawlik, J.; Wędrychowicz, A.; Nazim, J.; Starzyk, J. The incidence and causes of acute hospitalizations and emergency room visits in adolescents with type 1 diabetes mellitus prior to and during the COVID-19 pandemic: A single-centre experience. *Pediatr. Endocrinol. Diabetes Metab.* **2023**, *29*, 22–29.
168. Bui, H.; To, T.; Stein, R.; Fung, K.; Daneman, D. Is diabetic ketoacidosis at disease onset a result of missed diagnosis? *J. Pediatr.* **2010**, *156*, 472–477.
169. Wersäll, J.H.; Adolfsson, P.; Forsander, G.; Ricksten, S.E.; Hanas, R. Delayed referral is common even when new-onset diabetes is suspected in children. A Swedish prospective observational study of diabetic ketoacidosis at onset of type 1 diabetes. *Pediatr. Diabetes* **2021**, *22*, 900–908.
170. Keiner, E.S.; Slaughter, J.C.; Datye, K.A.; Cherrington, A.D.; Moore, D.J.; Gregory, J.M. COVID-19 Exacerbates Insulin Resistance During Diabetic Ketoacidosis in Pediatric Patients with Type 1 Diabetes. *Diabetes Care* **2022**, *45*, 2406–2411.
171. Piccolo, G.; De Rose, E.L.; Bassi, M.; Napoli, F.; Minuto, N.; Maghnie, M.; Patti, G.; D'annunzio, G. Infectious diseases associated with pediatric type 1 diabetes mellitus: A narrative review. *Front. Endocrinol.* **2022**, *13*, 966344. [CrossRef]
172. Ingrosso, D.M.F.; Primavera, M.; Samvelyan, S.; Tagi, V.M.; Chiarelli, F. Stress and Diabetes Mellitus: Pathogenetic Mechanisms and Clinical Outcome. *Horm. Res. Paediatr.* **2023**, *96*, 34–43.
173. Zorena, K.; Michalska, M.; Kurpas, M.; Jaskulak, M.; Murawska, A.; Rostami, S. Environmental Factors and the Risk of Developing Type 1 Diabetes-Old Disease and New Data. *Biology* **2022**, *11*, 608.
174. Lança, A.; Rodrigues, C.; Diamantino, C.; Fitas, A.L. COVID-19 in two children with new-onset diabetes: Case reports. *BMJ Case Rep.* **2022**, *15*, e247309.
175. Prosperi, S.; Chiarelli, F. COVID-19 and diabetes in children. *Ann. Pediatr. Endocrinol. Metab.* **2022**, *27*, 157–168.
176. Lammi, N.; Karvonen, M.; Tuomilehto, J. Do microbes have a causal role in type 1 diabetes? *Med. Sci. Monit.* **2005**, *11*, 63–69.
177. Rubino, F.; Amiel, S.A.; Zimmet, P.; Alberti, G.; Bornstein, S.; Eckel, R.H.; Mingrone, G.; Boehm, B.; Cooper, M.E.; Chai, Z.; et al. New-Onset Diabetes in Covid-19. *N. Engl. J. Med.* **2020**, *383*, 789–790.
178. Mine, K.; Nagafuchi, S.; Mori, H.; Takahashi, H.; Anzai, K. SARS-CoV-2 Infection and Pancreatic Cell Failure. *Biology* **2021**, *11*, 22.
179. Zubkiewicz-Kucharska, A.; Seifert, M.; Stepkowski, M.; Noczyńska, A. Diagnosis of type 1 diabetes during the SARS-CoV-2 pandemic: Does lockdown affect the incidence and clinical status of patients? *Adv. Clin. Exp. Med.* **2021**, *30*, 127–134.
180. Wang, Y.; Guo, H.; Wang, G.; Zhai, J.; Du, B. COVID-19 as a Trigger for type 1 diabetes. *J. Clin. Endocrinol. Metab.* **2023**, dgad165. [CrossRef]
181. Deinhardt-Emmer, S.; Wittschieber, D.; Sanft, J.; Kleemann, S.; Elschner, S.; Haupt, K.F.; Vau, V.; Haring, C.; Rödel, J.; Henke, A.; et al. Early postmortem mapping of SARS-CoV-2 RNA in patients with COVID-19 and the correlation with tissue damage. *Elife* **2021**, *10*, e60361.
182. Ding, Y.; He, L.; Zhang, Q.; Huang, Z.; Che, X.; Hou, J.; Wang, H.; Shen, H.; Qiu, L.; Li, Z.; et al. Organ distribution of severe acute respiratory syndrome (SARS) associated coronavirus (SARS-CoV) in SARS patients: Implications for pathogenesis and virus transmission pathways. *J. Pathol.* **2004**, *203*, 622–630.

183. Suwanwongse, K.; Shabarek, N. Newly diagnosed diabetes mellitus, DKA, and COVID-19: Causality or coincidence? A report of three cases. *J. Med. Virol.* **2021**, *93*, 1150–1153.
184. Kim, M. Is type 1 diabetes related to coronavirus disease 2019 in children? *Clin. Exp. Pediatr.* **2022**, *65*, 252–253.
185. Rewers, M.; Bonifacio, E.; Ewald, D.; Geno Rasmussen, C.; Jia, X.; Pyle, L.; Ziegler, A.-G.; ASK Study Group; Fr1da Study Group. SARS-CoV-2 Infections and Presymptomatic Type 1 Diabetes Autoimmunity in Children and Adolescents from Colorado, USA, and Bavaria, Germany. *JAMA* **2022**, *328*, 1252–1255.
186. Tekin, H.; Josefsen, K.; Krogvold, L.; Dahl-Jørgensen, K.; Gerling, I.; Pociot, F.; Buschard, K. PDE12 in type 1 diabetes. *Sci. Rep.* **2022**, *12*, 18149.
187. Calcaterra, V.; Bosoni, P.; Dilillo, D.; Mannarino, S.; Fiori, L.; Fabiano, V.; Carlucci, P.; Di Profio, E.; Verduci, E.; Mameli, C.; et al. Impaired Glucose-Insulin Metabolism in Multisystem Inflammatory Syndrome Related to SARS-CoV-2 in Children. *Children* **2021**, *8*, 384.
188. Calcaterra, V.; Zuccotti, G. Persistent insulin resistance at one year follow-up in multisystem inflammatory syndrome in children. *Diabetes Res. Clin. Pract.* **2023**, *202*, 110724. [CrossRef]

Disclaimer/Publisher's Note: The statements, opinions and data contained in all publications are solely those of the individual author(s) and contributor(s) and not of MDPI and/or the editor(s). MDPI and/or the editor(s) disclaim responsibility for any injury to people or property resulting from any ideas, methods, instructions or products referred to in the content.

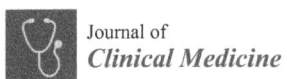

Review

Psychological and Cognitive Effects of Long COVID: A Narrative Review Focusing on the Assessment and Rehabilitative Approach

Rosaria De Luca, Mirjam Bonanno and Rocco Salvatore Calabrò *

IRCCS Centro Neurolesi "Bonino-Pulejo", Via Palermo, SS 113, C. da Casazza, 98124 Messina, Italy
* Correspondence: roccos.calabro@irccsme.it

Abstract: Long COVID is a clinical syndrome characterized by profound fatigue, neurocognitive difficulties, muscle pain, weakness, and depression, lasting beyond the 3–12 weeks following infection with SARS-CoV-2. Among the symptoms, neurocognitive and psychiatric sequelae, including attention and memory alterations, as well as anxiety and depression symptoms, have become major targets of current healthcare providers given the significant public health impact. In this context, assessment tools play a crucial role in the early screening of cognitive alterations due to Long COVID. Among others, the general cognitive assessment tools, such as the Montreal Cognitive assessment, and more specific ones, including the State Trait Inventory of Cognitive Fatigue and the Digit Span, may be of help in investigating the main neurocognitive alterations. Moreover, appropriate neurorehabilitative programs using specific methods and techniques (conventional and/or advanced) through a multidisciplinary team are required to treat COVID-19-related cognitive and behavioral abnormalities. In this narrative review, we sought to describe the main neurocognitive and psychiatric symptoms as well as to provide some clinical advice for the assessment and treatment of Long COVID.

Keywords: Long COVID syndrome; psychometric assessment; behavioral alterations; cognitive rehabilitation; conventional and advanced approaches

Citation: De Luca, R.; Bonanno, M.; Calabrò, R.S. Psychological and Cognitive Effects of Long COVID: A Narrative Review Focusing on the Assessment and Rehabilitative Approach. *J. Clin. Med.* 2022, 11, 6554. https://doi.org/10.3390/jcm11216554

Academic Editor: Giovanni Giordano

Received: 23 September 2022
Accepted: 3 November 2022
Published: 4 November 2022

Publisher's Note: MDPI stays neutral with regard to jurisdictional claims in published maps and institutional affiliations.

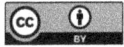

Copyright: © 2022 by the authors. Licensee MDPI, Basel, Switzerland. This article is an open access article distributed under the terms and conditions of the Creative Commons Attribution (CC BY) license (https://creativecommons.org/licenses/by/4.0/).

1. Introduction

Because of the COVID-19 pandemic, caused by SARS-CoV-2, many individuals experience post-infection long-lasting symptoms, namely post-COVID syndrome or Long COVID [1,2]. Long COVID is characterized by the persistence of exhausting fatigue, neurocognitive difficulties such as mental fog, muscle pain, and weakness, as well as depression, lasting beyond the 3–12 weeks following SARS-CoV-2 infection [3]. According to Naik et al., the most common symptoms are myalgia (10.9%), fatigue (5.5%), shortness of breath (6.1%), cough (2.1%), insomnia (1.4%), mood disturbances (0.48%), and anxiety (0.6%) [4,5]. The persistence of the symptoms seems to be linked to immune dysregulation due to harmful inflammation, although the exact causes are still unknown [6,7]. Recently, a huge number of studies have reported immune abnormalities, such as an increase in the innate immune system activity, chronic fatigue/myalgic syndrome, encephalomyelitis [8], fibromyalgia [9], cognitive dysfunction [10], depression, and other mental health disorders [11–13]. Concerning the latter disorders, neuroinflammation may play a key role in the onset of symptoms, through either an activation of microglia or auto-immune reactions [14,15]. Indeed, Long COVID often presents with "brain fog", which is characterized by low energy, concentration problems, disorientation, and difficulty finding the right words [16,17]. However, long-term psychological, cognitive, or adverse mental health consequences of COVID-19 have recently begun to be recognized. Hampshire et al. [18] showed that COVID-19 could have a multi-domain impact on human cognition, as assessed using psychometric subtests. In particular, people who had recovered from the infectious disease, including those no longer reporting symptoms, may exhibit significant cognitive deficits as compared to controls, when controlled for age, gender, education level, income, racial–ethnic group, pre-existing medical disorders, tiredness, depression, and anxiety. Moreover, Ocsovszky et al. [19] found a positive correlation between the level of depressive symptoms and anxiety in a Long COVID non-hospitalized cohort. Depression and anxiety have been shown to have a negative impact on symptom perception and also contribute to a higher number of symptoms in a non-hospitalized sample, suggesting a bi-directional interconnection between the clinical and psychological factors [20–23]. Therefore, multi-disciplinary rehabilitation interventions are necessary to better manage individuals with Long COVID. In fact, cognitive rehabilitation, including compensatory and metacognitive strategies, which are usually administered to patients with brain injury, can be also applied to the Long COVID population [24,25].

The aim of this narrative review is to describe Long COVID's neurological, cognitive and psychiatric sequelae and to give some clinical advice for assessment and cognitive rehabilitation of this long-lasting syndrome.

2. Search Methodology

The data were collected by searching on the following databases: Cochrane Library, PEDro, PubMed, and Google Scholar, using the following keywords: "long COVID symptoms" AND "long COVID cognitive manifestations" OR "long COVID neurological sequelae" AND "neuropsychiatric symptoms in long COVID" OR "depressive symptoms in long COVID" OR "anxiety symptoms in long COVID", AND "cognitive rehabilitation in long COVID" OR "rehabilitation in long COVID". Moreover, we also analyzed the references of the selected articles, including only English papers, in order to obtain a complete search. The articles were evaluated according to title, abstracts, and text, and selected based on their scientific validity, as per the authors' assessment. We include systematic and narrative reviews, randomized clinical trials (RCT), and pilot studies published between July 2020 and September 2022 which deal with the Long COVID psychological and cognitive symptoms in adult patients. Two reviewers (RDL and MB) screened 616 studies, of which 276 were selected, and after removing duplicates, we finally included 54 papers that addressed the main psychometric assessment tools and the neurorehabilitative approaches.

3. Neurological Manifestations of Long COVID

The neurological manifestations (NMs) of Long COVID remain an outstanding issue since the pathogenic mechanisms are poorly understood despite the high prevalence of the symptoms. The most commonly reported NMs are fatigue (72%), muscle aches/myalgia (57%), and headache (53%) [26]. Orrù G. et al. [27] also included loss of smell and loss of concentration, as well as insomnia and reduced quality of life. However, it has been pointed out that anosmia and dysgeusia are more commonly related to the acute COVID-19 infection as these specific symptoms generally resolve [28]. Conversely, symptoms such as headaches, anxiety, depression, brain fog, fatigue, and insomnia are more likely to belong to the post-infection syndrome. NM onset may be due to an association between biological and psychological factors. In fact, SARS-CoV-2 could remain in brain tissue long-term, affecting neuronal loss over time, in association with systemic inflammation and cerebrovascular changes, as recently demonstrated by Desai et al. [29]. Notably, inflammation may induce neuron injury/damage through the release of the cytotoxic and chemotactic mediators, activating the surrounding microglial cells and intensifying the microglia-mediated neuroinflammation [30]. This cytotoxins release causes neuronal loss and neurodegeneration, accounting for the cross-talk between the neurons and glial cells in the neuroinflammation status [31]. To overcome these negative implications, steroids have been successfully used, especially in the acute phase and in the most severely affected patients [32]. Moreover, to counteract prostaglandin-mediated inflammation, non-steroidal anti-inflammatory drugs may be used in different stages of the disease [33]. Some authors considered the use of Palmitoylethanolamide (PEA) in the treatment of Long COVID, showing that the compound could resolve these inflammatory processes, reducing the progression of chronic inflammation and promoting positive effects on the neurological system [34]. It has been highlighted that the peripheral activation of the trigemino-vascular system, through the inflammatory cytokine storm, is strictly involved in the development of headaches [35]. Headache, from continuous mild pain to severe migraine, seems to be one of the most common and persistent COVID-19 sequelae, and it is often accompanied with trigeminal neuralgia. Neuropathic pain due to Long COVID is underestimated compared to the other symptoms, although the main clinical features of neuropathic pain in COVID-19 patients, i.e., a prickling sensation (defined as a sensation of electric shock, burns, paresthesia, and hyperalgesia), have been well described [36,37].

Many patients complained of subtle cognitive impairment and behavioral changes that may be difficult for them to describe. These symptoms are often collectively referred to as "brain fog" or "mental clouding" [38]. However, the correlation between these self-reported symptoms and objective dysfunctions remains an unclear question. Di Stadio et al. [39] investigated the possible correlation between mental clouding and olfactory dysfunction: they found that the former might interfere with the capacity of the individual to identify odors, indirectly affecting olfactory function. In addition, subjects who suffered from mental clouding, headache, or both presented a more severe olfactory dysfunction compared to those patients without neurological complaints.

4. Cognitive Dysfunctions, Psychiatric Symptoms, and Behavioral Alterations

Cognitive dysfunctions are becoming the most popular symptoms in the research of Long COVID. In fact, cognitive symptoms have been reported in around 70% of the subjects [40,41]. Davis et al. [42] showed a high impact of post-COVID-19 cognitive dysfunction and/or memory impairment in daily working abilities, accounting for 86% of the sample affected. Guo et al. found a similar prevalence of cognitive symptoms: 77.8% of the patients presented difficulty in concentrating, 69% brain fog, 67.5% forgetfulness, 59.5% tip-of-the-tongue word-finding problems, and 43.7% semantic disfluency (saying or typing the wrong word) [43]. In addition, it has been shown that cognitive symptoms are more likely to develop in subjects affected by fatigue, cardiopulmonary, neurological, and autoimmune symptoms. However, in current clinical practice, it is very difficult to understand and define the "type and severity of the self-reported cognitive deficits", such as brain fog and difficulty concentrating, and consequently to more objectively measure cognitive performance. Indeed, most studies focused on the prevalence of cognitive alterations due to Long COVID, but not on the psychometric tools to measure the cognitive domains affected by the post-SARS-CoV-2 infection [44]. To overcome this issue, Alemanno et al. measured the cognitive abilities of patients in the COVID-19 post-acute phase that had experienced severe disease, using the Montreal Cognitive Assessment (MoCA). They have observed that 80% of patients reported cognitive alterations, especially in memory abilities, executive functioning, and language skills [45]. It has been observed that 33% of individuals in an intensive care unit showed a dysexecutive syndrome associated with inattention, disorientation, and reduced planning movements in response to the verbal indications [46]. Hosp et al. found a possible correlation between the cognitive dysfunctions and neurological abnormalities revealed with positron emission tomography, showing a predominant frontoparietal hypometabolism that correlated with poor MoCA scores [47], with lower scores in verbal memory and executive functions. However, these studies are limited to severely ill and old-age patients, and it is very challenging for clinicians to determine the nature of these dysfunctions and whether they are specific to COVID-19 or are more a-specific, such as a general consequence of acute respiratory distress. Indeed, some survivors of critical disease are recognized as experiencing long-term cognitive loss [48], particularly if they experience delirium [49,50].

In this context, it is important to know whether these deficits may also involve younger populations, as demonstrated by Almeria et al. in patients aged 24–60. This study reported that patients with neurological sequelae had lower performance in attention, memory, and executive function, suggesting an association between symptomatology and cognitive deficits [51].

Recent literature regarding the long-term neuropsychiatric sequelae of COVID-19 focused on self-reported symptoms through questionnaires administered either in-person or by telephone interviews [52–54]. Notably, Long COVID has been found to cause anxiety and depression symptoms as well as other neuropsychiatric and cognitive sequelae [55–59]. Indeed, the incidence of anxiety, depression, and post-traumatic stress was 42%, 31%, and 28%, respectively, in an Italian sample [60]. Considering the alarming impact of COVID-19 on mental health, Clemente et al. investigated the correlation between the psychological status of patients who had recovered from the SARS-CoV-2 infection and their inflammatory status, showing that survivors are at risk of developing psychiatric sequelae, such as anxiety, depression, and somatization symptoms, as well as sleep disorders [61–63]. An interesting association has also been demonstrated between high ferritin blood levels and sleep disturbances, stress, depression, and suicidal ideation [64,65].

To summarize, the SARS-CoV-2 epidemic was associated with psychiatric and cognitive complications, as confirmed by several researchers [66–69], and patients with preexisting psychiatric disorders reported the worsening of previous symptoms [70–73]. These findings could support the idea that those who have experienced the COVID-19 infection may be at a higher risk for neurodegeneration and dementia. In fact, COVID-19-related cardiovascular and cerebrovascular disease may also contribute to a higher long-term risk of cognitive decline and dementia in recovered individuals [74].

Moreover, a vast number of studies showed that obesity and diabetes have been associated with worse outcomes during the COVID-19 infection. In fact, people with obesity have an increased prevalence of diseases such as renal insufficiency, cardiovascular diseases, Type 2 diabetes mellitus, certain types of cancers, and a significant degree of endothelial dysfunction. These conditions are major risk factors for the disease severity and mortality associated with COVID-19 [75,76]. In particular, Vimercate et al. (2021) have shown that obesity is associated also with worse Long COVID symptoms such as respiratory diseases and hypertension, suggesting that being affected by overweight or obesity is associated with prolonged symptoms after resolution [77]. Today, limited evidence has shown that the clinical and socio-demographical features of the patients (such as the number of symptoms in the first week, age, and sex) before the COVID-19 infection play a key role in the prediction of Long COVID's duration [78]. Notably, Bellou et al. have investigated the association of 91 unique prognostic factors, divided into seven different categories, including demographic and anthropometric individual characteristics, biomarkers, symptoms, clinical signs, medical history and comorbid diseases, and medications, thus facilitating the selection of candidate predictors for a prognostic model [79]. In this context, Wang et al. found that psychological distress before the COVID-19 infection, including depression, anxiety, worry, perceived stress, and loneliness, was associated with a 32–46% increased risk of Long COVID [80]. For all these reasons, urgent in-person neuropsychological and neuropsychiatric assessments on Long COVID individuals are needed.

5. Psychometric Assessment and Neurorehabilitative Approach

In the rehabilitation of cognitive dysfunctions, assessment plays a crucial role, and even more so in patients with Long COVID. Few of the aforementioned studies have explored the long-term psychological, behavioral, and cognitive sequelae of this potentially disabling syndrome. In fact, only recently have researchers begun to more objectively address the specific cognitive domains affected by this disease through the use of proper clinical scales and psychometric batteries [81]. In this context, Holdsworth et al. demonstrated that systematic cognitive testing may offer a tool to 'rule in' objective neurocognitive insult in the wake of this prevalent disease [54]. However, administering psychometric tests overtime to the same subjects is useful to detect changes that may confirm either persistence or resolution of cognitive symptoms and deficits [82]. Specifically, some authors used the Montreal Cognitive Assessment (MoCA) to test general cognitive status in

COVID-19 patients at discharge [83]. Neuropsychological and cognitive symptoms due to Long COVID were evaluated by a complete psychometric battery to assess verbal fluency, nonverbal skills, memory abilities, executive functions, and reasoning [84–86]. In particular, researchers noticed that both Long COVID patients and healthy participants completed the tasks, but only the "No COVID" group completed a specific cognitive task referred to as the Test of 2D mental rotation, indicating a deficit in reasoning in the Long COVID patients' group [87].

O'Connor et al. have developed the COVID-19 Yorkshire Rehabilitation Scale (C19-YRS), a useful measure for examining an LCS's sample. C19-YRS is a 22-item patient-reported outcome measure designed to evaluate the long-term impact of COVID-19 across the domains of the activities and participation of the International Classification of Functioning, Disability, and Health and to evaluate the impact of LCS rehabilitation, including clinician-completed, self-report, and digital versions [88,89].

On the other hand, post-COVID-19 psychological and psychiatric symptoms have been investigated using numerous standardized questionnaires: the Hospital Anxiety and Depression Scale (HADS) [90] and the Generalized Anxiety Disorder-7 (GAD-7) [84], for anxiety and related symptoms. In detail, Monterrosa-Blanco recommended the use of GAD-7 during the COVID-19 pandemic; it is a widely used screening tool for anxiety with a cut-off score of 10, and it has been standardized in a sample of Colombian general practitioners [91], while the Patient Health Questionnaire-9 (PHQ-9) is for depression. The PHQ-9 is a commonly used screening tool for depression with a cut-off of 10 to consider the diagnosis. The bivariate meta-analysis of 18 validation studies identified cut-off scores between 8 and 11 as optimal means for detecting major depressive disorder [92], and the Zung Self-Rating Depression Scale (ZSDS) was used to investigate the depression symptoms in the COVID-19 pandemic among Colombian university workers [93]. Moreover, considering the high frequency of sleep alterations due to COVID-19, some authors have investigated sleep quality and insomnia using ad hoc clinical scales such as the Medical Outcomes Study Sleep Scale (MOS-SS) [94] and the Pittsburgh Sleep Quality Index (PSQI) [95]. In post-acute COVID-19 syndrome, the quality of life was investigated using the EuroQol-5 Dimension (EQ-5D) [96], while fatigue symptoms were evaluated through the FACIT-Fatigue scale, a self-report questionnaire to investigate symptoms on a five-point Likert-scale, with a sum score ranging from 0 (worst fatigue) to 52 (no fatigue) [97], as well as post-traumatic stress disorder checklist for DSM 5 (PCL-5) for post-traumatic stress symptoms [98,99].

Most of the preexisting tools to investigate mood, behavioral, and cognitive problems in other patient populations have been adapted to individuals with Long COVID, whilst only a few scales have been specifically developed to test this syndrome (Table 1). In particular, Klok et al. proposed the post-COVID-19 Functional Status Scale (PCFS) to measure the full spectrum of functional outcomes following COVID-19 [100]. Hughes et al. have validated a novel outcome measure for patients after COVID-19: the symptom burden questionnaire for Long COVID (SBQ-LC). The SBQ-LC includes 16 symptom scales, each measuring a different symptom domain and a single scale measuring symptom interference. Each scale measures a different symptom domain (e.g., breathing and circulation) and an "interference" scale measures the impact of a person's symptoms on everyday life. This was developed as a comprehensive measure of the symptom burden from Long COVID [101].

High-quality instruments to measure patients' reported outcomes are required to better understand the signs, symptoms, and underlying pathophysiology of Long COVID, to develop safe and effective interventions, and to meet the day-to-day needs of this growing patient group. There is at this time a lack of information in literature about the current effectiveness of motor and psychological repair in Long COVID subjects. However, growing evidence is demonstrating the importance of a targeted rehabilitation intervention of psychological sequelae and cognitive dysfunctions, using different techniques and systems focused on various methodological approaches, in addition to an early screening. Indeed, the treatment of Long COVID is not well defined, given that, until today, no drug therapy has been shown to improve the symptomatology.

Only a paper [102] by our group has demonstrated the potential efficacy of Palmitoylethanolamide (PEA), an endogenous lipid mediator that has an entourage effect on the endocannabinoid system mitigating the cytokine storm, in improving COVID-19-associated symptoms, as evaluated by the PCFS (a specific tool that investigates the physical and psychological symptoms following SARS Cov-2 infection). In fact, the anti-inflammatory properties of PEA are related to its ability to regulate several genes involved in the anti-inflammatory response, such as pro-inflammatory cytokines (tumor necrosis factor [TNF]-α and inter-leucine-1β), and also to counteract in the chronic inflammation status. Although some authors attempted to give indications on treating and managing this syndrome, no agreement has been reached about the best therapeutic strategy [103].

Compagno et al. reported the use of a multidisciplinary rehabilitation (MDR) program, including both physical training and psychological treatment, to stimulate psycho-motor parameters in patients with Long COVID. These authors suggested that the MDR program is safe and feasible in these patients and could reduce residual symptoms and promote physical and psychological recovery [104]. Fine et al. described the guidelines statement about the Long-COVID-related cognitive symptom assessment coupled with the specific cognitive disease, as well as the specific treatment recommendations [105].

Table 1. The neuropsychological and psychological measures used to assess cognitive and behavioral alterations in Long COVID, including the non-specific "adapted" tools and newly "designed" Long COVID ones.

Neuropsychological Measures	Domain	Short Description
Adapted assessment tools for Long COVID		
Mini Mental State Examination—MMSE (Fine et al., 2022) [105]	Global Cognitive Status in Long COVID subjects with moderate and severe cognitive deterioration.	MMSE is a psychometric test commonly used for screening global cognitive functioning. It consists of eleven questions and takes only 5–10 min to administer. It is a 30-point test used to measure some specific cognitive domains: − orientation to time and place (knowing where you are and the season or day of the week) − short-term memory (recall) − attention and ability to solve problems (such as spelling a simple word backwards) − language (identifying common objects by name) − comprehension and motor skills (drawing a slightly complicated shape such as two pentagons intersecting)
Montreal Cognitive Assessment—MoCA (Lynch et al., 2022) [83]	Global cognitive functioning in Long COVID subjects with mild–moderate and severe neuropsychological sequelae	The Montreal Cognitive Assessment (MoCA) is a widely used screening assessment for detecting cognitive impairment. It was validated as a highly sensitive tool for early detection of mild cognitive impairment (MCI) in 2000. MoCA accurately and quickly assesses: − Short-term memory − Visuo-spatial abilities − Executive functions − Attention, concentration, and working memory − Language − Orientation to time and place

Table 1. Cont.

Neuropsychological Measures	Domain	Short Description
Trail Making Test Part A and Part B—TMT A and B (Becker et al., 2021) [86]	Processing speed Executive functioning	TMT consists of 25 circles distributed over a sheet of paper. In Part A, the circles are numbered 1–25, and the patient should draw lines to connect the numbers in ascending order. In Part B, the circles include both numbers (1–13) and letters (A–L); as in Part A, the patient draws lines to connect the circles in an ascending pattern but with the added task of alternating between the numbers and letters (i.e., 1-A-2-B-3-C, etc.). The patient should be instructed to connect the circles as quickly as possible without lifting the pen or pencil from the paper. The patient is timed as he or she connects the "trail". Results for both TMT A and B are reported as the number of seconds required to complete the task; therefore, higher scores reveal greater impairment.
Saint Louis University Mental—SLUMS (Fine et al., 2022) [105]	Cognitive impairment	SLUMS measures diverse aspects of cognition. It consists of 11 questions that help a healthcare provider evaluate: — Orientation — Short-term memory — Calculations — Naming of animals — Clock drawing test — Recognition of geometric figures — Final scores range from 0 to 30.
Mini-Cog—MC (Fine et al., 2022) [105]	Short-term memory learning	The Mini-Cog is a 3 min instrument that can increase detection of cognitive impairment in older adults. It combines a short memory test with a simple clock-drawing test to enable fast screening for short-term memory problems, learning disabilities, and other cognitive functions that are reduced in dementia patients.
Short Test of Mental Status—STMS (Fine et al., 2022) [105]	Global cognition	The Short Test of Mental Status can be administered to patients in approximately 5 min, and it contains items that test orientation, attention, immediate recall, arithmetic, abstraction, construction, information, and delayed (approximately 3 min) recall.
Digit Span—DGS (Fine et al., 2022) [105] Number span forward and backward (Becker et al., 2021) [86]	Attention and working memory	Digit Span (DGS) is a measure of verbal short-term and working memory. DGS can be used in two formats, Forward Digit Span and Reverse Digit Span. This is a verbal task, with stimuli presented auditorily, and responses spoken by the participant and scored automatically by the software. Participants are presented with a random series of digits and are asked to repeat them in either the order presented (forward span) or in reverse order (backwards span).

Table 1. Cont.

Neuropsychological Measures	Domain	Short Description
Digit Vigilance Test—DVT (Fine et al., 2022) [105]	Sustained attention	The DVT is a simple task designed to measure vigilance during rapid visual tracking and accurate selection of target stimuli. It focuses on alertness and vigilance, while placing minimal demands on two other components of attention: selectivity and capacity.
Cancellation test (Albert's Test)—CT-AT (Fine et al., 2022) [105]	Unilateral spatial neglect (USN) visuo-spatial research	Albert's Test is commonly a visual neglect screen that requires patients to cross out lines on a single piece of paper.
Letter Fluency Test—LFT adapted tool (Fine et al., 2022) [105]	Phonemic verbal fluency	Verbal fluency tests are brief assessment tools with relatively simple administration and scoring procedures. Semantic and phonemic fluency are measures of non-motor processing speed, language production, and executive functions. In particular, the Phonemic Verbal Fluency Test was shown to be sensitive for assessment of functional communication skills, commonly used for aphasic patients. Letter fluency is also referred to as phonemic test fluency.
Category Fluency Test—CFT (Guo et al., 2022) [87]	Semantic/Category fluency	Verbal fluency tests are a kind of psychological test in which participants have to produce as many words as possible from a category in a given time (usually 60 s). This category can be semantic, including objects such as animals or fruits, or phonemic, including words beginning with a specified letter, such as p, for example. The semantic fluency test is sometimes described as the category fluency test or simply as "free listing".
Boston Naming Test—BNT (Fine et al., 2022) [105]	Denomination language abilities	The Boston Naming Test (BNT) is a widely used neuropsychological assessment tool to measure confrontational word retrieval in individuals with aphasia or other language disturbances caused by stroke, Alzheimer's disease, or other dementing disorders. The BNT contains 60 line drawings graded in difficulty. Patients with anomia often have greater difficulties with the naming of not only difficult and low-frequency objects but also easy and high-frequency objects.
Brief Visual Memory Test—BVMT (Fine et al., 2022) [105]	Visuo-spatial learning and memory	The brief visuo-spatial memory test-revised (BVMT-R) assesses visuo-spatial learning and memory in adults. It has equivalent forms that allow reassessing of patients.
Rey–Osterrieth Complex Figure Test—R-OCFT (Fine et al., 2022) [105]	Visuo-spatial abilities, memory, attention, planning, working memory, and executive functions	The Rey–Osterrieth complex figure (ROCF) is a neuropsychological assessment in which examinees are asked to reproduce a complicated line drawing, first by copying it freehand (recognition), and then drawing from memory (recall).

Table 1. Cont.

Neuropsychological Measures	Domain	Short Description
Wechsler Memory Scale-IV—WMS-IV (Fine et al., 2022) [105]	Memory functions	The Wechsler Memory Scale (WMS) is a neuropsychological test designed to measure different memory functions. A person's performance is reported as five index scores: Auditory Memory, Visual Memory, Visual Working Memory, Immediate Memory, and Delayed Memory.
State Trait Inventory of Cognitive Fatigue (STI-CF) (Fine et al., 2022) [105]	Cognitive fatigue	The STI-CF is a 32-item subjective measure of cognitive fatigue. It refers to low alertness and cognitive impairment.
Stroop Color Word—SCW (Fine et al., 2022) [105]	Executive functions	The Stroop Color and Word Test (SCWT) is a neuropsychological test extensively used to assess the ability to inhibit cognitive interference that occurs when the processing of a specific stimulus feature impedes the simultaneous processing of a second stimulus attribute, known well as the Stroop Effect.
Tower of London—TOL (Fine et al., 2022) [105]	Executive functions	The Tower of London test is a test used in applied clinical neuropsychology for the assessment of executive functioning, specifically to detect deficits in planning, which may occur due to a variety of medical and neuropsychiatric conditions.
Wisconsin Card Sorting Test—WCST (Guo et al., 2022) [87]	Executive functions	The Wisconsin Card Sorting Test (WCST) is a neuropsychological test that is frequently used to measure such higher-level cognitive processes as attention, perseverance, working memory, abstract thinking, category fluency, and set shifting. The WCST consists of two card packs with four stimulus cards and 64 response cards in each.
Word List Recognition Memory Test—WLRMT (Guo et al., 2022) [87]	Verbal memory learning	Wordlist memory tests are commonly used for cognitive assessment, particularly in Alzheimer's disease research and screening. Commonly used tests employ a variety of inherent features, such as list length, number of learning trials, order of presentation across trials, and inclusion of semantic categories.
Pictorial Associative Memory Test—PAMT (Guo et al., 2022) [87]	Visual associative memory	Picture Memory Impairment Screen for People with Intellectual Disability (PMIS-ID). The PMIS-ID consists of four-color photographs semantically unrelated in each quadrant. It includes four distinct parts: Identification (I), Learning (L), Immediate Recall (IR), and Delayed Recall (DR)
Mental Rotation Test—MRT (Guo et al., 2022) [87]	Spatial abilities/Mental rotation	The Mental Rotations Test is a test of spatial ability. Mental rotation time is defined as the time it takes someone to find out if a stimulus matches another stimulus through mental rotation.

Table 1. *Cont.*

Neuropsychological Measures	Domain	Short Description
Hospital Anxiety and Depression Scale (HADS) (Herrmann-Lingen et al., 2011) [90]	Depression and anxiety symptoms	HADS-A consists of 7 items assessing anxiety symptoms, whereas HADS-D consists of 7 items evaluating depressive symptoms. Each item is scored on a 4-point Likert scale (0–3), providing a maximum of 21 points for each subscale. It is a patient-reported outcome measure for evaluating the emotional consequences of SARS-CoV-2 in hospitalized COVID-19 survivors with Long COVID.
Generalized Anxiety Disorder-7 (GAD-7) (Spitzer et al. 2006; Monterrosa-Blanco et al., 2021) [84,91]	Anxiety and related symptoms	GAD-7 is a screening and monitoring test for Generalized Anxiety Disorder. It is not a replacement for a diagnosis from a doctor. The answers to each question are given a value from 0 to 3 depending on severity.
Patient Health Questionnaire-9, (PHQ-9) (Olanipekun et al., 2022) [92]	Depression symptoms	The PHQ-9 is the depression module, which scores each of the nine DSM-IV criteria as "0" (not at all) to "3" (nearly every day). It has been validated for use in primary care. It is not a screening tool for depression, but it is used to monitor the severity of depression and the response to treatment.
Zung Self-Rating Depression Scale (ZSDS) (García-Garro et al., 2022) [93]	Depression symptoms	Depression was assessed using the Zung Self-Rating Depression Scale (ZSDS). This instrument consists of 20 questions split into 10 positive and 10 negative questions related to the frequency of depressive symptoms (DS). Each question receives a score between 1 and 4 (a little of the time = 1; some of the time = 2; good part of the time = 3; most of the time = 4), which means that the total score can range between 20 and 80 points, where higher scores are related to the presence of DS. For dichotomization, a global score of 55 points was taken as the cut-off point, resulting in two categories: with DS (>55) and without DS ($\leq$55).
Medical Outcomes Study Sleep Scale (MOS-SS) (Scarpelli et al., 2021) [94]	Insomnia—Sleeping difficulty	The Medical Outcomes Study-Sleep Scale is a self-administered questionnaire with 12 items to assess sleep quality and quantity within 4 weeks (details in the online supporting information). Three variables were extracted from the MOS-SS for further analyses: (a) the Sleep Index II or sleep problem index, an aggregate measure of responses concerning four sleep domains (sleep disturbance, awakening with shortness of breath or with headache, sleep adequacy, and somnolence), as a synthetic measure of sleep quality; (b) sleep duration (item 2); and (c) self-reported evaluation of intrasleep wakefulness (item 8), dichotomized as follows: "high intrasleep wakefulness" (answer 3, 4, or 5) and "low intrasleep wakefulness" (answer 1 or 2).

Table 1. Cont.

Neuropsychological Measures	Domain	Short Description
Pittsburgh Sleep Quality Index (PSQI) (Taporoski et al., 2022) [95]	Sleep quality	The Pittsburgh Sleep Quality Index (PSQI) was used to assess the participants' sleep quality. The PSQI is composed of 24 questions and measures seven different domains: (i) sleep latency, (ii) subjective sleep quality, (iii) daytime dysfunctions, (iv) sleep duration, (v) sleep disturbances, (vi) habitual sleep efficiency, and (vii) use of sleep medications, generating a global score. Each domain can be scored between 0 and 3 points, resulting in a global score ranging from 0 to 21, where higher scores are related to worse sleep quality.
EuroQol-5 Dimension (EQ-5D) (Tabacof et al., 2022) [96]	Health-related quality of life	EQ-5D is an instrument which evaluates the generic quality of life developed in Europe and is widely used. The EQ-5D descriptive system is a preference-based HRQL measure with one question for each of the five dimensions, which include mobility, self-care, usual activities, pain/discomfort, and anxiety/depression.
FACIT-Fatigue scale (Sanchez-Ramirez et al., 2021) [97]	Fatigue	Fatigue was assessed using the 13-item FACIT fatigue scale, a widely used and validated self-report questionnaire to assess symptoms on a five-point Likert-scale with a sum score ranging from 0 (worst fatigue) to 52 (no fatigue). Clinically relevant fatigue was defined by scores ≤ 30, as suggested by the creators of the scale, based on general population data.
Checklist for DSM 5 (PCL-5) (Liyanage-Don et al., 2022; Bovin et al., 2016) [98,99]	Post-traumatic stress symptoms (PTSD)	The PCL-5 is a 20-item self-report measure of the 20 DSM-5 symptoms of Post-Traumatic Stress Disorder (PTSD). Included in the scale are four domains consistent with the four criteria of PTSD in DSM-5: Re-experiencing (criterion B) Avoidance (criterion C); Negative alterations in cognition and mood (criterion D); Hyper-arousal (criterion E). The PCL-5 can be used to monitor symptom change, to screen for PTSD, or to make a provisional PTSD diagnosis.
"Newly" Designed tools for Long COVID		
COVID-19 Yorkshire Rehabilitation Scale (C19-YRS) (O'Connor et al., 2022; Sivan et al., 2021) [88,89]	Persistent COVID-19 symptoms	The C19-YRS outcome measure is a clinically validated screening tool recommended for use, consisting of 22 items with each item rated on an 11-point numerical rating scale from 0 (none of this symptom) to 10 (extremely severe level or impact). The C19-YRS is divided into four subscales (range of total score for each subscale): symptom severity score (0–100), functional disability score (0–50), additional symptoms (0–60), and overall health (0–10).

Table 1. Cont.

Neuropsychological Measures	Domain	Short Description
Post-COVID-19 Functional Status scale (PCFS) (Klok et al., 2020) [100]	Post-COVID-19 functional symptoms	PCFS is a tool to measure functional status over time after COVID-19. The PCFS scale stratification is composed of five scale grades: grade 0 (No functional limitations); grade 1 (Negligible functional limitations); grade 2 (Slight functional limitations); grade 3 (Moderate functional limitations) and grade 4 (Severe functional limitations). The final scale grade 5 is 'death', which is required to be able to use the scale as an outcome measure in clinical trials, but was left out for this self-administered questionnaire.
Symptom burden questionnaire for Long COVID (SBQ-LC) (Hughes et al., 2021) [101]	Long COVID burden	The SBQ-LC includes 16 symptom scales, each measuring a different symptom domain and a single-scale measuring symptom interference. It is a patient-reported outcome (PRO) measure and a multi-domain item bank that has been developed according to international best-practice and regulatory guidance. The SBQ™-LC system measures symptom burden in adults (18+ years) with post-acute sequelae of COVID-19 (PASC), also known as "post COVID-19 condition" or "Long COVID".

Legend: MMSE (Mini Mental State Examination), MoCA (Montreal Cognitive Assessment), SLUMS (Saint Louis University Mental Status), MC (Mini-Cog), STMS (Short Test of Mental Status), DS (Digit Span), DVT (Digit Vigilance Test), CT–AT (Cancellation Test–Albert's Test), LFT (Letter Fluency Test), CFT (Category Fluency Test), BNT (Boston Naming Test), BVMT (Brief Visual Memory Test), R-OCFT (Rey–Osterrieth Complex Figure Test), WMS-IV (Wechsler Memory Scale-IV), STI-CF (State Trait Inventory of Cognitive Fatigue), SCW (Stroop Color Word), TOL (Tower of London), WCST (Wisconsin Card Sorting Test), WLRMT (Word List Recognition Memory Test), PAMT (Pictorial Associative Memory Test), MRT (Mental Rotation Test), GAD-7 (Generalized Anxiety Disorder-7), HADS (Hospital Anxiety and Depression Scale), ZSDS (Zung Self-Rating Depression Scale), MOS-SS (Medical Outcomes Study Sleep Scale), PSQI (Pittsburgh Sleep Quality Index), EQ-5D (EuroQol-5 Dimension), FACIT (Fatigue Scale), PCL-5 (Checklist for DSM 5), SBQ-LC (Symptom burden questionnaire for Long COVID).

Moreover, these authors reported an interesting classification of the main traditional therapeutic interventions or tasks to stimulate specific neuropsychological sub-domains, such as attention, processing speed, motor function/speed, language, memory, mental fatigue, executive function, and visuo-spatial or visuo-construction skills [105].

The main cognitive tasks and treatments, as reported in the current literature for Long COVID subjects, concerned attention process training, structured tasks for speech-language alterations, recording talks and lectures, semantic feature analysis, training in metacognitive strategies to promote self-awareness and self-monitoring, application of compensatory strategies/aids for writing and organization, use of language-mediated strategies such as self-talk or verbalization to solve problems or remember information, and cognitive behavioral therapy [106,107]. Recent evidence has shown that Long COVID patients at home will benefit from mindfulness-based cognitive therapy using different strategies that include prescribing memory-strengthening homework to address lack of concentration, inability to remember common words, and trouble recalling the events from the previous day, such as taking notes, using a planner to record information, and dividing a task into smaller increments to prevent brain fatigue, which are common strategies that can be used with pacing, endurance, and memory [108,109] (see Table 2).

These approaches are those commonly used to train patients with severe acquired brain injury (SABI) and play a role in cognitive rehabilitation following COVID-19, including the Long COVID condition.

In line with this rehabilitative prospective, Mathern et al. have emphasized the importance of a multidisciplinary team to realize some specific neurocognitive rehabilitation programs [109], such as physiatrists, neurologists, neuropsychologists, therapists of psychiatric rehabilitation, and speech therapists who can help COVID-19 patients (see Figure 1).

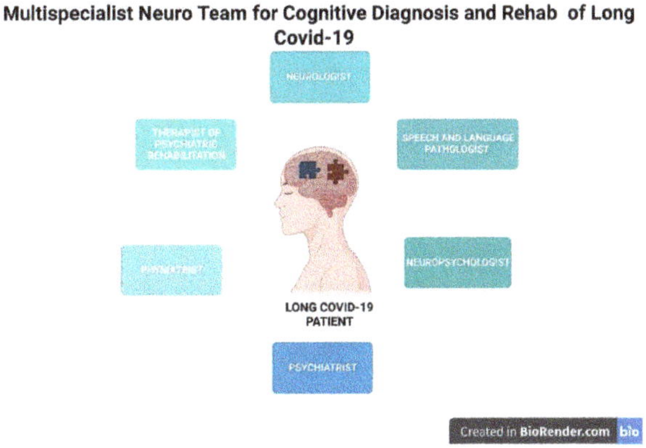

Figure 1. This represents the necessary healthcare figures for the cognitive diagnosis and rehabilitation of Long COVID patients. Created with BioRender.com https://biorender.com/ (accessed on 13 September 2022) [110].

In fact, according to our opinion, a multidisciplinary approach to both assess and treat the sequelae of COVID-19 is essential; this also confirmed by García-Molina et al. [111]. In addition, rehabilitation programs should also focus on developing an outpatient multidisciplinary programmatic approach to improve functional outcome and facilitate recovery [112,113]. In particular, rehabilitation programs based on endurance and balance training have yielded improvements in cognition [114], as have the use of virtual reality or PC-based tasks; VR gaming was perceived as a positive and motivating rehabilitation treatment after Long COVID, with benefits regarding stress reduction and cognitive functioning [115–117]. In this context, a plan for discharge should also be included to follow patients in the long-term, using psychological services. In fact, tele-rehabilitation allows us to perform home-based exercises tailored to the patients' needs, which can be implemented based on specific areas of cognitive deficit [118].

Patients could benefit from tele-therapy or tele-counseling to address emotional and mood disturbances [119], and some studies [120–123] have demonstrated improvement with on-line intervention for older adults with neurodegenerative disease and for caregivers of patients affected by severe acquired brain injury during the COVID-19 era.

Other technologies are available and approved for clinical use but have not been extensively studied in the treatment of the cytokine storm in COVID-19 patients [124]. Indeed, brain and immune response are bidirectionally correlated, acting throughout the body as potential targets for noninvasive neuromodulatory approaches [125]. In particular, an emergent and advanced approach to improve visual and cognitive impairments due to Long COVID is represented by neuromodulation, namely non-invasive brain stimulation (NIBS) using microcurrent. Considering that visual and cognitive symptoms in Long COVID may also be a neuro-vascular problem caused by a reduced blood flow (vascular dysregulation and deoxygenation) associated with neural hypometabolism, Sabel et al. hypothesized that the transorbital alternating current stimulation (tACS) might be able to reduce Long COVID symptoms [126]. However, there is no substantial evidence of treatment for this novel neuromodulatory approach to these impairments, except for that of Thams F. et al., who elaborated an innovative protocol about the combined use of transcranial direct current stimulation (tDCS) with concurrent cognitive training in post-COVID-19 infection, without publishing their results yet [127].

Table 2. The main conventional and advanced techniques used in the Long COVID treatment of psychological and cognitive sequelae, reporting major findings according to current evidence.

Task Domain–Specific	Conventional Approach Face to Face with Therapist Paper/Pencil Tasks		Advanced Approach PC-Based/Virtual Setting/Assistent Software Dedicated/Virtual Task	
	Reference	Training and Major Findings	Reference	Training and Major Findings
Attention processes Well-being	(Fine et al., 2022) [105]	Attention Process Training—APT (For verbal and nonverbal tasks, metacognitive strategies, timed structured activities, minimized distractions) was mentioned in the treatment recommendations, as possible therapeutic intervention strategy.	(Kolbe et al., 2021) [116]	Virtual Reality Rehabilitation The authors implemented a VR program for COVID-19 subjects. The rehabilitation unit for patients and healthcare providers was rated as highly satisfactory with perceived benefit for enhancing patient treatment and healthcare staff well-being, improving outcomes, such as mood, anxiety, sleep, pain, and feelings of isolation.
Coping, Cognition, and Mental Health	(Antonova et al., 2022) [106]	Mindfulness-based cognitive therapy These authors recommended the provision of mindfulness-based support during the COVID-19 pandemic to promote a more positive effect on well-being, as avoidance-type coping with stress and anxiety in COVID-19 context.	(O'Bryan et al., 2022) [107]	Mindfulness-based cognitive therapy via telehealth—MBCT According to these authors, MBCT (as an adjunctive treatment for anxiety via telehealth) can be considered a feasible and acceptable treatment and a promising treatment for reducing anxiety symptoms.
			(Sabel et al., 2022) [126]	Non-invasive brain stimulation using microcurrent (NIBS) NIBS can improve sensory and cognitive deficits in individuals suffering from Long COVID. Controlled trials are now needed to confirm these observations.
			(Czurra et al., 2022) [124]	Non invasive—Neuromodulation Strategies The authors have supported studies of NIBS in the current coronavirus pandemic. Neuromodulatory techniques provide a rationale for testing non-invasive neuromodulation to reduce an acute systemic inflammation and respiratory dysfunction caused by SARS-CoV-2, with beneficial role for psychological symptoms such as depression and anxiety.
Visuo-Research/Visuo-construction Skills Satisfaction Working Memory	(Fine et al., 2022) [105]	Visuo-spatial exercise programs (i.e., the use of visual cancellation tasks and strategies for visual organization, such as scanning from left to right, top to bottom, for symbols, shapes, numbers, etc.) were mentioned in the treatment recommendations, as therapeutic intervention strategies.	(Kolbe et al., 2021) [116]	Virtual Reality Rehabilitation The authors considered the use of VR that could be implemented within the context of clinical care for COVID-19 patients and both patients and staff members reported overall positive satisfaction and perceived benefit with VR as part of a comprehensive rehabilitation model.
			(Thams et al., 2022) [127]	Study protocol for a PROBE—phase IIb trial on brain stimulation-assisted cognitive training. Cognitive training group will additionally receive anodal tDCS, all other patients will receive sham tDCS (double-blinded, secondary intervention). Primary outcome: to improve working memory performance at the post-intervention assessment. Secondary outcomes: to increase health-related quality of life at post-assessment and follow-up Assessments (1 month after the end of the training).

Table 2. Cont.

Task Domain–Specific	Conventional Approach Face to Face with Therapist Paper/Pencil Tasks		Advanced Approach PC-Based/Virtual Setting/Assistent Software Dedicated/Virtual Task	
Executive Functions Social Functioning	(Fine et al., 2022) [105]	Metacognitive strategies Problem-solving training (examples of metacognitive strategies: Goal–Plan–Do–Review, Self-talk, Goal Management Training (Stop– Think–Plan), Predict–Perform Technique). These therapeutic interventions strategies are reported as treatment recommendations by the authors.	(Maggio et al., 2020) [117]	Cognitive tele-rehabilitation home-based exercises The authors analyzed the role of cognitive tele-rehabilitation following the journalistic '5W' (what, where, who, when, why), taking into account the growing interest in this matter in the 'COVID Era', and also promoting the practice of the human–technology interaction to improve social functioning and psychological well-being by also avoiding isolation.
			(Bernini et al., 2021) [119]	Tele-rehabilitation Home Cognitive Rehabilitation software (HomeCoRe). Authors suggested that HomeCoRe software could be incorporated as a valid support into clinical routine protocols as a complementary non-pharmacological therapy to support the continuum of care from the hospital to the patient's home.
Communication Pragmatic Language skills	(Fine et al., 2022) [105]	Compensatory strategies/aids; writing and organization, use of language-mediated strategies such as self-talk or verbalization to solve problems or remember information (i.e., structured tasks to address various domains, such as comprehension, recall, word finding, thought organization), were described as therapeutic intervention strategies, reported in treatment recommendations.	(De Luca et al., 2020) [118]	Tele-counseling In Italy, psychological tele-counseling has been an effective method of supporting the physical and psychosocial needs of all patients, regardless of their geographical locations. In this commentary, the authors promoted the use of telehealth as an effective tool for treating patients with mental health illness, specifically, as a growing need during the COVID era.
Emotions/Mood Quality of Life Caregiver Distress	(Skilbeck et al., 2022) [108]	Cognitive behavioral therapy (CBT) This study illustrated the use of patient-led CBT for managing symptoms of Long COVID with comorbid depression and anxiety in primary care, showing reliable change in somatic, depression, and anxiety symptoms and quality of life.	(Woodall et al., 2020) [120]	Telemedicine Service/Online therapy during COVID-19. This commentary explored the use of telemedicine in reaching under-served COVID-19 patients. The authors recommended the use of telemedicine that may be helpful to limit transportation, distance, or mobility challenges, reducing physical and psychological distances.
			(Liu et al., 2020) [123]	Online therapy The authors illustrated how the main online mental health services (including online mental health education with communication programmes and online psychological counseling services) being used for the COVID-19 epidemic are facilitating the development of Chinese public emergency interventions and eventually could improve the quality and effectiveness of emergency interventions.
			(De Luca et al., 2021) [121]	Skype therapy (OLST) The authors showed that OLST may be of support in favoring global cognitive and sensory-motorrecovery in Severe Acquired Brain Injury (SABI) patients and reducing caregiver distress during COVID-19 era.

Table 2. *Cont.*

Task Domain–Specific	Conventional Approach Face to Face with Therapist Paper/Pencil Tasks		Advanced Approach PC-Based/Virtual Setting/Assistent Software Dedicated/Virtual Task	
Neuropsychiatric sequelae	(Rolin et al., 2022) [112]	Rehabilitation Strategies Neuropsychiatric manifestation (psychoeducation, anxiety modulation psychotherapy, psychopharmacology, and peer support). These authors supported the idea that multidisciplinary rehabilitation of the cognitive and neuropsychiatric manifestations of COVID-19 during all levels of care is essential. An approach combining general medical, neurological, and neuropsychological intervention is recommended.	(Ghazanfarpour, et al., 2021) [122]	Tele-counseling The authors suggested that a systematic monitoring of the negative psychological impacts on medical staff is needed, as well as the implementation of appropriate tele-interventions to improve medical staff mental health of those working in hospitals and COVID-19 clinics.
Physical Function Cognition	(Daynes et al., 2021) [114]	Endurance and balance training The authors developed an adapted rehabilitation programme for individuals following COVID-19 that has demonstrated feasibility and promising improvements in clinical outcomes, with significant improvements in walking capacity, symptoms of fatigue, cognition, and respiratory symptoms.	(Groenveld et al., 2022) [115]	Virtual reality exercise at home The authors have investigated the feasibility of self-administered VR exercises at home for the post-COVID-19 condition, demonstrating that the use of VR for physical and self-administered mental exercising at home is well tolerated and appreciated in patients with a post–COVID-19 condition. Physical function outcomes registered positive health, and quality of life improved in time, whereas cognitive function seemed unaltered.

6. Discussion

Cognitive impairment in patients with Long COVID is an under-reported and challenging issue. Indeed, most patients suffer from subjective or subclinical deficits which may be under/misdiagnosed, negatively affecting patients' quality of life. Therefore, clinicians dealing with these "fragile" patients should be aware of their cognitive and behavioral symptoms and ask for them even when they are not spontaneously reported by the patients. Indeed, we found that psychological and cognitive alterations are common concerns of individuals with Long COVID and seem to be related to different causes as well as pre-existing conditions. The activation of the inflammation and immune response with the increase in cytokines and procoagulant molecules may account for either the acute or chronic consequences of the infection [102], especially fatigue and myalgia. Neuroinflammation and the related neural loss with the reduction in microcirculation are instead believed to subtend the neuropathological basis of the Long COVID-related cognitive impairment. Conversely, most of the behavioral and psychological alterations seem to not have a biological basis but are related to the reaction to the disease. In this sense, traits of personality, coping strategies, and premorbid conditions may worsen psychiatric symptoms [15]. With these premises, it appears fundamental to assess COVID-19-induced neuropsychiatric symptoms early in order to better manage this long-lasting syndrome.

In our opinion, psychologists and psychiatric therapists should be trained on which test they have to administer in specific conditions, taking into consideration the amount of clinical and psychometric tools available. This review is based on the presentation of the main psychological and cognitive measures used in the evaluation of Long COVID syndrome, illustrating the newly designed tools (i.e., C19-YRS, PCFS, and SBQ-LC) and the "older", adapted tools, which are commonly administered to patients with cognitive impairment due to different etiology (such as acquired brain injury and neurodegenerative disorders). In fact, although many tests, such as MMSE, MoCa, Digit Span, TMT, ZSDS, GAD- 7, etc., may be successfully used to investigate cognitive impairment as well as behavioral abnormalities in patients with Long COVID, newly specific tools are needed to better investigate these symptoms. Post-COVID-19 patients have several symptoms that may have features (duration, intensity, comorbidities, ...) which are different from other pathologies and should be specifically addressed and treated.

On the other hand, we analyzed evidence about the main rehabilitative approaches, including the conventional and the advanced, that are applied to this patient population. Notably, we observed that conventional rehabilitative interventions [105–108] and strategies [112] to treat the cognitive and neuropsychiatric manifestations of COVID-19 are based on adapted programs already performed in other neurological diseases [105,114]. According to Fine et al. [105], treatment recommendations for the management of acquired brain injury-related cognitive deficits may be helpful in implementing treatment as well as the education of patients with Long COVID. Otherwise, the use of innovative technology (i.e., the PC-based approach, tele-rehabilitation, and virtual reality training) is collecting considerable interest from researchers [116,119,121]. However, the evidence on the role of these innovative approaches in improving cognitive recovery and psychological well-being in the Long COVID population is still poor. For these reasons, more consistent studies and significant data are needed, according to specific inclusion criteria such as socio-demographic variables, the duration of Long COVID syndrome, the description of symptoms, and comorbidity [78,79]. Finally, non-invasive brain stimulation (NIBS) seems to play a key role in the improvement of psychological well-being, mood symptoms [124], and sensory–cognitive deficits [126] in individuals suffering from Long COVID syndrome. In the near future, the implementation of a combined approach of tDCS associated with cognitive training [127] will be useful as a non-pharmacological and complementary approach.

7. Conclusions

In conclusion, an early diagnosis of the neurocognitive and psychiatric symptoms due to Long COVID is essential in order to set up a specific rehabilitation program. The implementation in current clinical practice of early screening for the detection of post-COVID-19 could prevent enduring cognitive–behavioral alterations. The therapeutic programs must be addressed by a multidisciplinary team of experts that can give information to guide programs and public policies for the neurorehabilitation of this disabling long-term syndrome.

Author Contributions: Conceptualization, R.D.L.; methodology, M.B.; software, M.B.; validation, R.D.L., M.B. and R.S.C.; investigation, R.D.L., M.B. and R.S.C.; resources, R.S.C.; writing—original draft preparation, R.D.L. and M.B.; writing—review and editing, R.S.C.; visualization, R.D.L., M.B. and R.S.C.; supervision, R.S.C.; funding acquisition, R.S.C. All authors have read and agreed to the published version of the manuscript.

Funding: The funding was supported by the Italian Ministry of Health—Current Research 2022. This funding does not have an alphanumeric identification code.

Institutional Review Board Statement: Not applicable.

Informed Consent Statement: Not applicable.

Data Availability Statement: Not applicable.

Conflicts of Interest: The authors declare no conflict of interest.

References

1. Sarker, A.; Ge, Y. Mining long-COVID symptoms from Reddit: Characterizing post-COVID syndrome from patient reports. *JAMIA Open* **2021**, *4*, ooab075. [CrossRef] [PubMed]
2. Haran, J.P.; Bradley, E.; Zeamer, A.L.; Cincotta, L.; Salive, M.C.; Dutta, P.; Mutaawe, S.; Anya, O.; Meza-Segura, M.; Moormann, A. Inflammation-type dysbiosis of the oral microbiome associates with the duration of COVID-19 symptoms and long COVID. *JCI Insight.* **2021**, *6*, e152346. [CrossRef] [PubMed]
3. Mondelli, V.; Pariante, C.M. What can neuroimmunology teach us about the symptoms of long-COVID? *Oxford Open Immunol.* **2021**, *2*, iqab004. [CrossRef] [PubMed]

4. Naik, S.; Haldar, S.N.; Soneja, M.; Mundadan, N.G.; Garg, P.; Mittal, A.; Desai, D.; Trilangi, P.K.; Chakraborty, S.; Begam, N.N.; et al. Post COVID-19 sequelae: A prospective observational study from Northern India. *Drug Discov. Ther.* **2021**, *15*, 254–260. [CrossRef]
5. Dantzer, R.; O'Connor, J.C.; Freund, G.G.; Johnson, R.W.; Kelley, K.W. From inflammation to sickness and depression: When the immune system subjugates the brain. *Nat. Rev. Neurosci.* **2008**, *9*, 46–56. [CrossRef]
6. Raison, C.L.; Lin, J.M.; Reeves, W.C. Association of peripheral inflammatory markers with chronic fatigue in a population-based sample. *Brain Behav. Immun.* **2009**, *23*, 327–337. [CrossRef]
7. Mondelli, V.; Vernon, A.C.; Turkheimer, F.; Dazzan, P.; Pariante, C.M. Brain microglia in psychiatric disorders. *Lancet Psychiatry* **2017**, *4*, 563–572. [CrossRef]
8. Russell, A.; Hepgul, N.; Nikkheslat, N.; Borsini, A.; Zajkowska, Z.; Moll, N.; Forton, D.; Agarwal, K.; Chalder, T.; Mondelli, V.; et al. Persistent fatigue induced by interferon-alpha: A novel, inflammation-based, proxy model of chronic fatigue syndrome. *Psychoneuroendocrinology* **2019**, *100*, 276–285. [CrossRef]
9. Albrecht, D.S.; Forsberg, A.; Sandstrom, A.; Bergan, C.; Kadetoff, D.; Protsenko, E.; Lampa, J.; Lee, Y.C.; Höglund, C.O.; Catana, C.; et al. Brain glial activation in fibromyalgia—A multi-site positron emission tomography investigation. *Brain Behav. Immun.* **2019**, *75*, 72–83. [CrossRef]
10. Marsland, A.L.; Gianaros, P.J.; Kuan, D.C.; Sheu, L.K.; Krajina, K.; Manuck, S.B. Brain morphology links systemic inflammation to cognitive function in midlife adults. *Brain Behav. Immun.* **2015**, *48*, 195–204. [CrossRef]
11. Stefanou, M.I.; Palaiodimou, L.; Bakola, E.; Smyrnis, N.; Papadopoulou, M.; Paraskevas, G.P.; Rizos, E.; Boutati, E.; Grigoriadis, N.; Krogias, C.; et al. Neurological manifestations of long-COVID syndrome: A narrative review. *Ther. Adv. Chronic. Dis.* **2022**, *13*, 20406223221076890. [CrossRef] [PubMed]
12. Seeßle, J.; Waterboer, T.; Hippchen, T.; Simon, J.; Kirchner, M.; Lim, A.; Müller, B.; Merle, U. Persistent Symptoms in Adult Patients 1 Year After Coronavirus Disease 2019 (COVID-19): A Prospective Cohort Study. *Clin. Infect. Dis.* **2022**, *74*, 1191–1198. [CrossRef] [PubMed]
13. Hossain, M.A.; Hossain, K.M.A.; Saunders, K.; Uddin, Z.; Walton, L.M.; Raigangar, V.; Sakel, M.; Shafin, R.; Hossain, M.S.; Kabir, M.F.; et al. Prevalence of Long COVID symptoms in Bangladesh: A prospective Inception Cohort Study of COVID-19 survivors. *BMJ Glob. Health* **2021**, *6*, e006838. [CrossRef] [PubMed]
14. Martelletti, P.; Bentivegna, E.; Spuntarelli, V.; Luciani, M. Long-COVID Headache. *SN Compr. Clin. Med.* **2021**, *3*, 1704–1706. [CrossRef] [PubMed]
15. Castanares-Zapatero, D.; Chalon, P.; Kohn, L.; Dauvrin, M.; Detollenaere, J.; Maertens de Noordhout, C.; Primus-de Jong, C.; Cleemput, I.; Van den Heede, K. Pathophysiology and mechanism of long COVID: A comprehensive review. *Ann. Med.* **2022**, *54*, 1473–1487. [CrossRef] [PubMed]
16. Torjesen, I. COVID-19: Long COVID symptoms among hospital inpatients show little improvement after a year, data suggest. *BMJ* **2021**, *375*, n3092. [CrossRef]
17. Jennings, G.; Monaghan, A.; Xue, F.; Duggan, E.; Romero-Ortuño, R. Comprehensive Clinical Characterisation of Brain Fog in Adults Reporting Long COVID Symptoms. *J. Clin. Med.* **2022**, *11*, 3440. [CrossRef]
18. Hampshire, A.; Trender, W.; Chamberlain, S.R.; Jolly, A.E.; Grant, J.E.; Patrick, F.; Mazibuko, N.; Williams, S.C.; Barnby, J.M.; Hellyer, P.; et al. Cognitive deficits in people who have recovered from COVID-19. *EClinicalMedicine* **2021**, *39*, 101044. [CrossRef]
19. Ocsovszky, Z.; Otohal, J.; Berényi, B.; Juhász, V.; Skoda, R.; Bokor, L.; Dohy, Z.; Szabó, L.; Nagy, G.; Becker, D.; et al. The associations of long-COVID symptoms, clinical characteristics and affective psychological constructs in a non-hospitalized cohort. *Physiol. Int.* **2022**, *109*, 230–245. [CrossRef]
20. Yelin, D.; Margalit, I.; Nehme, M.; Bordas-Martínez, J.; Pistelli, F.; Yahav, D.; Guessous, I.; Durà-Miralles, X.; Carrozzi, L.; Shapira-Lichter, I.; et al. Patterns of Long COVID Symptoms: A Multicenter Cross Sectional Study. *J. Clin. Med.* **2022**, *11*, 898. [CrossRef]
21. Mariani, C.; Borgonovo, F.; Capetti, A.F.; Oreni, L.; Cossu, M.V.; Pellicciotta, M.; Armiento, L.; Bocchio, S.; Dedivitiis, G.; Lupo, A.; et al. Persistence of Long-COVID symptoms in a heterogenous prospective cohort. *J. Infect.* **2022**, *84*, 722–746. [CrossRef] [PubMed]
22. Burton, A.; Aughterson, H.; Fancourt, D.; Philip, K.E.J. Factors shaping the mental health and well-being of people experiencing persistent COVID-19 symptoms or 'long COVID': Qualitative study. *BJPsych Open* **2022**, *8*, e72. [CrossRef] [PubMed]
23. Yaksi, N.; Teker, A.G.; Imre, A. Long COVID in Hospitalized COVID-19 Patients: A Retrospective Cohort Study. *Iran J. Public Health* **2022**, *51*, 88–95. [CrossRef] [PubMed]
24. Cha, C.; Baek, G. Symptoms and management of long COVID: A scoping review. *J. Clin. Nurs.* **2021**, *online ahead of print*. [CrossRef]
25. Tang, S.W.; Leonard, B.E.; Helmeste, D.M. Long COVID, neuropsychiatric disorders, psychotropics, present and future. *Acta Neuropsychiatr.* **2022**, *34*, 109–126. [CrossRef]
26. Neurology, T.L. The Lancet Neurology. Long COVID: Understanding the Neurological Effects. *Lancet Neurol.* **2021**, *20*, 247. [CrossRef]
27. Orrù, G.; Bertelloni, D.; Diolaiuti, F.; Mucci, F.; Di Giuseppe, M.; Biella, M.; Gemignani, A.; Ciacchini, R.; Conversano, C. Long-COVID Syndrome? A Study on the Persistence of Neurological, Psychological and Physiological Symptoms. *Healthcare* **2021**, *9*, 575. [CrossRef]

28. Premraj, L.; Kannapadi, N.V.; Briggs, J.; Seal, S.M.; Battaglini, D.; Fanning, J.; Suen, J.; Robba, C.; Fraser, J.; Cho, S.M. Mid and long-term neurological and neuropsychiatric manifestations of post-COVID-19 syndrome: A meta-analysis. *J. Neurol. Sci.* **2022**, *434*, 120162. [CrossRef]
29. Desai, A.D.; Lavelle, M.; Boursiquot, B.C.; Wan, E.Y. Long-term complications of COVID-19. *Am. J. Physiol. Cell Physiol.* **2022**, *322*, C1–C11. [CrossRef]
30. Zhang, Z.J.; Jiang, B.C.; Gao, Y.J. Chemokines in neuron-glial cell interaction and pathogenesis of neuropathic pain. *Cell Mol. Life Sci.* **2017**, *74*, 3275–3291. [CrossRef]
31. Leitner, G.R.; Wenzel, T.J.; Marshall, N.; Gates, E.J.; Klegeris, A. Targeting toll-like receptor 4 to modulate neuroinflammation in central nervous system disorders. *Expert. Opin. Ther. Targets* **2019**, *23*, 865–882. [CrossRef] [PubMed]
32. Sen, S.; Singh, B.; Biswas, G. Corticosteroids: A boon or bane for COVID-19 patients? *Steroids* **2022**, *188*, 109102. [CrossRef] [PubMed]
33. Robb, C.T.; Goepp, M.; Rossi, A.G.; Yao, C. Non-steroidal anti-inflammatory drugs, prostaglandins, and COVID-19. *Br. J. Pharmacol.* **2020**, *177*, 4899–4920. [CrossRef] [PubMed]
34. Fonnesu, R.; Thunuguntla, V.B.S.C.; Veeramachaneni, G.K.; Bondili, J.S.; La Rocca, V.; Filipponi, C.; Spezia, P.G.; Sidoti, M.; Plicanti, E.; Quaranta, P.; et al. Palmitoylethanolamide (PEA) Inhibits SARS-CoV-2 Entry by Interacting with S Protein and ACE-2 Receptor. *Viruses* **2022**, *14*, 1080. [CrossRef]
35. Caronna, E.; Ballvé, A.; Llauradó, A.; Gallardo, V.J.; Ariton, D.M.; Lallana, S.; López Maza, S.; Olivé Gadea, M.; Quibus, L.; Restrepo, J.L.; et al. Headache: A striking prodromal and persistent symptom, predictive of COVID-19 clinical evolution. *Cephalalgia* **2020**, *40*, 1410–1421. [CrossRef] [PubMed]
36. Widyadharma, I.P.E.; Sari, N.N.S.P.; Pradnyaswari, K.E.; Yuwana, K.T.; Adikarya, I.P.G.D.; Tertia, C.; Wijayanti, I.; Indrayani, I.; Utami, D. Pain as clinical manifestations of COVID-19 infection and its management in the pandemic era: A literature review. *Egypt J. Neurol. Psychiatr. Neurosurg.* **2020**, *56*, 121. [CrossRef]
37. Research Accessibility Team (RAT). The microvascular hypothesis underlying neurologic manifestations of long COVID-19 and possible therapeutic strategies. *Cardiovasc. Endocrinol. Metab.* **2021**, *10*, 193–203. [CrossRef]
38. Grisanti, S.G.; Garbarino, S.; Barisione, E.; Aloè, T.; Grosso, M.; Schenone, C.; Pardini, M.; Biassoni, E.; Zaottini, F.; Picasso, R.; et al. Neurological long-COVID in the outpatient clinic: Two subtypes, two courses. *J. Neurol. Sci.* **2022**, *439*, 120315. [CrossRef]
39. Di Stadio, A.; Brenner, M.J.; De Luca, P.; Albanese, M.; D'Ascanio, L.; Ralli, M.; Roccamatisi, D.; Cingolani, C.; Vitelli, F.; Camaioni, A.; et al. Olfactory Dysfunction, Headache, and Mental Clouding in Adults with Long-COVID-19: What Is the Link between Cognition and Olfaction? A Cross-Sectional Study. *Brain Sci.* **2022**, *12*, 154. [CrossRef]
40. Cirulli, E.; Barrett, K.M.S.; Riffle, S.; Bolze, A.; Neveux, I.; Dabe, S.; Joseph, J.; James, T. Long-term COVID-19 symptoms in a large unselected population. *medRxiv* **2020**. [CrossRef]
41. Ziauddeen, N.; Gurdasani, D.; O'Hara, M.E.; Hastie, C.; Roderick, P.; Yao, G.; Alwan, N.A. Characteristics and impact of Long COVID: Findings from an online survey. *PLoS ONE* **2020**, *17*, e0264331. [CrossRef] [PubMed]
42. Davis, H.E.; Assaf, G.S.; McCorkell, L.; Wei, H.; Low, R.J.; Re'em, Y.; Redfield, S.; Austin, J.P.; Akrami, A. Characterizing long COVID in an international cohort: 7 months of symptoms and their impact. *EClin. Med.* **2021**, *38*, 3820561. [CrossRef]
43. Guo, P.; Ballesteros, A.B.; Yeung, S.P.; Liu, R.; Saha, A.; Curtis, L.; Kaser, M.; Haggard, M.P.; Cheke, L.G. COVCOG 1: Factors predicting cognitive symptoms in Long COVID. A first publication from the COVID and Cognition Study. *medRxiv* **2022**. [CrossRef]
44. Ferrucci, R.; Dini, M.; Rosci, C.; Capozza, A.; Groppo, E.; Reitano, M.R.; Allocco, E.; Poletti, B.; Brugnera, A.; Bai, F.; et al. One-year cognitive follow-up of COVID-19 hospitalized patients. *Eur. J. Neurol.* **2022**, *29*, 2006–2014. [CrossRef]
45. Alemanno, F.; Houdayer, E.; Parma, A.; Spina, A.; Del Forno, A.; Scatolini, A.; Angelone, S.; Brugliera, L.; Tettamanti, A.; Beretta, L.; et al. COVID-19 cognitive deficits after respiratory assistance in the subacute phase: A COVID-rehabilitation unit experience. *PLoS ONE* **2021**, *16*, e0246590. [CrossRef]
46. Ferrucci, R.; Dini, M.; Groppo, E.; Rosci, C.; Reitano, M.R.; Bai, F.; Poletti, B.; Brugnera, A.; Silani, V.; D'Arminio Monforte, A.; et al. Long-Lasting Cognitive Abnormalities after COVID-19. *Brain Sci.* **2021**, *11*, 235. [CrossRef]
47. Hosp, J.A.; Dressing, A.; Blazhenets, G.; Bormann, T.; Rau, A.; Schwabenland, M.; Thurow, J.; Wagner, D.; Waller, C.; Niesen, W.; et al. Cognitive impairment and altered cerebral glucose metabolism in the subacute stage of COVID-19. *Brain* **2021**, *144*, 1263–1276. [CrossRef]
48. Helms, J.; Kremer, S.; Merdji, H.; Clere-Jehl, R.; Schenck, M.; Kummerlen, C.; Collange, O.; Boulay, C.; Fafi-Kremer, S.; Ohana, M.; et al. Neurologic features in severe SARS-CoV-2 infection. *N. Engl. J. Med.* **2020**, *382*, 2268–2270. [CrossRef]
49. Iwashyna, T.J.; Ely, E.W.; Smith, D.M.; Langa, K.M. Long-term cognitive impairment and functional disability among survivors of severe sepsis. *JAMA* **2010**, *304*, 1787–1794. [CrossRef]
50. Pandharipande, P.P.; Girard, T.D.; Jackson, J.C.; Morandi, A.; Thompson, J.L.; Pun, B.T.; Brummel, N.E.; Hughes, C.G.; Vasilevskis, E.E.; Shintani, A.K.; et al. Long-term cognitive impairment after critical illness. *N. Engl. J. Med.* **2013**, *369*, 1306–1316. [CrossRef]
51. Almeria, M.; Cejudo, J.C.; Sotoca, J.; Deus, J.; Krupinski, J. Cognitive profile following COVID-19 infection: Clinical predictors leading to neuropsychological impairment. *Brain Behav. Immunity Health* **2020**, *9*, 100163. [CrossRef] [PubMed]
52. Chen, A.K.; Wang, X.; McCluskey, L.P.; Morgan, J.C.; Switzer, J.A.; Mehta, R.; Tingen, M.; Su, S.; Harris, R.A.; Hess, D.C.; et al. Neuropsychiatric sequelae of long COVID-19: Pilot results from the COVID-19 neurological and molecular prospective cohort study in Georgia, USA. *Brain Behav. Immun. Health* **2022**, *24*, 100491. [CrossRef] [PubMed]

53. Graham, E.L.; Clark, J.R.; Orban, Z.S.; Lim, P.H.; Szymanski, A.L.; Taylor, C.; DiBiase, R.M.; Jia, D.T.; Balabanov, R.; Ho, S.U.; et al. Persistent neurologic symptoms and cognitive dysfunction in non-hospitalized COVID-19 long haulers. *Ann. Clin. Transl. Neurol.* **2021**, *8*, 1073–1085. [CrossRef] [PubMed]
54. Taquet, M.; Geddes, J.R.; Husain, M.; Luciano, S.; Harrison, P.J. 6-month neurological and psychiatric outcomes in 236 379 survivors of COVID-19: A retrospective cohort study using electronic health records. *Lancet Psychiatry* **2021**, *8*, 416–427. [CrossRef]
55. Braga, L.W.; Oliveira, S.B.; Moreira, A.S.; Pereira, M.E.; Carneiro, V.S.; Serio, A.S.; Freitas, L.F.; Isidro, H.B.L.; Souza, L.M.N. Neuropsychological manifestations of long COVID in hospitalized and non-hospitalized Brazilian Patients. *NeuroRehabilitation* **2022**, *50*, 391–400. [CrossRef] [PubMed]
56. Nakamura, Z.M.; Nash, R.P.; Laughon, S.L.; Rosenstein, D.L. Neuropsychiatric complications of COVID-19. *Curr. Psychiatry Rep.* **2021**, *23*, 25. [CrossRef] [PubMed]
57. Taquet, M.; Luciano, S.; Geddes, J.R.; Harrison, P.J. Bidirectional associations between COVID-19 and psychiatric disorder: Retrospective cohort studies of 62 354 COVID-19 cases in the USA. *Lancet Psychiatry* **2021**, *8*, 130–140. [CrossRef]
58. Pistarini, C.; Fiabane, E.; Houdayer, E.; Vassallo, C.; Manera, M.R.; Alemanno, F. Cognitive and emotional disturbances due to COVID-19: An exploratory study in the rehabilitation setting. *Front. Neurol.* **2021**, *12*, 643646. [CrossRef]
59. Holdsworth, D.A.; Chamley, R.; Barker-Davies, R.; O'Sullivan, O.; Ladlow, P.; Mitchell, J.L.; Dewson, D.; Mills, D.; May, S.; Cranley, M.; et al. Comprehensive clinical assessment identifies specific neurocognitive deficits in working-age patients with long-COVID. *PLoS ONE* **2022**, *17*, e0267392. [CrossRef]
60. Mazza, M.G.; Palladini, M.; De Lorenzo, R.; Magnaghi, C.; Poletti, S.; Furlan, R.; Ciceri, F.; Rovere-Querini, P.; Benedetti, F.; COVID-19 BioB Outpatient Clinic Study Group. Persistent psychopathology and neurocognitive impairment in COVID-19 survivors: Effect of inflammatory biomarkers at three-month follow-up. *Brain Behav. Immun.* **2021**, *94*, 138–147. [CrossRef]
61. Clemente, I.; Sinatti, G.; Cirella, A.; Santini, S.J.; Balsano, C. Alteration of Inflammatory Parameters and Psychological Post-Traumatic Syndrome in Long-COVID Patients. *Int. J. Environ. Res. Public Health* **2020**, *19*, 7103. [CrossRef]
62. Gasnier, M.; Choucha, W.; Radiguer, F.; Faulet, T.; Chappell, K.; Bougarel, A.; Kondarjian, C.; Thorey, P.; Baldacci, A.; Ballerini, M.; et al. Comorbidity of long COVID and psychiatric disorders after a hospitalisation for COVID-19: A cross-sectional study. *J. Neurol. Neurosurg. Psychiatry* **2022**, *93*, 1091–1098. [CrossRef] [PubMed]
63. Vindegaard, N.; Benros, M.E. COVID-19 pandemic and mental health consequences: Systematic review of the current evidence. *Brain Behav. Immun.* **2020**, *89*, 531–542. [CrossRef] [PubMed]
64. Kim, K.M.; Hwang, H.R.; Kim, Y.J.; Lee, J.G.; Yi, Y.H.; Tak, Y.J.; Lee, S.H.; Chung, S.I. Association between Serum-Ferritin Levels and Sleep Duration, Stress, Depression, and Suicidal Ideation in Older Koreans: Fifth Korea National Health and Nutrition Examination Survey 2010. *Korean J. Fam. Med.* **2019**, *40*, 380–387. [CrossRef]
65. Sykes, D.L.; Holdsworth, L.; Jawad, N.; Gunasekera, P.; Morice, A.H.; Crooks, M.G. Post-COVID-19 Symptom Burden: What is Long-COVID and How Should We Manage It? *Lung* **2021**, *199*, 113–119. [CrossRef]
66. Rogers, J.P.; Chesney, E.; Oliver, D.; Pollak, T.A.; McGuire, P.; Fusar-Poli, P.; Zandi, M.S.; Lewis, G.; David, A.S. Psychiatric and neuropsychiatric presentations associated with severe coronavirus infections: A systematic review and meta-analysis with comparison to the COVID-19 pandemic. *Lancet Psychiatry* **2020**, *7*, 611–627. [CrossRef]
67. Mak, I.W.; Chu, C.M.; Pan, P.C.; Yiu, M.G.; Chan, V.L. Long-term psychiatric morbidities among SARS survivors. *Gen. Hosp. Psychiatry* **2009**, *31*, 318–326. [CrossRef]
68. Park, H.Y.; Park, W.B.; Lee, S.H.; Kim, J.L.; Lee, J.J.; Lee, H.; Shin, H.-S. Posttraumatic stress disorder and depression of survivors 12 months after the outbreak of Middle East respiratory syndrome in South Korea. *BMC Public Health* **2020**, *20*, 605. [CrossRef]
69. Naidu, S.B.; Shah, A.J.; Saigal, A.; Smith, C.; Brill, S.E.; Goldring, J.; Hurst, J.R.; Jarvis, H.; Lipman, M.; Mandal, S. The high mental health burden of "Long COVID" and its association with on-going physical and respiratory symptoms in all adults discharged from hospital. *Eur. Respir. J.* **2021**, *57*, 2004364. [CrossRef]
70. Li, D.; Wang, Q.; Jia, C.; Lv, Z.; Yang, J. An Overview of Neurological and Psychiatric Complications During Post-COVID Period: A Narrative Review. *J. Inflamm. Res.* **2022**, *15*, 4199–4215. [CrossRef]
71. Zeng, N.; Zhao, Y.M.; Yan, W.; Li, C.; Lu, Q.D.; Liu, L.; Ni, S.Y.; Mei, H.; Yuan, K.; Shi, L.; et al. A systematic review and meta-analysis of long term physical and mental sequelae of COVID-19 pandemic: Call for research priority and action. *Mol. Psychiatry* **2022**, 1–11. [CrossRef] [PubMed]
72. Douaud, G.; Lee, S.; Alfaro-Almagro, F.; Arthofer, C.; Wang, C.; McCarthy, P.; Lange, F.; Andersson, J.L.R.; Griffanti, L.; Duff, E.; et al. SARS-CoV-2 is associated with changes in brain structure in UK Biobank. *Nature* **2022**, *604*, 697–707. [CrossRef] [PubMed]
73. de Erausquin, G.A.; Snyder, H.; Carrillo, M.; Hosseini, A.A.; Brugha, T.S.; Seshadri, S. CNS SARS-CoV-2 Consortium. The chronic neuropsychiatric sequelae of COVID-19: The need for a prospective study of viral impact on brain functioning. *Alzheimers Dement.* **2021**, *17*, 1056–1065. [CrossRef] [PubMed]
74. Azeem, F.; Durrani, R.; Zerna, C.; Smith, E.E. Silent brain infarcts and cognitive decline: Systematic review and meta-analysis. *J. Neurol.* **2020**, *267*, 502–512. [CrossRef]
75. Hajifathalian, K.; Kumar, S.; Newberry, C.; Shah, S.; Fortune, B.; Krisko, T.; Ortiz-Pujols, S.; Zhou, X.K.; Dannenberg, A.J.; Kumar, R.; et al. Obesity is Associated with Worse Outcomes in COVID-19: Analysis of Early Data from New York City. *Obesity* **2000**, *28*, 1606–1612. [CrossRef]
76. Raveendran, A.V.; Misra, A. Post COVID-19 Syndrome ("Long COVID") and Diabetes: Challenges in Diagnosis and Management. *Diabetes Metab. Syndr.* **2021**, *15*, 102235. [CrossRef]

77. Vimercati, L.; De Maria, L.; Quarato, M.; Caputi, A.; Gesualdo, L.; Migliore, G.; Cavone, D.; Sponselli, S.; Pipoli, A.; Inchingolo, F.; et al. Association between Long COVID and Overweight/Obesity. *J. Clin. Med.* **2021**, *10*, 4143. [CrossRef]
78. Sudre, C.H.; Murray, B.; Varsavsky, T.; Graham, M.S.; Penfold, R.S.; Bowyer, R.C.; Pujol, J.C.; Klaser, K.; Antonelli, M.; Canas, L.S.; et al. Attributes and predictors of long COVID. *Nat. Med.* **2021**, *27*, 626–631. [CrossRef]
79. Bellou, V.; Tzoulaki, I.; van Smeden, M.; Moons, K.; Evangelou, E.; Belbasis, L. Prognostic factors for adverse outcomes in patients with COVID-19: A field-wide systematic review and meta-analysis. *Eur. Respir. J.* **2022**, *59*, 2002964. [CrossRef]
80. Wang, S.; Quan, L.; Chavarro, J.E.; Slopen, N.; Kubzansky, L.D.; Koenen, K.C.; Kang, J.H.; Weisskopf, M.G.; Branch-Elliman, W.; Roberts, A.L. Associations of Depression, Anxiety, Worry, Perceived Stress, and Loneliness Prior to Infection With Risk of Post–COVID-19 Conditions. *JAMA Psychiatry* **2022**, *79*, 1081–1091. [CrossRef]
81. Whiteside, D.M.; Basso, M.R.; Naini, S.M.; Porter, J.; Holker, E.; Waldron, E.J.; Melnik, T.E.; Niskanen, N.; Taylor, S.E. Outcomes in post-acute sequelae of COVID-19 (PASC) at 6 months post-infection Part 1: Cognitive functioning. *Clin. Neuropsychol.* **2022**, *36*, 806–828. [CrossRef] [PubMed]
82. Nasserie, T.; Hittle, M.; Goodman, S.N. Assessment of the Frequency and Variety of Persistent Symptoms Among Patients With COVID-19: A Systematic Review. *JAMA Netw. Open* **2021**, *4*, e2111417. [CrossRef] [PubMed]
83. Lynch, S.; Ferrando, S.J.; Dornbush, R.; Shahar, S.; Smiley, A.; Klepacz, L. Screening for brain fog: Is the Montreal cognitive assessment an effective screening tool for neurocognitive complaints post-COVID-19? *Gen. Hosp. Psychiatry* **2022**, *78*, 80–86. [CrossRef]
84. Spitzer, R.L.; Kroenke, K.; Williams, J.B.; Löwe, B. A brief measure for assessing generalized anxiety disorder: The GAD-7. *Arch. Intern. Med.* **2006**, *166*, 1092–1097. [CrossRef] [PubMed]
85. Manea, L.; Gilbody, S.; McMillan, D. Optimal cut-off score for diagnosing depression with the Patient Health Questionnaire (PHQ-9): A meta-analysis. *CMAJ* **2012**, *184*, E191–E196. [CrossRef] [PubMed]
86. Becker, J.H.; Lin, J.J.; Doernberg, M.; Stone, K.; Navis, A.; Festa, J.R.; Wisnivesky, J.P. Assessment of Cognitive Function in Patients After COVID-19 Infection. *JAMA Netw. Open* **2021**, *4*, e2130645. [CrossRef]
87. Guo, P.; Benito Ballesteros, A.; Yeung, S.P.; Liu, R.; Saha, A.; Curtis, L.; Kaser, M.; Haggard, M.P.; Cheke, L.G. COVCOG 2: Cognitive and Memory Deficits in Long COVID: A Second Publication From the COVID and Cognition Study. *Front. Aging Neurosci.* **2022**, *14*, 804937. [CrossRef] [PubMed]
88. O'Connor, R.J.; Preston, N.; Parkin, A.; Makower, S.; Ross, D.; Gee, J.; Halpin, S.J.; Horton, M.; Sivan, M. The COVID-19 Yorkshire Rehabilitation Scale (C19-YRS): Application and psychometric analysis in a post-COVID-19 syndrome cohort. *J. Med. Virol.* **2022**, *94*, 1027–1034. [CrossRef]
89. Sivan, M.; Halpin, S.; Gee, J.; Makower, S.; Parkin, A.; Ross, D.; Horton, M.; O'Connor, R. The self-report version and digital format of the COVID-19 Yorkshire Rehabilitation Scale (C19-YRS) for Long COVID or Post-COVID syndrome assessment and monitoring. *Adv. Clin. Neurosci. Rehabil.* **2021**, *20*, 2–5. [CrossRef]
90. Herrmann-Lingen, C.; Buss, U.; Snaith, R.P. *Hospital Anxiety and Depression Scale–Deutsche Version (HADS-D)*; Verlag Hans Huber: Bern, Switzerland, 2011.
91. Monterrosa-Blanco, A.; Cassiani-Miranda, C.A.; Scoppetta, O.; Monterrosa-Castro, A. Generalized anxiety disorder scale (GAD-7) has adequate psychometric properties in Colombian general practitioners during COVID-19 pandemic. *Gen. Hosp. Psychiatry* **2021**, *70*, 147–148. [CrossRef]
92. Olanipekun, T.; Abe, T.; Effoe, V.; Westney, G.; Snyder, R. Incidence and Severity of Depression Among Recovered African Americans with COVID-19-Associated Respiratory Failure. *J. Racial Ethn. Health Disparities* **2022**, *9*, 954–959. [CrossRef] [PubMed]
93. García-Garro, P.A.; Aibar-Almazán, A.; Rivas-Campo, Y.; Vega-Ávila, G.C.; Afanador-Restrepo, D.F.; Hita-Contreras, F. Influence of the COVID-19 Pandemic on Quality of Life, Mental Health, and Level of Physical Activity in Colombian University Workers: A Longitudinal Study. *J. Clin. Med.* **2022**, *11*, 4104. [CrossRef] [PubMed]
94. Scarpelli, S.; Alfonsi, V.; Mangiaruga, A.; Musetti, A.; Quattropani, M.C.; Lenzo, V.; Freda, M.F.; Lemmo, D.; Vegni, E.; Borghi, L.; et al. Pandemic nightmares: Effects on dream activity of the COVID-19 lockdown in Italy. *J. Sleep Res.* **2021**, *30*, e13300. [CrossRef] [PubMed]
95. Taporoski, T.P.; Beijamini, F.; Gómez, L.M.; Ruiz, F.S.; Ahmed, S.S.; von Schantz, M.; Pereira, A.C.; Knutson, K.L. Subjective sleep quality before and during the COVID-19 pandemic in a Brazilian rural population. *Sleep Health* **2022**, *8*, 167–174. [CrossRef]
96. Tabacof, L.; Tosto-Mancuso, J.; Wood, J.; Cortes, M.; Kontorovich, A.; McCarthy, D.; Rizk, D.; Rozanski, G.; Breyman, E.; Nasr, L.; et al. Post-acute COVID-19 syndrome negatively impacts physical function, cognitive function, health-related quality of life and participation. *Am. J. Phys. Med. Rehabil.* **2022**, *101*, 48. [CrossRef]
97. Sanchez-Ramirez, D.C.; Normand, K.; Zhaoyun, Y.; Torres-Castro, R. Long-Term Impact of COVID-19: A Systematic Review of Literature and Meta-Analysis. *Biomedicines* **2021**, *9*, 900. [CrossRef]
98. Liyanage-Don, N.A.; Winawer, M.R.; Hamberger, M.J.; Agarwal, S.; Trainor, A.R.; Quispe, K.A.; Kronish, I.M. Association of depression and COVID-induced PTSD with cognitive symptoms after COVID-19 illness. *Gen. Hosp. Psychiatry* **2022**, *76*, 45–48. [CrossRef]
99. Bovin, M.J.; Marx, B.P.; Weathers, F.W.; Gallagher, M.W.; Rodriguez, P.; Schnurr, P.P.; Keane, T.M. Psychometric properties of the PTSD Checklist for Diagnostic and Statistical Manual of Mental Disorders-Fifth Edition (PCL-5) in veterans. *Psychol. Assess* **2016**, *28*, 1379–1391. [CrossRef]

100. Klok, F.A.; Boon, G.J.A.M.; Barco, S.; Endres, M.; Geelhoed, J.J.M.; Knauss, S.; Rezek, S.A.; Spruit, M.A.; Vehreschild, J.; Siegerink, B. The Post-COVID-19 Functional Status scale: A tool to measure functional status over time after COVID-19. *Eur. Respir. J.* **2020**, *56*, 2001494. [CrossRef]
101. Hughes, S.E.; Haroon, S.; Subramanian, A.; McMullan, C.; Aiyegbusi, O.L.; Turner, G.M.; Jackson, L.; Davies, E.H.; Frost, C.; McNamara, G.; et al. Development and validation of the symptom burden questionnaire for long COVID (SBQ-LC): Rasch analysis. *BMJ* **2022**, *377*, e070230. [CrossRef]
102. Raciti, L.; Arcadi, F.A.; Calabrò, R.S. Could Palmitoylethanolamide Be an Effective Treatment for Long-COVID-19? Hypothesis and Insights in Potential Mechanisms of Action and Clinical Applications. *Innov. Clin. Neurosci.* **2022**, *19*, 19–25. [PubMed]
103. Nurek, M.; Rayner, C.; Freyer, A.; Taylor, S.; Järte, L.; MacDermott, N.; Delaney, B.C.; Panellists, D. Recommendations for the recognition, diagnosis, and management of long COVID: A Delphi study. *Br. J. Gen. Pract. J. R. Coll. Gen. Pract.* **2021**, *71*, e815–e825. [CrossRef] [PubMed]
104. Compagno, S.; Palermi, S.; Pescatore, V.; Brugin, E.; Sarto, M.; Marin, R.; Calzavara, V.; Nizzetto, M.; Scevola, M.; Aloi, A.; et al. Physical and psychological reconditioning in long COVID syndrome: Results of an out-of-hospital exercise and psychological—Based rehabilitation program. *Int. J. Cardiology. Heart Vasc.* **2022**, *41*, 101080. [CrossRef] [PubMed]
105. Fine, J.S.; Ambrose, A.F.; Didehbani, N.; Fleming, T.K.; Glashan, L.; Longo, M.; Merlino, A.; Ng, R.; Nora, G.J.; Rolin, S.; et al. Multi-disciplinary collaborative consensus guidance statement on the assessment and treatment of cognitive symptoms in patients with post-acute sequelae of SARS-CoV-2 infection (PASC). *PMR J. Inj. Funct. Rehabil.* **2022**, *14*, 96–111. [CrossRef] [PubMed]
106. Antonova, E.; Schlosser, K.; Pandey, R.; Kumari, V. Coping With COVID-19: Mindfulness-Based Approaches for Mitigating Mental Health Crisis. *Front. Psychiatry* **2021**, *12*, 563417. [CrossRef]
107. O'Bryan, E.M.; Davis, E.; Beadel, J.R.; Tolin, D.F. Brief adjunctive mindfulness-based cognitive therapy via Telehealth for anxiety during the COVID-19 pandemic. *Anxiety Stress Coping* **2022**, *2022*, e2117305. [CrossRef]
108. Skilbeck, L. Patient-led integrated cognitive behavioral therapy for management of long COVID with comorbid depression and anxiety in primary care—A case study. *Chronic Illn.* **2022**, *18*, 691–701. [CrossRef]
109. Mathern, R.; Senthil, P.; Vu, N.; Thiyagarajan, T. Neurocognitive Rehabilitation in COVID-19 Patients: A Clinical Review. *South. Med. J.* **2022**, *115*, 227–231. [CrossRef]
110. Illustration Created by. Available online: https://biorender.com/ (accessed on 13 September 2022).
111. García-Molina, A.; Espiña-Bou, M.; Rodríguez-Rajo, P.; Sánchez-Carrión, R.; Enseñat-Cantallops, A. Neuropsychological rehabilitation program for patients with post-COVID-19 syndrome: A clinical experience. *Neurologia* **2021**, *36*, 565–566. [CrossRef]
112. Rolin, S.; Chakales, A.; Verduzco-Gutierrez, M. Rehabilitation Strategies for Cognitive and Neuropsychiatric Manifestations of COVID-19. *Curr. Phys. Med. Rehabil. Rep.* **2022**, *10*, 182–187. [CrossRef]
113. Herrera, J.E.; Niehaus, W.N.; Whiteson, J.; Azola, A.; Baratta, J.M.; Fleming, T.K.; Kim, S.Y.; Naqvi, H.; Sampsel, S.; Silver, J.K.; et al. Multidisciplinary collaborative consensus guidance statement on the assessment and treatment of fatigue in postacute sequelae of SARS-COV-2 infection (PASC) patients. *PM&R* **2021**, *13*, 1027–1043. [CrossRef]
114. Daynes, E.; Gerlis, C.; Chaplin, E.; Gardiner, N.; Singh, S.J. Early experiences of rehabilitation for individuals post-COVID to improve fatigue, breathlessness, exercise capacity and cognition-a cohort study. *Chron. Respir. Dis.* **2021**, *18*, 147997312110156. [CrossRef] [PubMed]
115. Groenveld, T.; Achttien, R.; Smits, M.; de Vries, M.; van Heerde, R.; Staal, B.; van Goor, H.; COVID Rehab Group. Feasibility of Virtual Reality Exercises at Home for Post-COVID-19 Condition: Cohort Study. *JMIR Rehabil. Assist. Technol.* **2022**, *9*, e36836. [CrossRef] [PubMed]
116. Kolbe, L.; Jaywant, A.; Gupta, A.; Vanderlind, W.M.; Jabbour, G. Use of virtual reality in the inpatient rehabilitation of COVID-19 patients. *Gen. Hosp. Psychiatry* **2021**, *71*, 76–81. [CrossRef]
117. Maggio, M.G.; De Luca, R.; Manuli, A.; Calabrò, R.S. The five 'W' of cognitive telerehabilitation in the COVID-19 ERA. *Expert Rev. Med. Devices.* **2020**, *17*, 473–475. [CrossRef]
118. De Luca, R.; Calabrò, R.S. How the COVID-19 Pandemic is Changing Mental Health Disease Management: The Growing Need of Telecounseling in Italy. *Innov. Clin. Neurosci.* **2020**, *17*, 16–17.
119. Bernini, S.; Stasolla, F.; Panzarasa, S.; Quaglini, S.; Sinforiani, E.; Sandrini, G.; Vecchi, T.; Tassorelli, C.; Bottiroli, S. Cognitive Telerehabilitation for Older Adults With Neurodegenerative Diseases in the COVID-19 Era: A Perspective Study. *Front. Neurol.* **2021**, *11*, 623933. [CrossRef]
120. Woodall, T.; Ramage, M.; LaBruyere, J.T.; McLean, W.; Tak, C.R. Telemedicine Services during COVID-19: Considerations for medically underserved populations. *J. Rural. Health* **2020**, *37*, 231–234. [CrossRef]
121. De Luca, R.; Rifici, C.; Pollicino, P.; Di Cara, M.; Miceli, S.; Sergi, G.; Sorrenti, L.; Romano, M.; Naro, A.; Billeri, L.; et al. 'Online therapy' to reduce caregiver's distress and to stimulate post-severe acquired brain injury motor and cognitive recovery: A Sicilian hospital experience in the COVID era. *J. Telemed. Telecare* **2021**. [CrossRef]
122. Ghazanfarpour, M.; Ashrafinia, F.; Zolala, S.; Ahmadi, A.; Jahani, Y.; Hosseininasab, A. Investigating the effectiveness of telecounseling for the mental health of staff in hospitals and COVID-19 clinics: A clinical control trial. *Trends Psychiatry Psychother.* **2021**, *44*, 1–9. [CrossRef]
123. Liu, S.; Yang, L.; Zhang, C.; Xiang, Y.T.; Liu, Z.; Hu, S.; Zhang, B. Online mental health services in China during the COVID-19 outbreak. *Lancet Psychiatry* **2020**, *7*, e17–e18. [CrossRef]

124. Czura, C.J.; Bikson, M.; Charvet, L.; Chen, J.; Franke, M.; Fudim, M.; Grigsby, E.; Hamner, S.; Huston, J.M.; Khodaparast, N.; et al. Neuromodulation Strategies to Reduce Inflammation and Improve Lung Complications in COVID-19 Patients. *Front. Neurol.* **2022**, *13*, 897124. [CrossRef] [PubMed]
125. Dantzer, R. Neuroimmune interactions: From the brain to the immune system and vice versa. *Physiol. Rev.* **2018**, *98*, 477–504. [CrossRef] [PubMed]
126. Sabel, B.A.; Zhou, W.; Huber, F.; Schmidt, F.; Sabel, K.; Gonschorek, A.; Bilc, M. Non-invasive brain microcurrent stimulation therapy of long-COVID-19 reduces vascular dysregulation and improves visual and cognitive impairment. *Restor. Neurol. Neurosci.* **2021**, *39*, 393–408. [CrossRef] [PubMed]
127. Thams, F.; Antonenko, D.; Fleischmann, R.; Meinzer, M.; Grittner, U.; Schmidt, S.; Brakemeier, E.L.; Steinmetz, A.; Flöel, A. Neuromodulation through brain stimulation-assisted cognitive training in patients with post-COVID-19 cognitive impairment (Neuromod-COV): Study protocol for a PROBE phase IIb trial. *BMJ Open* **2020**, *12*, e055038. [CrossRef] [PubMed]

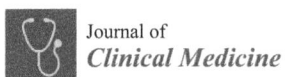

Systematic Review

The Impact of COVID-19 on Carotid–Femoral Pulse Wave Velocity: A Systematic Review and Meta-Analysis

Iwona Jannasz [1], Michal Pruc [2,3], Mansur Rahnama-Hezavah [4], Tomasz Targowski [1], Robert Olszewski [5], Stepan Feduniw [6,7], Karolina Petryka [8] and Lukasz Szarpak [9,10,11,*]

1. Department of Geriatrics, National Institute of Geriatrics, Rheumatology and Rehabilitation, 02-637 Warsaw, Poland
2. Research Unit, Polish Society of Disaster Medicine, 05-806 Warsaw, Poland
3. Department of Public Health, International Academy of Ecology and Medicine, 02-091 Kyiv, Ukraine
4. Chair and Department of Oral Surgery, Medical University of Lublin, 20-093 Lublin, Poland
5. Department of Gerontology, Public Health and Education, National Institute of Geriatrics Rheumatology and Rehabilitation, 02-637 Warsaw, Poland
6. Department of Gynecology, University Hospital Zurich, 8091 Zurich, Switzerland
7. Department of Obstetrics, University Hospital Zurich, 8091 Zurich, Switzerland
8. Research Unit, Internal Medicine Clinic, 03-003 Warsaw, Poland; karolinapetryka2001@gmail.com
9. Henry JN Taub Department of Emergency Medicine, Baylor College of Medicine, Houston, TX 77030, USA
10. Institute of Outcomes Research, Maria Sklodowska-Curie Medical Academy in Warsaw, 00-136 Warsaw, Poland
11. Research Unit, Maria Sklodowska-Curie Bialystok Oncology Center, 15-027 Bialystok, Poland
* Correspondence: lukasz.szarpak@gmail.com; Tel.: +48-500186225

Abstract: COVID-19 is a complex multisystemic disease that can result in long-term complications and, in severe cases, death. This study investigated the effect of COVID-19 on carotid–femoral pulse wave velocity (cfPWV) as a measurement to evaluate its impact on arterial stiffness and might help predict COVID-19-related cardiovascular (CV) complications. PubMed, Web of Science, Embase, and the Cochrane Library were searched for relevant studies, and meta-analysis was performed. The study protocol was registered in PROSPERO (nr. CRD42023434326). The Newcastle–Ottawa Quality Scale was used to evaluate the quality of the included studies. Nine studies reported cfPWV among COVID-19 patients and control groups. The pooled analysis showed that cfPWV in COVID-19 patients was 9.5 ± 3.7, compared to 8.2 ± 2.2 in control groups (MD = 1.32; 95% CI: 0.38–2.26; $p = 0.006$). A strong association between COVID-19 infection and increased cfPWV suggests a potential link between the virus and increased arterial stiffness. A marked increase in arterial stiffness, a known indicator of CV risk, clearly illustrates the cardiovascular implications of COVID-19 infection. However, further research is required to provide a clearer understanding of the connection between COVID-19 infection, arterial compliance, and subsequent CV events.

Keywords: COVID-19; SARS-CoV-2; pulse wave velocity; PWV; cfPWV; arterial stiffness

1. Introduction

The COVID-19 pandemic has had wide-ranging global effects, affecting a substantial proportion of the population worldwide. By June 2023, there were over 765 million confirmed cases, and almost 7 million people died as a result of the severe acute respiratory syndrome coronavirus 2 (SARS-CoV-2) [1,2]. Initially, there was limited information about COVID-19, and the disease was thought to be simply an acute respiratory condition. Since then, research has shown that COVID-19 is a complicated multisystemic disease that can lead to death or long-term complications after recovery [3,4]. One significant concern is the close link between COVID-19 and cardiovascular (CV) complications. Patients with pre-existing CV conditions are at a higher risk of an unfavorable prognosis for COVID-19 infection. Moreover, COVID-19 itself may directly or indirectly cause significant CV complications [5], which persist even after recovering from the virus [6,7]. Not only the severity of COVID-19 in the acute phase but also the duration of symptoms might have an effect on vascular function [8]. Long COVID-19 is described as a condition that can arise after recovery from the primary infection or an unresolved COVID-19 infection, which presents with ongoing symptoms that cannot be attributed to any other disease or condition. Using a conservative 10% estimate, at least 76 million people worldwide are affected by long COVID-19. Furthermore, studies suggest that 10–30% of non-hospitalized and 50–70% of hospitalized individuals experience long COVID-19 symptoms [9]. However, the actual numbers might be higher due to the vast number of unreported cases [10].

COVID-19's cardiovascular (CV) manifestations include arrhythmias, asymptomatic myocardial damage, overt congestive heart failure, and thromboembolic events [5,11,12] and result from the virus's direct cytotoxic effect or the subsequent systemic inflammatory cytokine storm. Endothelial dysfunction seems to be a crucial driver and mediator of the COVID-19 pathophysiologic pathways [13]. Vascular endothelial cells have the angiotensin-converting enzyme 2 cellular receptors (ACE2-R) and the transmembrane serine protease 2 (TMPRSS2), synergistically facilitating SARS-CoV-2 entry into host cells. Infected endothelial cells increase the production of cytokines, promoting inflammation and thrombosis [14]. The resulting vasculitis, which may affect different parts of the body, contributes to the multiorgan failure seen in some COVID-19 patients [15]. There is evidence suggesting that COVID-19 accelerates vascular aging on a macrovascular level [16]. Other proposed mechanisms contributing to cellular senescence and vascular stiffness include COVID-19-induced mitochondrial dysfunction, increased local formation of reactive oxygen species (ROS), and resulting oxidative telomere shortening [17]. Both endothelial dysfunction and continuous subintimal inflammation contribute to the rapid fragmentation of elastin fibers in the arterial wall and their substitution with stiff, fibrous tissue. Given that COVID-19-induced pulmonary fibrosis can only be reversed to a certain level, it has been proposed that arterial stiffness might be a long-term CV consequence in most patients, irrespective of the severity of the initial infection [15,18]. Notably, vascular changes, especially endothelial function and arterial stiffness, may last for a long time after the COVID-19 infection [19].

Arterial stiffness may serve as a reliable indicator reflecting the vascular system's age and the comprehensive health of the CV system. It is an integrated biomarker that evaluates the cumulative detrimental effect on the arteries of genetic and environmental exposures, as well as the influence of established CV risk factors [20]. Numerous studies have established the correlations between arterial stiffness, as measured by pulse wave velocity (PWV), and the elevated risk of CV disease [21]. This correlation is independent of other traditional risk variables that are often considered to be risk factors [22,23]. In order to confirm the arterial stiffness in COVID-19 patients, other tests such as the augmentation index (Aix), the cardio-ankle vascular index (CAVI), the arterial stiffness index (ASI), Young's modulus of elasticity, and pulse pressure (PP) were performed [24–27].

PWV is essential in assessing vascular age and may have a stronger correlation with CV disease onset than metrical age [28]. PWV is a technique that is noninvasive and reproducible, and carotid–femoral pulse wave velocity (cfPWV) is now regarded as the gold standard in assessing arterial stiffness. The progressive stiffening of the arteries adversely affects arterial–ventricular interactions, decreasing the vessel's capacity to alter volume in response to changes in blood pressure, which in turn might lead to heart failure. CfPWV has a high prognostic value since it may help identify individuals who are at a higher risk not just for future CV events, but also for all-cause mortality [19,29].

The purpose of this research is to investigate the effect of COVID-19 on carotid–femoral pulse wave velocity (cfPWV) as a measurement of the complications of COVID-19 on arterial stiffness and subsequent CV complications.

2. Materials and Methods

2.1. Study Design

This study is a systematic review and meta-analysis conducted in adherence to the Preferred Reporting Items for Systematic Reviews and Meta-Analyses (PRISMA) standards [30] (Table S1). The research protocol was pre-approved by all co-authors registered in the PROSPERO registry (International Prospective Registry of Systematic Reviews) under registration number CRD42023434326.

2.2. Search Strategy

Two independent reviewers (I.J. and M.P.) evaluated potential papers. Discrepancies were resolved via further discussion or arbitration by a third reviewer (L.S.). The literature search covered the period between January 2020 and June 2023, covering the following databases: PubMed, Web of Science, Embase, the Cochrane Library, as well as Google Scholar. The search included the combination of keywords: "pulse wave velocity" OR "PWV" OR "arterial stiffness" AND "COVID-19" OR "SARS-CoV-2" OR "severe acute respiratory syndrome coronavirus-2". Citations of listed studies were examined for further relevant literature. Only the most recent and comprehensive articles from identical authors were included to avoid duplicates. Furthermore, reference lists of relevant publications and systematic reviews were reviewed for potential inclusions. All references were consolidated in Endnote (version X9), duplicated entries were removed, and finally, Rayyan, a software screening tool, was used.

2.3. Inclusion and Exclusion Criteria

Studies qualified if they met the following inclusion criteria: research comparing cfPWV in patients with current or previous COVID-19 infection to a control group, as cfPWV is now regarded as the gold standard in assessing arterial stiffness. This method has a high prognostic value since it may help identify individuals who are at a higher risk not just for future outcomes as motioned in the introduction [19,29]. We excluded studies not detailing desired outcomes, other than cfPWV measurement of arterial stiffness, studies with unclear descriptions of COVID-19 infection, and studies that did not include a comparable group, non-English publications, and other types of publications such as the following: editorials, conference papers, reviews, and letters to the editor. In assessed studies, the study group was people who had been diagnosed with COVID-19 and had recovered. The control group was patients who had never had a positive COVID-19 test.

2.4. Data Extraction and Quality Assessment

Using a pre-defined data extraction form that was designed by L.S., the two independent reviewers (I.J. and M.P.) extracted the data from the research, and disagreements were mediated by the third reviewer (L.S.). The following information was extracted from the relevant publications: study characteristics (including first author, publication year, country of origin, study design, and research groups), and patient data (participant count, age, and carotid–femoral pulse wave velocity across groups). The Newcastle–Ottawa Quality Scale (NOS) was used in order to evaluate the level of methodological rigor that was present in each of the studies that were included in the analysis. Based on the selection, comparability, and exposure criteria, NOS allocates a potential four, two, and three stars, respectively. Studies achieving a NOS score ≥ 7 were deemed high quality [31].

2.5. Statistical Analysis

Statistical analyses used Review Manager (version 5.4, Nordic Cochrane Centre, Cochrane Collaboration, Odense, Denmark) and Stata (version 14, StataCorp, College Station, TX, USA) were used. The odds ratios (ORs) with 95% confidence intervals (CIs) were employed for dichotomous data, whereas mean differences (MDs) with 95% CIs were used for continuous data. Every statistical test was conducted using a two-sided approach, with a significance threshold of $p < 0.05$. For continuous outcomes presented as median, range, and interquartile range, the means and standard deviations were estimated using the methodology delineated by Hozo et al. [32]. The I^2 statistic was used to determine the degree of heterogeneity, with values of 25% indicating low heterogeneity, values of 25–50% indicating moderate heterogeneity, and values more than 50% showing high heterogeneity [33]. If I^2 was greater than 50%, a fixed-effects model was employed; otherwise, a random-effects model was used. Potential publication bias in the included studies was assessed via Egger's test and funnel plots.

3. Results

3.1. Study Selection and Characteristics

The bibliographic search results and selection process are shown in the PRISMA flow diagram (Figure 1). We identified 837 initial records, which were reduced to 612 after the elimination of duplicates. Titles and abstracts were screened, leading to the exclusion of 564 records. After assessing the remaining 48 articles for eligibility, we excluded 39 articles. As a result, nine studies were selected for qualitative synthesis and meta-analysis [34–42].

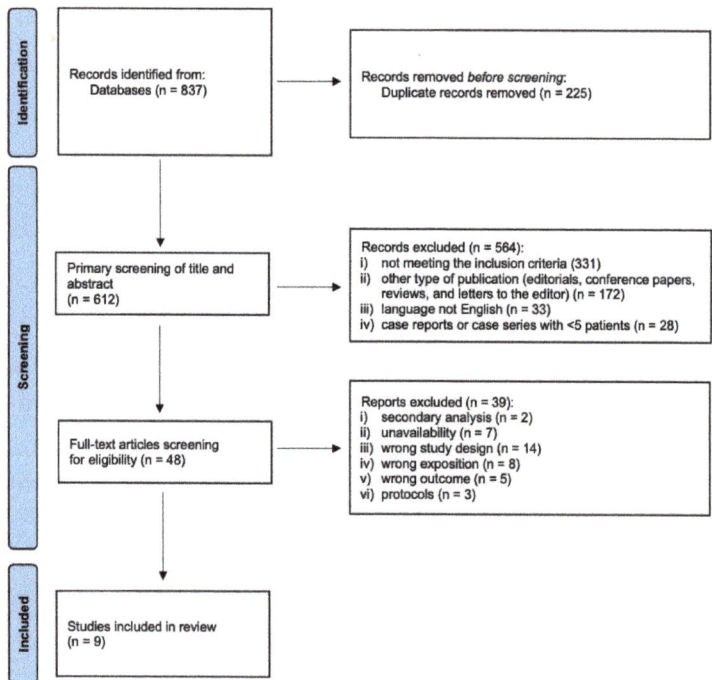

Figure 1. PRISMA systematic review flow diagram.

The essential characteristics of the included studies are outlined in Table 1. A total of nine studies that involved 536 patients were included in this meta-analysis. The mean age of the COVID-19 patient cohort was 50.8 ± 15.1 years, as compared to 51.3 ± 15.0 years in the control groups. Geographically, three studies were conducted in the United States, two in Greece, and the rest in Brazil, Austria, Romania, and the Netherlands. The sample size varied and ranged from 23 to 140 patients. Notably, the NOS scores of all the included studies were ≥7.

Table 1. Characteristics of included studies.

Study	Country	Study Group	No. of Patients	Age	Sex, Male	NOS Scale
Faria et al., 2023 [34]	Brazil	COVID-19	19	47 ± 8	12 (63.2%)	8
		Control	19	43 ± 10	11 (57.9%)	
Tudoran et al., 2023 [35]	Romania	COVID-19	54	47.76 ± 5.43	NS	7
		Control	40	49.47 ± 5.14	NS	
Nandadeva et al., 2023 [36]	United States	COVID-19	12	48 ± 9	NS	7
		Control	11	50 ± 13	NS	
Oikonomou et al., 2023 [37]	Greece	COVID-19	34	57.2 ± 12.9	26 (76.5%)	8
		Control	34	57.4 ± 12.8	23 (67.6%)	
Van der Sluijs et al., 2023 [38]	The Netherlands	COVID-19	31	57.5 ± 3.0	17 (54.8%)	7
		Control	31	56.5 ± 3.0	17 (54.8%)	
Skow et al., 2022 [39]	United States	COVID-19	23	23 ± 3	9 (39.1%)	8
		Control	13	26 ± 4	6 (46.2%)	
Lambadiari et al., 2021 [40]	Greece	COVID-19	70	54.53 ± 9.07	44 (62.85%)	9
		Control	70	54.77 ± 8.95	44 (62.85%)	
		Control	34	57.4 ± 12.8	23 (67.6%)	
Ratchford et al., 2021 [41]	United States	COVID-19	11	20.1 ± 1.1	NS	9
		Control	20	23.0 ± 1.3	NS	
Schnaubelt et al., 2021 [42]	Austria	COVID-19	22	76.0 ± 4.25	11 (50.0%)	8
		Control	22	75.8 ± 4.0	10 (45.5%)	

3.2. Meta-Analysis

All nine studies provided data on cfPWV values among COVID-19 patients and their respective control groups. The pooled analysis showed that cfPWV in COVID-19 patients was 9.5 ± 3.7, compared to 8.2 ± 2.2 in the control groups (MD = 1.32; 95% CI: 0.38 to 2.26; p = 0.006; Figure 2). It is important to note that the results from the sensitivity analysis did not alter the direction of the initial findings.

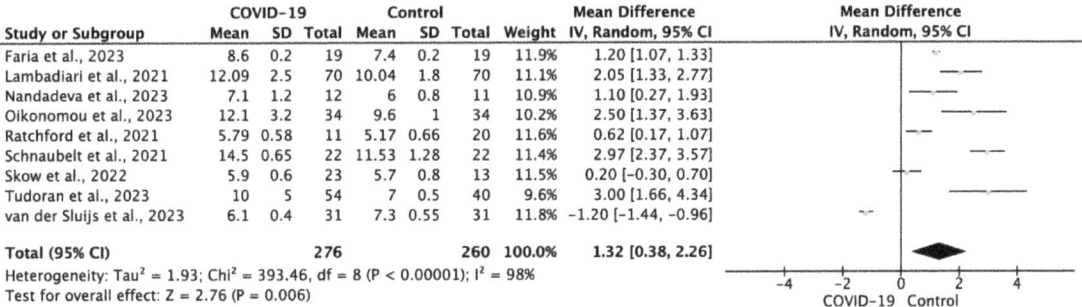

Figure 2. Forest plot of cfPWV in COVID-19 patients vs. non-COVID-19 controls [34–42]. The mean differences for individual studies are represented by the central point of each square, and the associated horizontal line indicates a 95% confidence range. The diamond shapes indicate the consolidated results.

4. Discussion

Our meta-analysis revealed a significant correlation between COVID-19 infection and an increase in cfPWV [34–42]. However, it is worth noting that Van der Sluijs et al. did not observe such a correlation of cfPWV in their research [38], while Skow et al. found a positive, yet insignificant correlation [39]. Nevertheless, the remaining seven analyzed studies demonstrated a clear correlation between cfPWV and COVID-19 infection [34–37,40–42]. These findings suggest that COVID-19 may be responsible for the observed rise in arterial stiffness, which is a well-known marker of cardiovascular (CV) risk [43]. Arterial stiffness reflects changes in blood pressure, flow, as well as vascular diameter, and serves as an indicator of both the mechanical and functional properties of arterial walls. While the degradation of elastic fibers is the primary factor influencing arterial stiffness, other factors, such as fibrosis on replacement, collagen, elastin cross-linking, and medial calcifications also play important roles.

Studies by Townsend et al. and Lambadiari et al. highlighted that multiple factors contribute to arterial stiffness, including endothelial dysfunction, inflammation, oxidative stress, the turnover of extracellular matrix, and the regulation of smooth muscle tone in muscular arteries [40,44]. SARS-CoV-2 virus targets endothelial cells, entering the cell as soon as it binds to ACE2 receptors, decreasing the number of ACE2 receptors on the cell surface, leading to endothelial cell dysfunction [15,45]. The decreased endothelial function observed in COVID-19 patients results from viral infiltration and increased systemic inflammatory responses [46]. Cytokine storm targets specific receptors located on the surface of endothelial cells, leading to the activation of a number of different mediators, resulting in the activation of platelets and the release of leukocytes into circulation [47]. Uncontrolled systemic inflammation may directly stimulate arterial remodeling or cause adrenoceptor hyporeactivity, impairing vascular responsiveness. Additionally, nitric oxide (NO) deficiency in COVID-19 patients can exacerbate endothelial dysfunction and lead to increased arterial stiffness, impaired smooth muscle relaxation, and increased oxidative stress (further exacerbated by the cytokine storm) [48]. Changes in NO bioavailability, combined with SARS-CoV-2's direct action on endothelial cells after binding to ACE2 receptors, can influence the functions of vascular smooth muscle cells and induce structural alterations in the vascular wall's extracellular matrix, promoting arterial stiffness [49].

This arterial stiffness raises the risk of CV complications, including high blood pressure, heart attacks, and strokes, exerting additional strain on the heart. People with pre-existing CV conditions are particularly susceptible. A study by Faria et al. showed that COVID-19 patients, compared to their healthy counterparts, experienced over-activation of the sympathetic nervous system, vascular dysfunction, decreased physical fitness, and elevated cfPWV values (higher by 1.12 m per second) [34]. This is concerning, considering that previously published studies established PWV as a strong predictor of future CV events and all-cause mortality, and showed that the predictive power of arterial stiffness is higher in subjects with a higher baseline CV risk. This in turn suggests that an increase in arterial stiffness contributes to the elevated CV risk observed in COVID-19 survivors [29]. Elevated risks of stroke are consequences of both COVID-19 and increased arterial stiffness [50]. It is concerning that the effects of COVID-19 seem to last beyond the acute phase of the disease, as the virus may induce post-acute sequelae from COVID-19 (PASC). Nandadev et al. highlighted heightened arterial pressure and cfPWV values in PASC patients, suggesting they could develop CV problems at a faster rate [36]. It is interesting to note that a meta-analysis by Menezes et al. demonstrated that CV disease in COVID-19 patients had both cardioembolic and cryptogenic etiology [51], while factors like atherosclerosis were not directly linked to a COVID-19 positive result. Atrial fibrillation, coronary artery disease, diabetes, and hypertension were shown to be the most prevalent risk factors among COVID-19-positive individuals, increasing the risk of CV disease [51,52].

Ratchford et al. demonstrated a strong association between increased cfPWV and mortality among COVID-19 patients, particularly those with pre-existing chronic conditions, including CV disease [41]. Furthermore, a study by Schnaubelt et al. found that cfPWV among COVID-19 patients who survived the disease was significantly lower than in healthy patients, indicating a potential link with long-term complications [42]. Additionally, Kumar et al. showed increased cfPWV in severe COVID-19 cases as compared to non-severe cases [53]. We can assume that COVID-19 influences arterial stiffness, and this effect correlates with the severity of symptoms.

Research also shows that pre-existing conditions are also major factors that can accelerate arterial aging in the course of COVID-19. Tudoran et al. demonstrated a correlation between aortic and arterial stiffness, as well as diastolic dysfunction, in seemingly healthy individuals with post-acute COVID-19 syndrome patients. Their findings showed that women with a history of PASC and metabolic syndrome showed elevated cfPWV values and metrics of worsening of their diastolic dysfunction [35]. Throughout a six-month observation period, the values showed improvement; however, they did not revert fully. Oikonomou et al. evaluated cfPWV as well as the impairment of the left ventricle function measured by global longitudinal strain in the 6-month observation. While improvement was noted in both parameters, the values are still worse than in the control group, which may support the hypothesis that after recovering from COVID-19, and there is an increase in both arterial stiffness and the risk of adverse CV events in comparison to the general population [37]. Similarly, a 12-month follow-up study by Iconomidis and their team found COVID-19 survivors to still possess higher cfPWV values compared to controls at the 12-month follow-up evaluation. The authors showed considerable improvements in oxidative stress (levels of MDA), CFR, and myocardial work measures, in addition to a borderline improvement in left ventricular strain, which, nevertheless, continued to be impaired in comparison to the controls [54].

Another crucial area of research pertains to the management of post-COVID complications, including chronic arterial stiffness. While arterial stiffness is not easily reversible with medication or surgical interventions, additional therapies can be explored. One potential approach is the implementation of post-COVID-19 rehabilitation, which could help alleviate symptoms and improve overall outcomes. Comprehensive rehabilitation strategies, including exercise, physiotherapy, lifestyle changes, and cardiovascular rehabilitation, might help combat the long-term implications of arterial stiffness and increase the patient's quality of life post-COVID. Gounaridi et al.'s research showed that a three-month cardiopulmonary post-acute COVID-19 rehabilitation significantly improved PWV, reducing it from 8.2 ± 1.3 m/s to 6.6 ± 1.0 m/s. Thus, rehabilitation could facilitate the recovery of endothelium-dependent vasodilation and arteriosclerosis [55]. Furthermore, exercise training conducted at home lowered cfPWV by a mean of -2.0 ± 0.6 m/s and has the potential to be an invaluable supplement to post-COVID rehabilitation [56].

However, it is essential to consider that the effect of COVID-19 may be dependent on the mutation of the virus. Skow et al. conducted their research on individuals during the Omicron wave of infections and found that arterial stiffness did not differ significantly between groups of individuals who had the Omicron variant of COVID-19 and controls who had never been exposed to COVID-19. According to these findings, the Omicron variant does not pose a threat to the CV health of young, vaccinated individuals who are otherwise healthy [39]. Nevertheless, there are no studies assessing other subtypes and mutations of COVID-19. Therefore, the correlation between the specific COVID-19 types and arterial stiffens remains inconclusive. Future research could provide us with more precise insights.

The measurement of cfPWV has significant clinical implications in terms of risk assessment and timely medical interventions to prevent COVID-19-related mortality and CV complications, particularly in hospitalized patients, patients with a severe disease course, or those who simply struggled with COVID-19. The timely identification of patients with increased arterial stiffness allows for the implementation of appropriate early medical interventions, including aggressive blood pressure management, optimization of medication regimens, and lifestyle changes, such as dietary changes, regular exercise, and smoking cessation. By implementing these interventions early on, healthcare providers can potentially mitigate the adverse CV effects of COVID-19 and improve patient outcomes. Moreover, longitudinal cfPWV monitoring in hospitalized COVID-19 patients can provide valuable information on the progression of arterial stiffness over time, enabling healthcare professionals to implement personalized treatment strategies, make necessary adjustments, and evaluate the effectiveness of interventions. By closely monitoring cfPWV, clinicians can track the response to treatment, identify any worsening of arterial stiffness, and promptly modify the management plan accordingly.

While our study brings valuable insights, it is essential to acknowledge its limitations. To the best of our knowledge, this is the first meta-analysis examining the influence of

COVID-19 disease on arterial stiffness evaluated by cfPWV. The available research on studies investigating the connection between cfPWV and COVID-19 remains limited, both in terms of the number of studies and participant numbers. Furthermore, the observation window is short, covering the period between 2021 and 2023.

5. Conclusions

There is a strong association between COVID-19 infection and an elevated cfPWV, indicating a potential link between the virus and increased arterial stiffness. The substantial rise in arterial stiffness, an established indicator of CV risk, clearly shows the profound impact of COVID-19 on both immediate and long-term health outcomes. By accurately identifying individuals with augmented arterial stiffness, clinicians can tailor interventions and implement strategies that are more targeted toward lowering the CV risks associated with COVID-19. This will also facilitate timely medical and rehabilitation interventions for patients. However, further research is required in order to provide a clearer understanding of the connection between COVID-19 infection, arterial stiffness, and subsequent CV events. Thus, cfPWV measurements will be more useful as a diagnostic and prognostic instrument.

Supplementary Materials: The following supporting information can be downloaded at the following link: https://www.mdpi.com/article/10.3390/jcm12175747/s1. Table S1: PRISMA 2020 Checklist.

Author Contributions: Conceptualization, I.J.; methodology, I.J., M.P. and L.S.; software, I.J. and L.S.; validation, I.J., M.P., M.R.-H., T.T. and R.O.; formal analysis, I.J. and L.S.; investigation, I.J., M.P. and L.S.; resources, I.J., M.P. and L.S.; data curation, I.J., M.P., S.F. and L.S.; writing—original draft preparation, I.J., M.P. and S.F.; writing—review and editing, I.J., M.P., M.R.-H., T.T., R.O., S.F., K.P. and L.S.; visualization, I.J. and T.T.; supervision, L.S.; project administration, I.J.; funding acquisition, I.J. All authors have read and agreed to the published version of the manuscript.

Funding: Study was supported by the National Institute of Geriatrics, Rheumatology, and Rehabilitation, Warsaw, Poland (project number: S.99).

Institutional Review Board Statement: Not applicable.

Informed Consent Statement: Not applicable.

Data Availability Statement: The data that support the findings of this study are available on request from the corresponding author (L.S.).

Conflicts of Interest: The authors declare no conflict of interest.

References

1. World Health Organisation. WHO Coronavirus Disease Dashboard. 2021. Available online: https://covid19.who.int/ (accessed on 12 June 2023).
2. Smereka, J.; Szarpak, L.; Filipiak, K.J. Modern Medicine in the COVID-19 Era. *Disaster Emerg. Med. J.* **2020**, *5*, 103–105. [CrossRef]
3. Berry, C.; Mangion, K. Multisystem Involvement Is Common in Post-COVID-19 Syndrome. *Nat. Med.* **2022**, *28*, 1139–1140. [CrossRef]
4. Gasecka, A.; Pruc, M.; Kukula, K.; Gilis-Malinowska, N.; Filipiak, K.J.; Jaguszewski, M.J.; Szarpak, L. Post-Covid-19 Heart Syndrome. *Cardiol. J.* **2021**, *28*, 353–354. [CrossRef] [PubMed]
5. Guzik, T.J.; Mohiddin, S.A.; Dimarco, A.; Patel, V.; Savvatis, K.; Marelli-Berg, F.M.; Madhur, M.S.; Tomaszewski, M.; Maffia, P.; D'Acquisto, F.; et al. COVID-19 and the Cardiovascular System: Implications for Risk Assessment, Diagnosis, and Treatment Options. *Cardiovasc. Res.* **2020**, *116*, 1666–1687. [CrossRef]
6. Wang, W.; Wang, C.Y.; Wang, S.I.; Wei, J.C.C. Long-Term Cardiovascular Outcomes in COVID-19 Survivors among Non-Vaccinated Population: A Retrospective Cohort Study from the TriNetX US Collaborative Networks. *eClinicalMedicine* **2022**, *53*, 101619. [CrossRef]
7. Szarpak, L.; Pruc, M.; Filipiak, K.J.; Popieluch, J.; Bielski, A.; Jaguszewski, M.J.; Gilis-Malinowska, N.; Chirico, F.; Rafique, Z.; Peacock, F.W. Myocarditis: A Complication of COVID-19 and Long-COVID-19 Syndrome as a Serious Threat in Modern Cardiology. *Cardiol. J.* **2022**, *29*, 178–179. [CrossRef]
8. Zanoli, L.; Gaudio, A.; Mikhailidis, D.P.; Katsiki, N.; Castellino, N.; Lo Cicero, L.; Geraci, G.; Sessa, C.; Fiorito, L.; Marino, F.; et al. Vascular Dysfunction of COVID-19 Is Partially Reverted in the Long-Term. *Circ. Res.* **2022**, *130*, 1276–1285. [CrossRef]

9. Davis, H.E.; McCorkell, L.; Vogel, J.M.; Topol, E.J. Author Correction: Long COVID: Major Findings, Mechanisms and Recommendations (Nature Reviews Microbiology, (2023), 21, 3, (133-146), 10.1038/S41579-022-00846-2). *Nat. Rev. Microbiol.* **2023**, *21*, 408. [CrossRef]
10. Ballering, A.V.; van Zon, S.K.R.; olde Hartman, T.C.; Rosmalen, J.G.M. Persistence of Somatic Symptoms after COVID-19 in the Netherlands: An Observational Cohort Study. *Lancet* **2022**, *400*, 452–461. [CrossRef]
11. Szarpak, L.; Filipiak, K.J.; Skwarek, A.; Pruc, M.; Rahnama, M.; Denegri, A.; Jachowicz, M.; Dawidowska, M.; Gasecka, A.; Jaguszewski, M.J.; et al. Outcomes and Mortality Associated with Atrial Arrhythmias among Patients Hospitalized with COVID-19: A Systematic Review and Meta-Analysis. *Cardiol. J.* **2022**, *29*, 33–43. [CrossRef]
12. Szarpak, L.; Mierzejewska, M.; Jurek, J.; Kochanowska, A.; Gasecka, A.; Truszewski, Z.; Pruc, M.; Blek, N.; Rafique, Z.; Filipiak, K.J.; et al. Effect of Coronary Artery Disease on COVID-19—Prognosis and Risk Assessment: A Systematic Review and Meta-Analysis. *Biology* **2022**, *11*, 221. [CrossRef] [PubMed]
13. Libby, P.; Lüscher, T. COVID-19 Is, in the End, an Endothelial Disease. *Eur. Heart J.* **2020**, *41*, 3038–3044. [CrossRef] [PubMed]
14. Hoffmann, M.; Kleine-Weber, H.; Schroeder, S.; Krüger, N.; Herrler, T.; Erichsen, S.; Schiergens, T.S.; Herrler, G.; Wu, N.H.; Nitsche, A.; et al. SARS-CoV-2 Cell Entry Depends on ACE2 and TMPRSS2 and Is Blocked by a Clinically Proven Protease Inhibitor. *Cell* **2020**, *181*, 271–280.e8. [CrossRef]
15. Varga, Z.; Flammer, A.J.; Steiger, P.; Haberecker, M.; Andermatt, R.; Zinkernagel, A.S.; Mehra, M.R.; Schuepbach, R.A.; Ruschitzka, F.; Moch, H. Endothelial Cell Infection and Endotheliitis in COVID-19. *Lancet* **2020**, *395*, 1417–1418. [CrossRef]
16. Çiftel, M.; Ateş, N.; Yılmaz, O. Investigation of Endothelial Dysfunction and Arterial Stiffness in Multisystem Inflammatory Syndrome in Children. *Eur. J. Pediatr.* **2022**, *181*, 91–97. [CrossRef] [PubMed]
17. Chang, R.; Mamun, A.; Dominic, A.; Le, N.T. SARS-CoV-2 Mediated Endothelial Dysfunction: The Potential Role of Chronic Oxidative Stress. *Front. Physiol.* **2021**, *11*, 605908. [CrossRef]
18. Ambardar, S.R.; Hightower, S.L.; Huprikar, N.A.; Chung, K.K.; Singhal, A.; Collen, J.F. Post-COVID-19 Pulmonary Fibrosis: Novel Sequelae of the Current Pandemic. *J. Clin. Med.* **2021**, *10*, 2452. [CrossRef]
19. Thijssen, D.H.J.; Bruno, R.M.; Van Mil, A.C.C.M.; Holder, S.M.; Faita, F.; Greyling, A.; Zock, P.L.; Taddei, S.; Deanfield, J.E.; Luscher, T.; et al. Expert Consensus and Evidence-Based Recommendations for the Assessment of Flow-Mediated Dilation in Humans. *Eur. Heart J.* **2019**, *40*, 2534–2547. [CrossRef]
20. Laurent, S.; Boutouyrie, P.; Cunha, P.G.; Lacolley, P.; Nilsson, P.M. Concept of Extremes in Vascular Aging: From Early Vascular Aging to Supernormal Vascular Aging. *Hypertension* **2019**, *74*, 218–228. [CrossRef]
21. Williams, B.; Mancia, G.; Spiering, W.; Rosei, E.A.; Azizi, M.; Burnier, M.; Clement, D.L.; Coca, A.; De Simone, G.; Dominiczak, A.; et al. 2018 ESC/ESH Guidelines for Themanagement of Arterial Hypertension. *Eur. Heart J.* **2018**, *39*, 3021–3104. [CrossRef]
22. Ben-Shlomo, Y.; Spears, M.; Boustred, C.; May, M.; Anderson, S.G.; Benjamin, E.J.; Boutouyrie, P.; Cameron, J.; Chen, C.H.; Cruickshank, J.K.; et al. Aortic Pulse Wave Velocity Improves Cardiovascular Event Prediction: An Individual Participant Meta-Analysis of Prospective Observational Data from 17,635 Subjects. *J. Am. Coll. Cardiol.* **2014**, *63*, 636–646. [CrossRef] [PubMed]
23. Van Bortel, L.M.; Laurent, S.; Boutouyrie, P.; Chowienczyk, P.; Cruickshank, J.K.; De Backer, T.; Filipovsky, J.; Huybrechts, S.; Mattace-Raso, F.U.; Protogerou, A.D.; et al. Expert consensus document on the Measurement of Aortic Stiffness in Daily Practice Using Carotid-Femoral Pulse Wave Velocity. *J. Hypertens.* **2012**, *30*, 445–448. [CrossRef] [PubMed]
24. Raisi-Estabragh, Z.; McCracken, C.; Cooper, J.; Fung, K.; Paiva, J.M.; Khanji, M.Y.; Rauseo, E.; Biasiolli, L.; Raman, B.; Piechnik, S.K.; et al. Adverse Cardiovascular Magnetic Resonance Phenotypes Are Associated with Greater Likelihood of Incident Coronavirus Disease 2019: Findings from the UK Biobank. *Aging Clin. Exp. Res.* **2021**, *33*, 1133–1144. [CrossRef] [PubMed]
25. Szeghy, R.E.; Province, V.M.; Stute, N.L.; Augenreich, M.A.; Koontz, L.K.; Stickford, J.L.; Stickford, A.S.L.; Ratchford, S.M. Carotid Stiffness, Intima–Media Thickness and Aortic Augmentation Index among Adults with SARS-CoV-2. *Exp. Physiol.* **2022**, *107*, 694–707. [CrossRef] [PubMed]
26. Rodilla, E.; López-Carmona, M.D.; Cortes, X.; Cobos-Palacios, L.; Canales, S.; Sáez, M.C.; Campos Escudero, S.; Rubio-Rivas, M.; Díez Manglano, J.; Freire Castro, S.J.; et al. Impact of Arterial Stiffness on All-Cause Mortality in Patients Hospitalized With COVID-19 in Spain. *Hypertension* **2021**, *77*, 856–867. [CrossRef]
27. Aydın, E.; Kant, A.; Yilmaz, G. Evaluation of the Cardio-Ankle Vascular Index in COVID-19 Patients. *Rev. Assoc. Med. Bras.* **2022**, *68*, 73–76. [CrossRef]
28. Bruno, R.M.; Nilsson, P.M.; Engström, G.; Wadström, B.N.; Empana, J.P.; Boutouyrie, P.; Laurent, S. Early and Supernormal Vascular Aging: Clinical Characteristics and Association With Incident Cardiovascular Events. *Hypertension* **2020**, *76*, 1616–1624. [CrossRef]
29. Vlachopoulos, C.; Aznaouridis, K.; Stefanadis, C. Prediction of Cardiovascular Events and All-Cause Mortality With Arterial Stiffness. A Systematic Review and Meta-Analysis. *J. Am. Coll. Cardiol.* **2010**, *55*, 1318–1327. [CrossRef]
30. Page, M.J.; McKenzie, J.E.; Bossuyt, P.M.; Boutron, I.; Hoffmann, T.C.; Mulrow, C.D.; Shamseer, L.; Tetzlaff, J.M.; Akl, E.A.; Brennan, S.E.; et al. The PRISMA 2020 Statement: An Updated Guideline for Reporting Systematic Reviews. *BMJ* **2021**, *372*, n71. [CrossRef]
31. Stang, A. Critical Evaluation of the Newcastle-Ottawa Scale for the Assessment of the Quality of Nonrandomized Studies in Meta-Analyses. *Eur. J. Epidemiol.* **2010**, *25*, 603–605. [CrossRef]

32. Hozo, S.P.; Djulbegovic, B.; Hozo, I. Estimating the Mean and Variance from the Median, Range, and the Size of a Sample. *BMC Med. Res. Methodol.* **2005**, *5*, 13. [CrossRef]
33. Higgins, J.P.T.; Thompson, S.G.; Deeks, J.J.; Altman, D.G. Measuring Inconsistency in Meta-Analyses. *Br. Med. J.* **2003**, *327*, 557–560. [CrossRef] [PubMed]
34. Faria, D.; Moll-Bernardes, R.J.; Testa, L.; Moniz, C.M.V.; Rodrigues, E.C.; Rodrigues, A.G.; Araujo, A.; Alves, M.J.N.N.; Ono, B.E.; Izaias, J.E.; et al. Sympathetic Neural Overdrive, Aortic Stiffening, Endothelial Dysfunction, and Impaired Exercise Capacity in Severe COVID-19 Survivors: A Mid-Term Study of Cardiovascular Sequelae. *Hypertension* **2023**, *80*, 470–481. [CrossRef] [PubMed]
35. Tudoran, C.; Bende, F.; Bende, R.; Giurgi-Oncu, C.; Dumache, R.; Tudoran, M. Correspondence between Aortic and Arterial Stiffness, and Diastolic Dysfunction in Apparently Healthy Female Patients with Post-Acute COVID-19 Syndrome. *Biomedicines* **2023**, *11*, 492. [CrossRef] [PubMed]
36. Nandadeva, D.; Skow, R.J.; Stephens, B.Y.; Grotle, A.K.; Georgoudiou, S.; Barshikar, S.; Seo, Y.; Fadel, P.J. Cardiovascular and Cerebral Vascular Health in Females with Postacute Sequelae of COVID-19. *Am. J. Physiol. Heart Circ. Physiol.* **2023**, *324*, H713–H720. [CrossRef]
37. Oikonomou, E.; Lampsas, S.; Theofilis, P.; Souvaliotis, N.; Papamikroulis, G.A.; Katsarou, O.; Kalogeras, K.; Pantelidis, P.; Papaioannou, T.G.; Tsatsaragkou, A.; et al. Impaired Left Ventricular Deformation and Ventricular-Arterial Coupling in Post-COVID-19: Association with Autonomic Dysregulation. *Heart Vessels* **2023**, *38*, 381–393. [CrossRef]
38. van der Sluijs, K.M.; Bakker, E.A.; Schuijt, T.J.; Joseph, J.; Kavousi, M.; Geersing, G.J.; Rutten, F.H.; Hartman, Y.A.W.; Thijssen, D.H.J.; Eijsvogels, T.M.H. Long-Term Cardiovascular Health Status and Physical Functioning of Nonhospitalized Patients with COVID-19 Compared with Non-COVID-19 Controls. *Am. J. Physiol.—Heart Circ. Physiol.* **2023**, *324*, H47–H56. [CrossRef]
39. Skow, R.J.; Nandadeva, D.; Grotle, A.K.; Stephens, B.Y.; Wright, A.N.; Fadel, P.J. Impact of Breakthrough COVID-19 Cases during the Omicron Wave on Vascular Health and Cardiac Autonomic Function in Young Adults. *Am. J. Physiol.—Heart Circ. Physiol.* **2022**, *323*, H59–H64. [CrossRef]
40. Lambadiari, V.; Mitrakou, A.; Kountouri, A.; Thymis, J.; Katogiannis, K.; Korakas, E.; Varlamos, C.; Andreadou, I.; Tsoumani, M.; Triantafyllidi, H.; et al. Association of COVID-19 with Impaired Endothelial Glycocalyx, Vascular Function and Myocardial Deformation 4 Months after Infection. *Eur. J. Heart Fail.* **2021**, *23*, 1916–1926. [CrossRef]
41. Ratchford, S.M.; Stickford, J.L.; Province, V.M.; Stute, N.; Augenreich, M.A.; Koontz, L.K.; Bobo, L.K.; Stickford, A.S.L. Vascular Alterations among Young Adults with SARS-CoV-2. *Am. J. Physiol.—Heart Circ. Physiol.* **2021**, *320*, H404–H410. [CrossRef]
42. Schnaubelt, S.; Oppenauer, J.; Tihanyi, D.; Mueller, M.; Maldonado-Gonzalez, E.; Zejnilovic, S.; Haslacher, H.; Perkmann, T.; Strassl, R.; Anders, S.; et al. Arterial Stiffness in Acute COVID-19 and Potential Associations with Clinical Outcome. *J. Intern. Med.* **2021**, *290*, 437–443. [CrossRef]
43. Oliveira, A.C.; Cunha, P.M.G.M.; Vitorino, P.V.d.O.; Souza, A.L.L.; Deus, G.D.; Feitosa, A.; Barbosa, E.C.D.; Gomes, M.M.; Jardim, P.C.B.V.; Barroso, W.K.S. Vascular Aging and Arterial Stiffness. *Arq. Bras. Cardiol.* **2022**, *119*, 604–615. [CrossRef]
44. Townsend, R.R. Arterial Stiffness: Recommendations and Standardization. *Pulse* **2016**, *4*, 3–7. [CrossRef]
45. Vrints, C.J.M.; Krychtiuk, K.A.; Van Craenenbroeck, E.M.; Segers, V.F.; Price, S.; Heidbuchel, H. Endothelialitis Plays a Central Role in the Pathophysiology of Severe COVID-19 and Its Cardiovascular Complications. *Acta Cardiol.* **2021**, *76*, 109–124. [CrossRef]
46. Montazersaheb, S.; Hosseiniyan Khatibi, S.M.; Hejazi, M.S.; Tarhriz, V.; Farjami, A.; Ghasemian Sorbeni, F.; Farahzadi, R.; Ghasemnejad, T. COVID-19 Infection: An Overview on Cytokine Storm and Related Interventions. *Virol. J.* **2022**, *19*, 92. [CrossRef]
47. Merad, M.; Martin, J.C. Pathological Inflammation in Patients with COVID-19: A Key Role for Monocytes and Macrophages. *Nat. Rev. Immunol.* **2020**, *20*, 355–362. [CrossRef]
48. Martel, J.; Ko, Y.F.; Young, J.D.; Ojcius, D.M. Could Nasal Nitric Oxide Help to Mitigate the Severity of COVID-19? *Microbes Infect.* **2020**, *22*, 168–171. [CrossRef]
49. Vlachopoulos, C.; Dima, I.; Aznaouridis, K.; Vasiliadou, C.; Ioakeimidis, N.; Aggeli, C.; Toutouza, M.; Stefanadis, C. Acute Systemic Inflammation Increases Arterial Stiffness and Decreases Wave Reflections in Healthy Individuals. *Circulation* **2005**, *112*, 2193–2200. [CrossRef]
50. Van Sloten, T.T.; Sedaghat, S.; Laurent, S.; London, G.M.; Pannier, B.; Ikram, M.A.; Kavousi, M.; Mattace-Raso, F.; Franco, O.H.; Boutouyrie, P.; et al. Carotid Stiffness Is Associated with Incident Stroke A Systematic Review and Individual Participant Data Meta-Analysis. *J. Am. Coll. Cardiol.* **2015**, *66*, 2116–2125. [CrossRef]
51. Menezes, R.G.; Alabduladhem, T.O.; Siddiqi, A.K.; Maniya, M.T.; Al Dahlawi, A.M.; Almulhim, M.W.A.; Almulhim, H.W.; Saeed, Y.A.A.; Alotaibi, M.S.; Alarifi, S.S.; et al. Infezioni in Medicina. *Infez. Med.* **2023**, *31*, 140–150. [CrossRef]
52. Maruhashi, T.; Higashi, Y. Pathophysiological Association of Endothelial Dysfunction with Fatal Outcome in Covid-19. *Int. J. Mol. Sci.* **2021**, *22*, 5131. [CrossRef]
53. Kumar, N.; Kumar, S.; Kumar, A.; Bhushan, D.; Kumar, A.; Kumar, A.; Singh, V.; Singh, P.K. The Cosevast Study Outcome: Evidence of Covid-19 Severity Proportionate to Surge in Arterial Stiffness. *Indian J. Crit. Care Med.* **2021**, *25*, 1111–1117. [CrossRef]
54. Ikonomidis, I.; Lambadiari, V.; Mitrakou, A.; Kountouri, A.; Katogiannis, K.; Thymis, J.; Korakas, E.; Pavlidis, G.; Kazakou, P.; Panagopoulos, G.; et al. Myocardial Work and Vascular Dysfunction Are Partially Improved at 12 Months after COVID-19 Infection. *Eur. J. Heart Fail.* **2022**, *24*, 727–729. [CrossRef]

55. Gounaridi, M.I.; Vontetsianos, A.; Oikonomou, E.; Theofilis, P.; Chynkiamis, N.; Lampsas, S.; Anastasiou, A.; Papamikroulis, G.A.; Katsianos, E.; Kalogeras, K.; et al. The Role of Rehabilitation in Arterial Function Properties of Convalescent COVID-19 Patients. *J. Clin. Med.* **2023**, *12*, 2233. [CrossRef]
56. Teixeira Do Amaral, V.; Viana, A.A.; Heubel, A.D.; Linares, S.N.; Martinelli, B.; Witzler, P.H.C.; Orikassa De Oliveira, G.Y.; Zanini, G.D.S.; Borghi Silva, A.; Mendes, R.G.; et al. Cardiovascular, Respiratory, and Functional Effects of Home-Based Exercise Training after COVID-19 Hospitalization. *Med. Sci. Sports Exerc.* **2022**, *54*, 1795–1803. [CrossRef]

Disclaimer/Publisher's Note: The statements, opinions and data contained in all publications are solely those of the individual author(s) and contributor(s) and not of MDPI and/or the editor(s). MDPI and/or the editor(s) disclaim responsibility for any injury to people or property resulting from any ideas, methods, instructions or products referred to in the content.

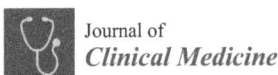

Case Report

The Implications of SARS-CoV-2 Infection in a Series of Neuro-Ophthalmological Manifestations—Case Series and Literature Review

Nicoleta Anton [1,2,*], Camelia Margareta Bogdănici [1,2,*], Daniel Constantin Brănișteanu [1], Ovidiu-Dumitru Ilie [3], Irina Andreea Pavel [1,2] and Bogdan Doroftei [1]

[1] Surgery Department, Faculty of Medicine, University of Medicine and Pharmacy, 700115 Iasi, Romania; dbranisteanu@yahoo.com (D.C.B.); irinaandreea.pavel@gmail.com (I.A.P.); bogdandoroftei@gmail.com (B.D.)
[2] Ophthalmology Clinic, St. Spiridon County Emergency Hospital, 700111 Iasi, Romania
[3] Department of Biology, Faculty of Biology, Alexandru Ioan Cuza University, 700505 Iasi, Romania; ovidiuilie90@yahoo.com
* Correspondence: anton.nicoleta1@umfiasi.ro (N.A.); camelia.bogdanici@umfiasi.ro (C.M.B.)

Citation: Anton, N.; Bogdănici, C.M.; Brănișteanu, D.C.; Ilie, O.-D.; Pavel, I.A.; Doroftei, B. The Implications of SARS-CoV-2 Infection in a Series of Neuro-Ophthalmological Manifestations—Case Series and Literature Review. *J. Clin. Med.* **2023**, *12*, 3795. https://doi.org/10.3390/jcm12113795

Academic Editors: Francesco Pugliese, Francesco Alessandri and Giovanni Giordano

Received: 30 April 2023
Revised: 22 May 2023
Accepted: 30 May 2023
Published: 31 May 2023

Copyright: © 2023 by the authors. Licensee MDPI, Basel, Switzerland. This article is an open access article distributed under the terms and conditions of the Creative Commons Attribution (CC BY) license (https://creativecommons.org/licenses/by/4.0/).

Abstract: The global pandemic impact of the COVID-19 infection included clinical manifestations that affected several organs and systems, with various neuro-ophthalmological manifestations associated with the infection. These are rare and occur either secondary to the presence of the virus or by an autoimmune mechanism secondary to viral antigens. The manifestations are atypical, being present even in the absence of the systemic symptoms typical of a SARS-CoV-2 infection. In this article, we introduce a series of three clinical cases with neuro-ophthalmological manifestations associated with COVID infection that were shown in Ophthalmology Clinic of St. Spiridon Emergency Hospital. Case 1 is that of a 45-year-old male patient with no personal history of general pathology or ophthalmology, with binocular diplopia, painful red eyes, and lacrimal hypersecretion with a sudden onset of about 4 days. Based on the evaluations, a positive diagnosis of orbital cellulitis in both eyes is made. Case 2 is that of a 52-year-old female patient with general PPA (personal pathological antecedents) of SARS-CoV-2 infection 1 month prior to presentation with decreased visual acuity in the right eye and a positive central scotoma, preceded by photopsia and vertigo with balance disorders. The diagnosis is made at the right eye for retrobulbar optic neuritis and post-SARS-CoV-2 infection status. The last clinical case is that of a 55-year-old male patient known to have high blood pressure (HBP) with a sudden, painless decrease in VARE approximately 3 weeks post-SARS-CoV-2 immunization (Pfizer vaccine first dose). The diagnosis is made after consulting all the RE results for central retinal vein thrombosis. Conclusions: Although the cases were quickly and efficiently investigated and the treatment was administered adequately by a multidisciplinary team (cases 1 and 3), the evolution was not favorable in all three situations. Atypical neuro-ophthalmological manifestations can also be present in the absence of systemic symptoms typical of SARS-CoV-2 infection.

Keywords: optic neuritis; orbital cellulitis; anterior ischemic optic neuropathy; venous thrombosis; ocular pathology; SARS-CoV-2; ocular manifestations in COVID infections

1. Introduction

The emergence of COVID-19 at the end of 2019 determined a particular series of cases that, in addition to respiratory manifestations, also had neurological manifestations, the virus being able to produce a wide range of systemic manifestations. In a 2022 review regarding the neurological changes associated with COVID infection in case series and group studies, Matthew K. et al. reported neurological manifestations in 14–57% of hospitalized patients with COVID-19, with taste and smell disturbances reported in many patients with milder disease. In this study, the incidence of ocular manifestations among patients with COVID-19 varies between groups, with an estimated incidence of up to 30%

in hospitalized patients [1]. Presentations range from completely asymptomatic carriers to multiple organ failure and death. The virus can affect the eye in several ways, and there is a wide range of ocular manifestations, with symptoms including irritation (chemosis), excessive lacrimation (epiphora), and ocular secretions showing conjunctivitis up to severe types with cranial nerve damage and neuro-ophthalmological manifestations. In a series of 38 hospitalized patients with COVID-19 in China, 12 (31.6%) patients had ocular symptoms before systemic symptoms [1–6].

Cases of patients who, within the context of the COVID-19 infection or secondary to immunization, were diagnosed with optic neuritis, cranial neuropathies, or optic neuromyelitis are cited in the literature. They have been reported in various studies as dysfunctions of the optic nerve, movement anomalies of the eyeballs, and visual field defects. Studies show that these neuro-ophthalmological manifestations can occur in isolation or in association with neurological syndromes. Manifestations include headache, eye pain, visual disturbances, diplopia, cranial nerve palsies secondary to Miller-Fisher syndrome, Guillain-Barré syndrome, or encephalitis, and nystagmus. The authors consider that some of the ocular and neuro-ophthalmological changes were not detected in time due to the general severity of the COVID-19 virus infection, which did not allow a complete ophthalmic evaluation in the anesthesia and intensive care departments [1,2].

As related to vaccination against the coronavirus disease 2019 (COVID-19), this was implemented to eliminate the SARS-CoV-2 pandemic, providing significant protection against infection and the development of multi-organ acute respiratory distress syndrome. However, subsequent studies have demonstrated potential adverse events in vaccinated patients, including ocular complications: non-arteritic anterior ischemic optic neuropathy (NAION), central serous chorioretinopathy (CSC), and Vogt-Koyanagi-Harada (VKH) disease have been reported [2–5,7].

Regarding these cases cited in the literature that occur after the COVID immunization, they are not highly numerous. Several mechanisms that are associated with secondary ophthalmological manifestations have been reported: the receptor for angiotensin 2, which is found in the central nervous system but also inside the retinal vessels [5], through a direct mechanism that leads to the dysfunction of endothelial cells, causing ischemia and coagulopathy [5,8–10].

Likewise, other studies claim that the neurological manifestations occur secondary to viremia crossing the blood-brain barrier or through infected leukocytes [5,9–11].

This study reports a series of three clinical cases of patients with neuro-ophthalmic diseases that occurred within the context of the COVID-19 pandemic and immunization against COVID.

2. Presentation of Cases

General Information about Patients

We introduce a series of three patients who presented themselves in the Ophthalmology Clinic of St. Spiridon Hospital with neuro-ophthalmic manifestations associated with the COVID infection in 2021, when vaccination was also possible: a 45-year-old male patient with bilateral orbital cellulitis, which occurred as a result of the SARS-CoV-2 infection; a 52-year-old female patient with post-SARS-CoV-2 optic neuritis; and a 55-year-old male patient with secondary ischemic optic neuropathy prior to SARS-CoV-2 immunization. All patients were fully evaluated and signed informed consent in order to carry out all investigations and appropriate treatment. The ophthalmic evaluation consisted of: visual acuity measurement, IOP determination, chromatic sense, visual field determination, ocular motility examination, interdisciplinary examinations, and brain imaging.

Case 1 is that of a 45-year-old male patient with no personal history of general pathology or ophthalmology who presented with BE binocular diplopia to the eye emergency department, painful red eyes, and lacrimal hypersecretion with a sudden onset of approx. 4 days (Figure 1) in April 2021. The functional ophthalmic examination reveals an VA BE (visual acuity both eyes) of 0.4 with correction cc (−2.75 sf) and an IOP (intraocular pressure) RE of 24 mmHg and an IOP LE of 23 mmHg. Biomicroscopic examination of the anterior segment reveals significant conjunctival congestion, dilated episcleral vessels, corneal epithelial edema 2+, and periocular skin congestion. The fundus is normal. Ocular motility: BE (both eyes) slight limitation of abduction. According to the protocol, the patient tested positive for SARS-CoV-2 virus infection. We mention the fact that the patient was asymptomatic while being isolated in a special room. Blood tests reveal leukocytosis with neutrophilia, thrombocytosis, and an inflammatory syndrome with elevated ESR and CRP; the OCT examination reveals a normal visual field without systematic changes or thinning of the retinal nerve fiber layers (Figure 2). The tests for HBV, HCV, HIV, TPHA, FT4, and TSH were negative. Craniocerebral computer tomography (CT) with contrast material diagnoses bilateral orbital cellulitis with infiltrating appearance of intra- and extraconal fat, infiltration of bilateral malar and palpebral subcutaneous cellular tissue, and discreet infiltrative appearance of the internal rectus muscles (RE 4.7 mm, LE 5.4 mm). The examination of infectious diseases, otolaryngology (ENT), and maxillofacial surgery (MFS) does not identify etiologies responsible for the clinical picture. Based on the evaluations, a positive diagnosis of BE orbital cellulitis is made. The evolution is slowly favorable, with gradual remission of clinical signs and recovery of visual acuity under treatment with Ceftriaxone (generally 2 g/day), Vancomycin, Aerius (desloratadine 5 mg), Moxifloxacin, Betabioptal (betamethasone 0.2 g), chloramphenicol 0.5 g, and Naabak (Sodium isospaglumate) (topical administration, initially six times a day). Thus, after 1 month, an improvement in eye movements, a reduction in periocular inflammation, a normal visual field, an OCT examination, and an improvement in visual acuity can be seen, indicating a favorable prognosis.

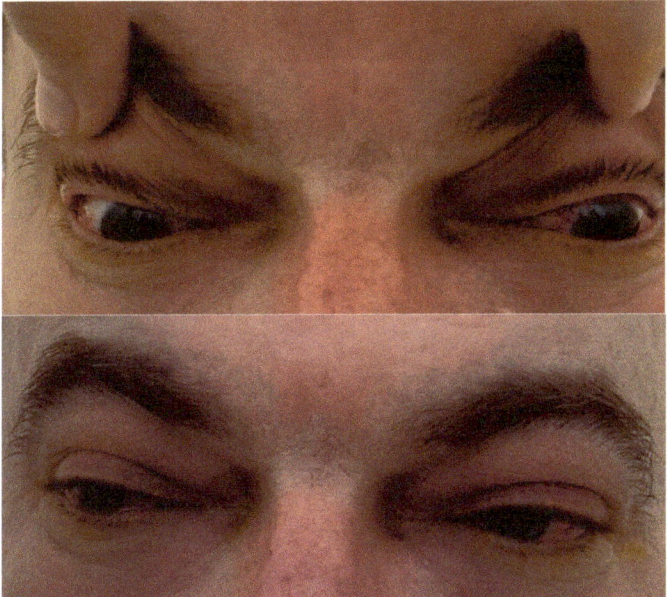

Figure 1. *Cont.*

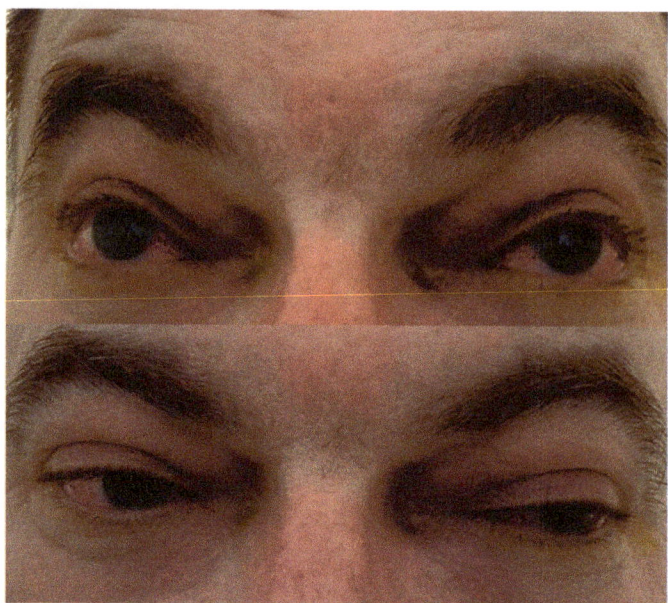

Figure 1. Examination of ocular motility and the segment prior to admission, case 1, slight limitation of abduction (COVID-19 isolation area).

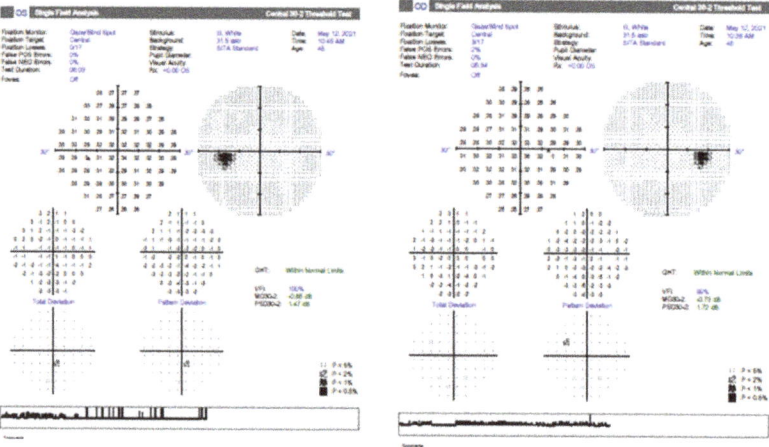

Figure 2. Cont.

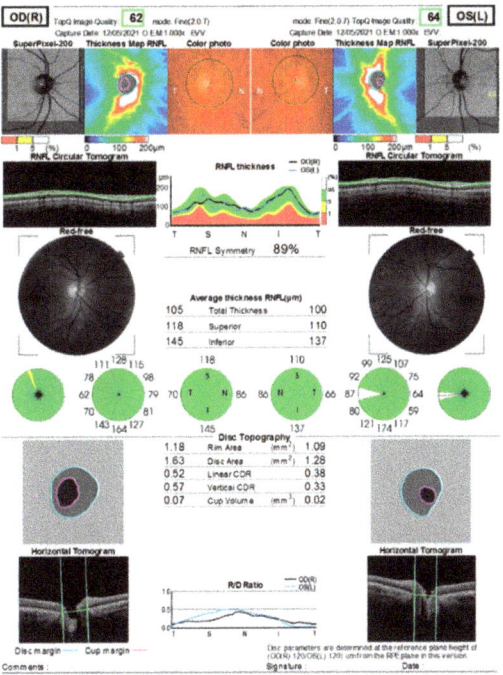

Figure 2. Visual field and OCT examination in both eyes 1 month after the presentation (12 may 2021) of case 1 (not possible immediately due to the COVID infection).

Case 2 is that of a 52-year-old female patient with general APP of SARS-CoV-2 infection 1 month prior to presentation in September 2021. She complained of decreased VARE and a positive central scotoma, preceded by photopsia and vertigo with balance disorders. After the functional examination revealed the VA RE is 1, VA LE is 1.2, IOP RE is 13 mmHg, and IOP LE is 12 mmHg, the anterior segment examination is within normal limits, without Relative Afferent Pupillary Defect (RAPD), and color sense and ocular motility are normal. The OF RE (ocular fundus) optic nerve papilla has an erased contour in the nasal sector. Blood tests are within normal limits: negative HIV, negative RPR, normal rheumatoid factor, liver and kidney samples, HLG, and normal coagulation. A contrast-enhanced MRI is normal. VF RE (visual field right eye) centrocecal scotoma (Figure 3) and normal LE (left eye); OCT macula and optic nerve normal; X-ray chest aortic atheromatous; normal bilateral X-ray of sacroiliac joints. After gathering the data, the diagnosis is made at the RE (right eye) of retrobulbar optic neuritis and post-SARS-CoV-2 infection status. The therapy is initiated with metilprednisolon iv (intravenous route) for 3 days at 1 g (1000 mg) per day and then decreased to 1 mg/kg/body for 11 days. Under treatment, the general condition of the patient gradually recovered with the gradual remission of changes in the visual field. At the 3-month evaluation, the optic nerve OCT examination reveals the sequelae of optic neuritis, namely a moderate thinning of the retinal nerve fiber layers in the superior and nasal sectors without affecting the visual acuity (Figure 4).

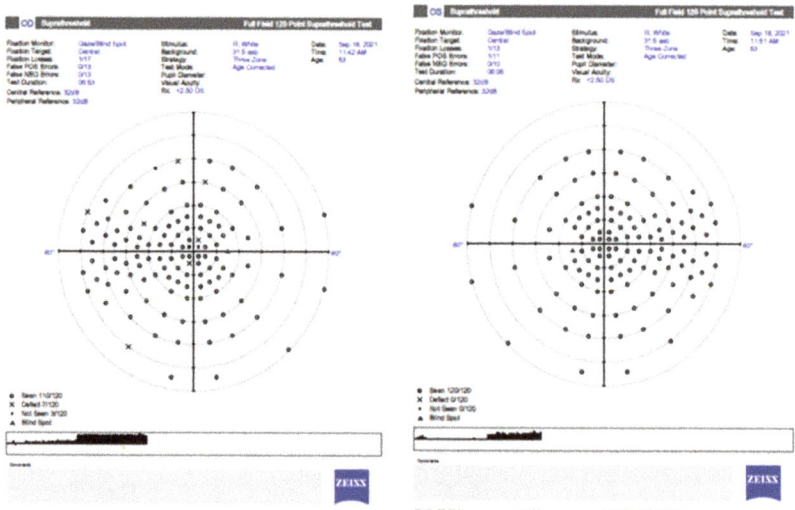

Figure 3. The RE visual field with a centrocecal scotoma at hospitalization (Full Field 120 points Suprathreshold). LE normal (case 2).

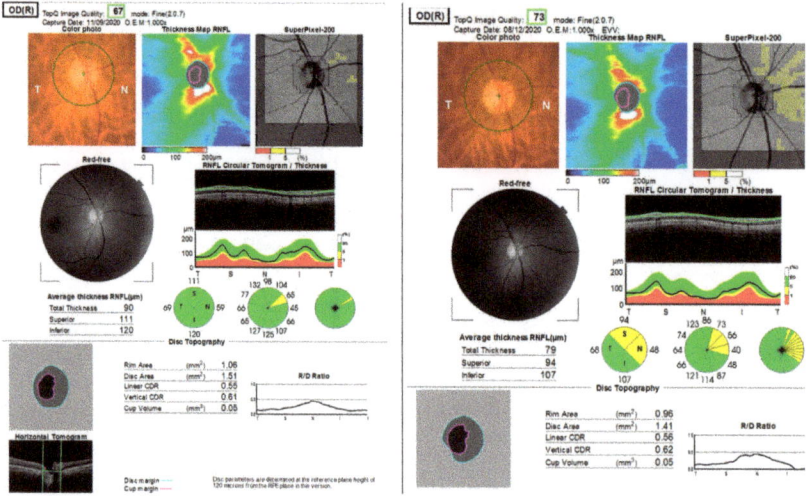

Figure 4. OCT at hospitalization (11 September 2020) vs. 3 months after treatment (8 December 2020) (thin RE superior and nasal SNFR, 136 vs. 94 and 66 vs. 48 μm) if there is also a visual field at discharge (case 2).

Case 3 is that of a 55-year-old male patient known to suffer from hypertension. He suffers from a sudden, painless decrease in VA RE approximately 3 weeks post-SARS-CoV-2 immunization (Pfizer vaccine first dose). VA RE PL uncertain, VA LE 0.7 fc, 1 corrected, IOP BE with normal values. Biomicroscopic examination of the LE anterior pole for conjunctival melanosis, crystalline transparency disorders, and otherwise normal. OF RE papillary edema, peripapillary hemorrhages in the flame, dilated veins due to the emergency, and at normal LE of the optic nerve (Figure 5).

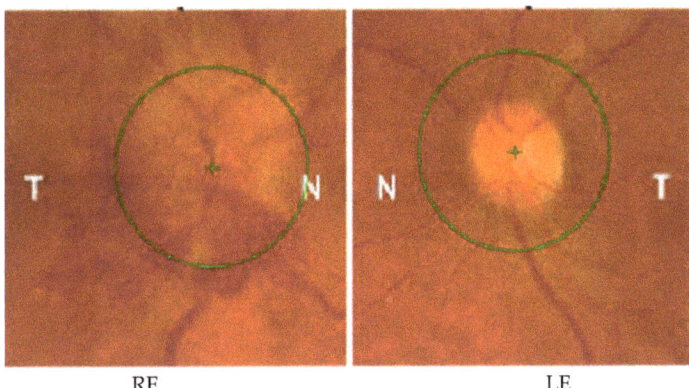

RE   LE

Figure 5. The optic nerve during the fundus examination with papillary edema revealed in the RE, normal aspect in the LE.

Blood tests revealed mild hypercholesterolemia and inflammatory markers within normal limits. ANA, RPR, and Ac anti-HIV tests within normal limits (antinuclear antibodies, rapid plasma reagin test for treponema pallidum, and acquired immune deficiency syndrome). The inter-clinical examinations of cardiology, dermatology, ENT (otorhinolaryngology), maxillofacial surgery (MFS), hematology, and neurology did not raise the suspicion of another etiology. Contrast-enhanced MRI examination: right optic nerve 10 mm with moderate contrast uptake. Normal chest X-ray. The visual field (Full Field 120 points Suprathreshold test) of the LE upon hospitalization (June 2021) and after 2 months (August 2021) shows relative scotoma without systematization (Figure 6). The OCT examination reveals a significant diffuse thickening of the optic nerve and a normal aspect of the LE. A normal visual field of the LE, while this is not possible due to poor visual acuity in the RE (Figure 7).

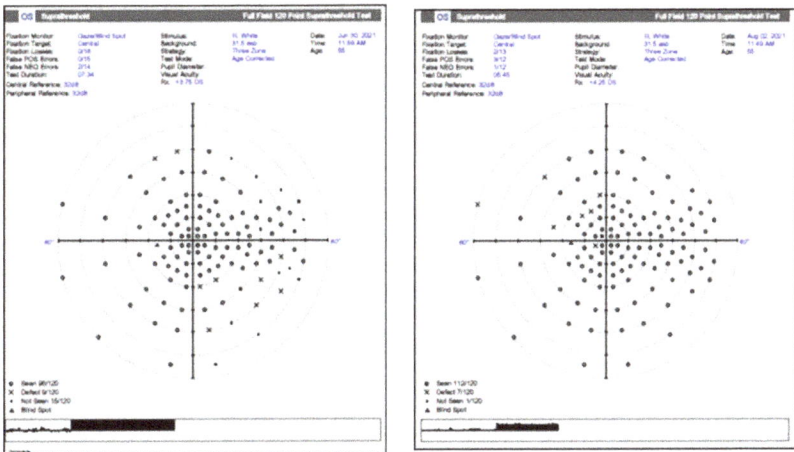

Figure 6. The visual field (Full Field 120 points Suprathreshold test) of the LE upon hospitalization (June 2021) and after 2 months (August 2021), relative scotoma without systematization.

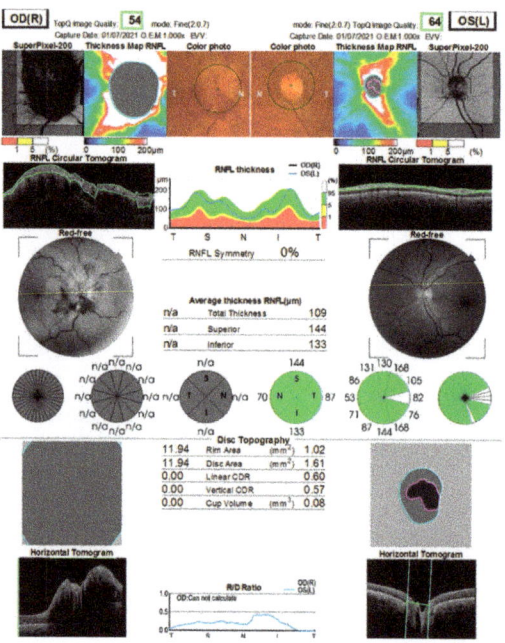

Figure 7. OCT of the optic nerve. RE diffusely thickens SNFR in all sectors (papilar edema); LE normal.

Furthermore, in order to establish the etiology, thus preventing an episodic event in the left eye, the patient is directed again to the laboratory to perform the thrombophilic profile, which reveals the presence of factor XIII, homozygous mutant PAI gene, heterozygous mutant factor V, heterozygous mutant MTHFR C677T, MTHFR A1298C homozygous mutant, and homocysteine with values above 21.2 µmol/mL (ideally <10 µmol/mL). The hematological examination confirmed the diagnosis of hereditary thrombophilia and hyperhomocysteinemia with a recommendation of Clexane (enoxaparin sodium) 0.4×2/day (anticoagulant), acetylsalicylic acid (75 mg/day) 1 pc/day, and natalvit (vitamin complex) 1 pc/day for 30 days and subsequent reevaluation. Thus, the diagnosis is made after consulting all the RE results of central retinal vein thrombosis within the context of the COVID-19 infection, with hereditary thrombophilia and hypermocysteinemia as aggravating factors. Under general treatment with Metilprednisolon, Pentoxifylline, Ceftriaxone, enoxaparin sodium 0.4×2, aspenter 1 pc per day, and natalvit, no favorable result is obtained, with the visual acuity evolving towards no light perception (NLP).

3. Results and Discussions

In the present study, we report two cases that were associated with COVID-19 infection (one case of orbital cellulitis and one of retrobulbar optic neuritis) and one case that was registered after vaccination against COVID-19 with central vein thrombosis of the retina, which had presented a favorable evolution except for the last case, which evolved towards the loss of visual function in the respective eye.

Coronavirus disease (COVID)-19 is caused by the novel severe acute respiratory syndrome coronavirus 2 (SARS-CoV-2) (as described by the Coronaviridae Study Group of the International Committee on Taxonomy of Viruses 2020) and has a predominant clinical presentation with respiratory disease [6]. Up to 21% of patients with COVID-19 may have systemic neurological signs, and 0.4% have cranial nerve involvement. Potential neuro-ophthalmic associations with COVID-19 include optic neuritis and myelitis, ischemic optic neuropathy, Guillain-Barre syndrome, Miller-Fisher syndrome, and cranial neuropathies such as cranial nerve III or VI palsies [6,9–14]. Most studies present cases with an association of ocular manifestations, representing 6–12% of patients with COVID-19. Ocular manifestations may precede systemic symptoms by 3 h to 5 days in 13% of patients [1,13]. In addition to the already known changes at the level of the anterior segment, the studies show the changes that can occur at the level of the posterior eye segment. As happened in our cases, the occlusion of the central vein of the retina and the central artery are two of the several vascular manifestations of COVID-19. Patients with COVID-19 have hypercoagulability, as evidenced by higher levels of fibrinogen, prothrombin time (PT), prothrombin dimer, and activated partial thromboplastin time (aPTT). A literature review showed that COVID-19 was associated with an 8.86-fold risk of retinal vascular microvasculopathy [13]. Another major complication is papillophlebitis, a rare condition characterized by venous congestion and optic disc edema; it manifests as a consequence of inflammation of the retinal veins or, possibly, of the optic capillaries, which occurs in healthy young people and has a benign evolution [14]. Neurological complications reported in studies include optic neuritis and myelitis, ischemic optic neuropathy, Guillain-Barre syndrome, Miller-Fisher syndrome, CNIII or CNVI palsy-like cranial neuropathies, and neuromyelitis optica spectrum disorder. Optic neuritis is an uncommon manifestation of the SARS-CoV-2 infection. One contextual mechanism in which viral antigens would induce an immune response against self-proteins, or direct SARS-CoV-2 infection of the central nervous system, may be involved in the optic nerve damage. A delay in the diagnosis of neuro-ophthalmic manifestations of COVID-19 can lead to irreversible optic atrophy [10,15]. There are few publications in the literature that refer strictly to cases with posterior segment pathology associated with the COVID-19 infection. Between 2020 and 2022 while carrying out a search through the specific research literature by accessing PubMed/Medline, ISI Web of Knowledge, ScienceDirect, and Scopus databases and by using keywords such as: optic neuritis, orbital cellulitis, anterior ischemic optic neuropathy, venous thrombosis, ocular pathology, SARS-CoV-2, ocular manifestations in COVID infections, we identified a number of 665 articles (review, case report, original article) that refer to eye diseases and the COVID infection, of these 127 review articles and open access and 41 case reports with eye pathologies associated with the COVID infection and selected case reports with eye damage after the vaccine, some of which are presented in Figure 8, Tables 1 and 2.

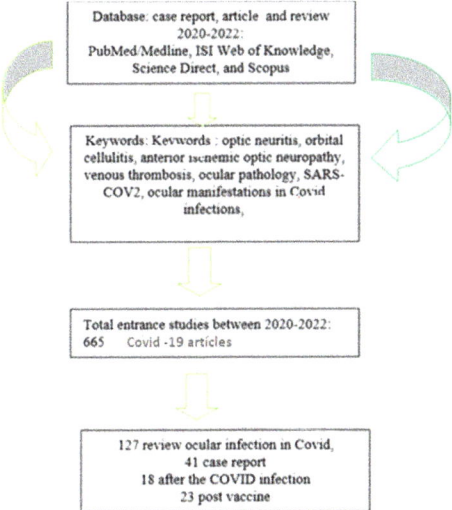

Figure 8. A flowchart of the current survey design, strategy, results, and current studies selected according to the selection criteria.

Table 1. Summary of the previous case reports (ocular pathology and COVID infections).

Study	Country	Design	Intervention	Population	Result
1. Mohammed A. Azab et al., 2021 [16]	Egypt	Case reports and meta-analysis	One-gram intravenous methylprednisolone for three days, followed by 60 mg oral prednisone, were prescribed for a week with gradual tapering.	A 32-year-old male patient with unilateral optic neuritis, 2 weeks after COVID infection.	The VA improved, but not like before the COVID infection.
2. Jaydeep A. Walinjkar et al., 2020 [17]	India	Report cases	Tree Intravitreal injection of Ranibizumab 0.05 mL of 10 mg/mL concentration with due precautions. The second dose is after 1 month.	A 17-year-old girl with unilateral OVCR 2 days after COVID infections.	Significant improvement in edema and VA after the first doses (from 6/18 to 6/12)
3. Davide Romano et al., 2022 [18]	Italy	Report cases	Intravenous (IV) methylprednisolone 1 g once daily for 5 days.	A 35-year-old female with a positive anamnesis of COVID-19 infection, visual disorders, and neurological symptoms.	Improving symptoms.
4. Rodríguez-Rodríguez M.S. et al., 2021 [10]	Mexico City	Report cases	One g/day of intravenous methylprednisolone for 5 days, followed by an oral prednisone taper.	A 55-year-old woman examined on 25 April 2020, for a 12-day history of headache and unilateral optic neuritis.	At a follow-up visit 3 months later, the ocular pain decreased. Nevertheless, left-eye vision did not improve, so the optical atrophy still manifested despite the treatment.
5. Anuradha Raj et al., 2021 [19]	India	Case report and review	The first intravenous (IV) injection of remdesivir in the dose of 200 mg, followed by daily IV maintenance doses of 100 mg for the next 5 days, azithromycin 500 mg/day IV infusion, and tocilizumab 400 mg IV.	A 37-year-old man, cavernous sinus thrombosis with central retinal artery or secondary to COVID-19 infection occlusion.	Proptosis, ptosis, and ophthalmoplegia recovered completely within 1 month of treatment.
6. Tsu Hong Lim et al., 2021 [20]	China	Report cases	Intravenous (IV) ganciclovir 225 mg twice a day (10 mg/kg/day) for 2 weeks.	A 33-year-old Malay with frosted branch angiitis (FBA) in the right eye 1 month after COVID with acquired immunodeficiency syndrome (AIDS).	It was noted that his FBA in his right eye had improved gradually and that his best corrected visual acuity had recovered to 6/12.
7. Helio F. Shiroma et al., 2022 [21]	Brazil	Report cases	Nine patients received intravitreal injections of anti-angiogenic drugs, and one received ketorolac. Tromethamine drops for the management of secondary macular edema; four were untreated.	Fourteen cases of retinal vascular occlusion within 3 months of laboratory-confirmed COVID-19 infections were identified.	Improving visual acuity and reducing macular edema.

Table 2. Summary of the previous case reports (ocular pathology and COVID vaccine).

Study	Country	Design	Intervention	Population	Result
1. Gustavo Savino, et.al, 2022 [22]	Italy	Case report series	Patients were females, 64, 58, and 45 years old, respectively. MRI showed enlargement of all right rectus muscles, with both belly muscle and insertion involvement in the first case associated with right scleritis.	The first and second patients were treated, respectively, with oral and topical glucocorticoids with a complete clinical response. Two cycles of oral non-steroidal anti-inflammatory drugs were administered to the third patient with a partial response.	A rapid clinical improvement after 2–4 days reported improvement of pain and diplopia, but no change in the proptosis
2. Sonia Valsero Franco et al., 2022 [23]	Spain	Case report series	No specific treatment was given.	A 53-year-old man who presented a visual field defect in the right eye 7 days after the first vaccine dose. A 65-year-old man who presented anterior optic disc neuropathy 12 days after his first vaccination.	Case 1: The OCT showed a slight loss of ganglion cells in both eyes, and the RNFL showed atrophy. Case 2: OCT showed atrophy of the temporal quadrants of the RNFL and a general loss of ganglion cells in the affected eye.
3. Wumeng Jin et al., 2021 [24]	China	Report cases	under chronic treatment with methylprednisolone (Medrol) 10 mg/d, mycophenolate mofetil (Cycopin) 1 g/d, tacrolimus (Prograf) 1.5 mg/d, and perindopril (Acertil) 4 mg/d. The patient was symptomatically treated with levofloxacin eye drops on the third day after the symptom onset, when the conjunctival congestion was already significant in the left eye. Diclofenac sodium eye drops and ganciclovir ophthalmic gel were added to the treatment.	A 28-year-old female suffering from SLE for six years. The patient received an inactivated COVID-19 vaccine on 6 April 2021.	Finally, the patient reported that the lesions faded ten days after symptom onset.
4. Rachna Subramony et al., 2021 [25]	California	Report cases	She underwent bilateral vitrectomies for simultaneous rhegmatogenous retinal detachments.	A 22-year-old woman with myopia but no ocular trauma or other major medical history presented to the emergency department with 5 days of progressive, painless vision loss in her right eye.	She had follow-up visits with ophthalmology on postoperative days 1, 6, and 13, with reportedly improved field of vision and acuity in the right eye.
5. Kyohei Tsuda et al., 2019 [26]	Japan	Report cases	No specific treatment was given.	A healthy 18-year-old Japanese female noticed a floater in the left eye 1 day after the second vaccination for coronavirus disease 2019. Fundus examination revealed retinal and optic disc hemorrhage.	The hemorrhage resolved spontaneously within 5 months.
6. Ruyi Han et al., 2022 [7]	China	Case report and review	Systemic prednisone was administered, Complicated CSC may develop in the eyes with vaccine-related VKH after steroid treatment. By gradually replacing prednisone with cyclosporine within 2 months, the subretinal fluid was completely absorbed at the last visit.	A 62-year-old Chinese man who developed Vogt-Koyanagi-Harada (VKH) disease six days after his third dose of an inactivated COVID-19 vaccine, with a preceding severe headache and tinnitus. Another three and a half months later, the visual acuity of his right eye slightly decreased due to complications of the central serous chorioretinopathy (CSC) disease.	Completely relieved inflammation and improved visual acuity.

During the active period of COVID (March 2020–May 2020), when there were restrictions and only urgent cases were admitted, we carried out an analysis in our clinic that included adults. Only 61 of the 616 patients who presented themselves for evaluation were hospitalized, and in most cases, the eye damage was not related to the COVID infection (most frequently, patients were hospitalized with retinal detachment (29.5%), trauma (24.6%), and corneal sclerosis (13.1%), most cases being surgical) [27]. Furthermore, in a similar study that we carried out, including both the non-pandemic period (2016–2019) and the pandemic period (2020), we found out that there were practically no significant differences between the two periods, both in terms of the number of presentations and in the type of pathology, with trauma showing a significant percentage of patients [28]. This can be explained by the fact that, when admitted to the ATI department during the pandemic, most of the patients with serious respiratory damage could not be evaluated from an ophthalmological point of view, making it practically impossible to identify possible eye contact caused by the COVID infection. The cases presented in this case report were identified in 2021, practically 1 year after the top outbreak, in the case of mild types of COVID infection that resulted in severe eye damage in the absence of respiratory symptoms in young people.

From what we have identified as cases, there is no case of bilateral orbital cellulitis recorded in the literature within the context of COVID infection in a young person without general pathological antecedents—a case that had a favorable evolution under treatment with remission of symptoms.

The second case with optic neuritis, with a rather rare association with COVID, as studies say, that usually occurs in multiple sclerosis, brings into discussion that complete multidisciplinary evaluation and imaging play a key role in the diagnostic process. According to other studies, we also recommend that the patient be periodically followed up by both ophthalmologists and neurologists to rule out any other later medical conditions [18,20]. Failing to diagnose the neuro-ophthalmic manifestations of the SARS-CoV-2 infection can lead to treatment delays, additional eye damage, and irreversible vision loss.

Also, the case of central vein thrombosis of the retina within the context of the vaccine in a young person who was unaware of hereditary thrombophilia brings into question the hypothesis that the immune response of the human body to the COVID-19 vaccinations may be involved in the pathogenesis of post-vaccination ocular side effects.

4. Conclusions

Neuro-ophthalmological manifestations secondary to contact with the SARS-CoV-2 virus/immunization are rare but must be known. There are three clinical cases with favorable clinical evolution (cases 1 and 2) but also unfavorable within the context of the patient's presentation at an increased time interval compared to the onset of the symptoms (case 3). Although the cases were quickly and efficiently investigated and the treatment was administered adequately by a multidisciplinary team (cases 1 and 3), the evolution was not favorable in all three situations. Atypical neuro-ophthalmological manifestations may also be present in the absence of systemic symptoms typical of SARS-CoV-2 infection, sometimes preceding respiratory manifestations. An early diagnosis, a multidisciplinary evaluation, and a fast dose of anticoagulant medication when required could have led, especially in case 3, to a favorable evolution and preservation of visual function.

Author Contributions: Conceptualization, N.A., C.M.B. and B.D.; methodology N.A., C.M.B. and B.D.; software I.A.P. and O.-D.I.; validation, N.A., C.M.B. and B.D.; formal analysis, D.C.B., I.A.P. and O.-D.I. investigation, N.A. and D.C.B.; resources N.A.; data curation, N.A., C.M.B. and B.D.; writing—original draft preparation, N.A., C.M.B. and B.D.; writing-review and editing, N.A., C.M.B. and B.D.; visualization, N.A. and B.D.; supervision N.A. and C.M.B.; project administration N.A. and C.M.B.; funding acquisition B.D. All authors have read and agreed to the published version of the manuscript.

Funding: This research received no external funding.

Institutional Review Board Statement: The study was approved by the Ethics Commission of the University Hospital Sf. Spiridon Iasi, approval no. 5657/7 March 2020, in compliance with ethical and deontological rules for medical and research practice. The study was conducted in accordance with the Helsinki Declaration.

Informed Consent Statement: Informed consent was obtained from all subjects involved in the study.

Data Availability Statement: The data published in this research are available on request from the first author and corresponding authors.

Conflicts of Interest: The authors declare no conflict of interest.

References

1. Matthew; Hensley, K.; Markantone, D.; Prescott, H.C. Annual Review of Medicine Neurologic Manifestations and Complications of COVID-19. www.annualreviews.org • Neurologic Manifestations of COVID-19. *Annu. Rev. Med.* **2022**, *73*, 113–127.
2. Luís, M.E.; Hipólito-Fernandes, D.; Mota, C.; Maleita, D.; Xavier, C.; Maio, T.; Cunha, J.P.; Ferreira, J.T. A Review of Neuro-Ophthalmological Manifestations of Human Coronavirus Infection. *Eye Brain* **2020**, *12*, 129–137. [CrossRef] [PubMed]
3. Betsch, D.; Paul, R. Neuro-Ophthalmologic Manifestations of Novel Coronavirus. *Adv. Ophthalmol. Optom.* **2021**, *6*, 275–288. [CrossRef]
4. Bolletta, E.; Iannetta, D.; Mastrofilippo, V.; De Simone, L.; Gozzi, F.; Bonacini, M.; Belloni, L.; Zerbini, A.; Adani, C.; Salvarani, C.; et al. Uveitis and Other Ocular Complications Following COVID-19 Vaccination. *J. Clin. Med.* **2021**, *10*, 5960. [CrossRef] [PubMed]
5. Schrage, N.; Blomet, J.; Holzer, F.; Tromme, A.; Ectors, F.; Desmecht, D. Eye Infection with SARS-CoV-2 as a Route to Systemic Immunization? *Viruses* **2022**, *14*, 1447. [CrossRef] [PubMed]
6. Leung, E.H.; Fan, J.; Flynn, H.W.; Albini, T.A. Ocular and Systemic Complications of COVID-19: Impact on Patients and Healthcare. *Clin. Ophthalmol.* **2022**, *16*, 1–13. [CrossRef]
7. Han, R.; Xu, G.; Ding, X. COVID-19 Vaccine-Related Vogt–Koyanagi–Harada Disease Complicated by Central Serous Chorioretinopathy during Treatment Course: Case Report and Literature Review. *Vaccines* **2022**, *10*, 1792. [CrossRef]
8. Burgos-Blasco, B.; Güemes-Villahoz, N.; Donate-Lopez, J.; Vidal-Villegas, B.; García-Feijóo, J. Optic nerve analysis in COVID-19 patients. *J. Med. Virol.* **2021**, *93*, 190–191. [CrossRef]
9. Sawalha, K.; Adeodokun, S.; Kamoga, G.-R. COVID-19-Induced acute bilateral optic neuritis. *J. Investig. Med. High. Impact Case Rep.* **2020**, *8*, 2324709620976018. [CrossRef]
10. Rodríguez-Rodríguez, M.S.; Romero-Castro, R.M.; Alvarado-de la Barrera, C.; González-Cannata, M.G.; García-Morales, A.K.; Ávila-Ríos, S. Optic neuritis following SARS-CoV-2 infection. *J. Neurovirol.* **2021**, *27*, 359–363. [CrossRef]
11. Mabrouki, F.Z.; Sekhsoukh, R.; Aziouaz, F.; Mebrouk, Y. Acute Blindness as a Complication of Severe Acute Respiratory Syndrome Coronavirus-2. *Cureus* **2021**, *13*, e16857. [CrossRef] [PubMed]
12. Ellul, M.A.; Benjamin, L.; Singh, B.; Lant, S.; Michael, B.D.; Easton, A.; Kneen, R.; Defres, S.; Sejvar, J.; Solomon, T. Neurological associations of COVID-19. *Lancet Neurol.* **2020**, *19*, 767–783. [CrossRef] [PubMed]
13. Lukiw, W.J.; Pogue, A.; Hill, J.M. SARS-CoV-2 Infectivity and Neurological Targets in the Brain. *Cell. Mol. Neurobiol.* **2022**, *42*, 217–224. [CrossRef]
14. Taha, M.J.J.; Abuawwad, M.T.; Alrubasy, W.A.; Sameer, S.K.; Alsafi, Y.; Al-Busataji, Y.; Abu-Ismail, L.; Nashwan, A.J. Ocular manifestations of recent viral pandemics: A literature review. *Front. Med.* **2022**, *9*, 1011335. [CrossRef] [PubMed]
15. Insausti-García, A.; Reche-Sainz, J.A.; Ruiz-Arranz, C.; Vázque, Á.L.; Ferro-Osuna, M. Papillophlebitis in a COVID-19 patient Inflammation and hypercoagulable state. *Eur. J. Ophthalmol.* **2022**, *32*, NP168–NP172. [CrossRef]
16. Azab, M.A.; Hasaneen, S.F.; Hanifa, H.; Azzam, A.Y. Optic neuritis post-COVID-19 infection. A case report with meta-analysis. *Interdisciplinary Neurosurgery. Adv. Techn. Case Manag.* **2021**, *26*, 101320.
17. Makhija, S.C.; Walinjkar, J.A.; Sharma, H.R.; Morekar, S.R.; Natarajan, S. Central retinal vein occlusion with COVID-19 infection as the presumptive etiology. *Indian J. Ophthalmol.* **2020**, *68*, 2572–2574. [CrossRef]
18. Romano, D.; Macerollo, A.; Giannaccare, G.; Mazzuca, D.; Borgia, A.; Romano, V.; Semeraro, F.; Ellis, R. COVID-19 and Clinically Isolated Syndrome: Coincidence or Causative Link? A 12-Month Follow-Up Case Report. *Appl. Sci.* **2022**, *12*, 11531. [CrossRef]
19. Raj, A.; Kaur, N.; Kaur, N. Cavernous sinus thrombosis with central retinal artey occlusion in COVID-19: A case report and review of literature. *Indian J. Ophthalmol.* **2021**, *69*, 1327–1329. [CrossRef]
20. Lim, T.H.; Wai, Y.Z.; Chong, J.C. Unilateral frosted branch angiitis in an human immunodeficiency virus-infected patient with concurrent COVID-19 infection: A case report. *J. Med. Case Rep.* **2021**, *15*, 267. [CrossRef]
21. Shiroma, H.F.; Lima, L.H.; Shiroma, Y.B.; Kanadani, T.C.; Nobrega, M.J.; Andrade, G.; de Moraes Filho, M.N.; Penha, F.M. Retinal vascular occlusion in patients with the COVID-19 virus. *Int. J. Retin. Vitr.* **2022**, *8*, 45.
22. Savino, G.; Gambini, G.; Scorcia, G.; Comi, N.; Fossataro, C.; Rizzo, S. Orbital myositis and scleritis after anti-SARS-CoV-2 mRNA vaccines: A report of three cases. *Eur. J. Ophthalmol.* **2022**, 1–6. [CrossRef] [PubMed]
23. Franco, S.V.; Fonollosa, A. IOptic Neuropathy After Administration of a SARS-CoV-2 Vaccine: A Report of 2 Cases. *Am. J. Case Rep.* **2022**, *23*, e935095. [CrossRef]

24. Jin, W.; Tang, Y.; Wen, C. An ocular adverse event in temporal association with COVID-19 vaccination in a patient with systemic lupus erythematosus: A case report. *Hum. Vaccines Immunother.* **2021**, *17*, 4102–4104. [CrossRef] [PubMed]
25. Subramony, R.; Lin, L.C.; Darren, K.; Knight, D.K.; Aminlari, A.; Belovarski, I. Bilateral Retinal Detachments in a Healthy 22-year-old Woman After Moderna SARS-CoV-2 Vaccination. *J. Emerg. Med.* **2021**, *16*, e146–e150. [CrossRef]
26. Tsuda, K.; Oishi, A.; Kitaoka, T. Optic disc hemorrhage in a young female following mRNA coronavirus disease 2019 vaccination: A case report. *J. Med. Case Rep.* **2022**, *16*, 462. [CrossRef]
27. Camelia, B.M.; Iuliana, A.A.; Elena, C.R.; Giurgica, M.; Anca, P.; Grigoras, C.; Otilia, O.; Ionela, N.D.; Nicoleta, A. Ophthalmoic Pathology Treated During COVID-19 at the Ophthalmology Clinic of "SF. Spiridon" County Clinical Emergency Hospital in Iasi, Romania. *Med. Surg. J.* **2021**, *125*, 93–101.
28. Andronic, D.G.; Anton, N.; Niagu, I.A.; Bogdanici, C.M. The incidence of pediatric eye injuries—Before and during the SARS-CoV-2 pandemic. *Med. Surg. J. Rev. Med. Chir. Soc. Med. Nat. Iași* **2021**, *125*, 521–530. [CrossRef]

Disclaimer/Publisher's Note: The statements, opinions and data contained in all publications are solely those of the individual author(s) and contributor(s) and not of MDPI and/or the editor(s). MDPI and/or the editor(s) disclaim responsibility for any injury to people or property resulting from any ideas, methods, instructions or products referred to in the content.

MDPI
St. Alban-Anlage 66
4052 Basel
Switzerland
www.mdpi.com

Journal of Clinical Medicine Editorial Office
E-mail: jcm@mdpi.com
www.mdpi.com/journal/jcm

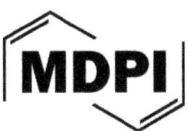

Disclaimer/Publisher's Note: The statements, opinions and data contained in all publications are solely those of the individual author(s) and contributor(s) and not of MDPI and/or the editor(s). MDPI and/or the editor(s) disclaim responsibility for any injury to people or property resulting from any ideas, methods, instructions or products referred to in the content.

www.ingramcontent.com/pod-product-compliance
Lightning Source LLC
LaVergne TN
LVHW070414100526
838202LV00014B/1454